Intracranial Pressure III

Edited by
J.W.F. BEKS, D.A. BOSCH, and
M. BROCK

With 131 Figures and 86 Tables

Springer-Verlag
Berlin Heidelberg New York 1976

Prof. Dr. Johannes W.F. Beks

Dr. D. Andries Bosch

Kliniek voor Neuro-Chirurgie, Akademisch Ziekenhuis,
Oostersingel 59, Groningen (The Netherlands)

Prof. Dr. Mario Brock

MHH Neurochirurgische Klinik, Postfach 180
D-3000 Hannover-Kleefeld (Federal Republic of Germany)

ISBN-13: 978-3-642-66510-3 e-ISBN-13: 978-3-642-66508-0
DOI: 10.1007/978-3-642-66508-0

Library of Congress Cataloging in Publication Data. International Symposium on Intracranial Pressure, 3d, Groningen, 1976. Intracranial Pressure III. Includes bibliographies and index. 1. Intracranial pressure--Congresses. I. Beks, J.W.F. II. Bosch, Dirk A., 1942-. III. Brock, Mario. IV. Title. [DNLM: 1. Intracranial pressure--Congresses. W3 IN995] RC386.2.I57 1976 616.8 76-46339.

Softcover reprint of the hardcover 1st edition 1976

Preface

The papers presented at the Third International Symposium on Intracranial Pressure that was held at the University of Groningen, June 1–3, 1976 are brought together in this volume.

After the successful meetings in Hannover and Lund the feeling of the Advisory Board was, that the third meeting should have more clinical implications, and therefore 7 out of the 10 Sessions deal with clinical problems.

That there is still a growing interest in the problems of the intracranial pressure appears from the fact that 152 papers were submitted. Unfortunately only 56 could be read, due to lack of time. The selection was made by the members of the Advisory Board. It is a pity that so many good papers had to be rejected because they did not fit in the program.

It was decided in a meeting of chairmen and co-chairmen during the symposium that the next congress will take place in 1979, to keep away from the CBF-meeting in June 1977 in Copenhagen and the "Brain-Edema" meeting in 1978 in Bethesda. This fourth symposium will be held in Williamsburg (USA) and prepared by Donald P. Becker, Douglas Miller, Gerald M. Hochwald and Kenneth Shulman.

The organizers want to thank the Advisory Board for the work they did and the chairmen and co-chairmen for their contribution in the success. Moreover, the editors wish to express their gratitude to Mrs. Kuipers, Mrs. Meijer and Mr. Meinders for the enormous amount of work they managed and to all the others who did their job behind the scenes.

We are grateful to Springer-Verlag for technical aid in the preparation of this book and for its prompt publication.

The editors

Contents

Session A: Basic Concepts I

Chairman: N.N. Zwetnow; *Co-chairman:* F. Isamat

Session B: Basic Concepts II

Chairman: K. Shulman; *Co-chairman:* J. Hoff

Session C: Trauma I

Chairman: T.W. LANGFITT; *Co-chairman:* H. NORNES

Session D: Trauma II

Chairman: M. BROCK; *Co-chairman:* D.P. BECKER

Session E: Subarachnoid Hemorrhage

Chairman: L. SYMON: *Co-chairman:* E. PASZTOR

Session F: Hydrocephalus

Chairman: U. PONTÉN; *Co-chairman:* G.M. HOCHWALD

Session G: Drugs and Anaesthetica

Chairman: J.D. MILLER; *Co-chairman:* H.J. REULEN

Session H: Patient Management

Chairman: H. Troupp; *Co-chairman:* D.G. McDowall

Session I: Data Handling

Chairman: R. Cooper; *Co-chairman:* J. de Rougemont

Session J: Pediatric Aspects

Chairman: N. LUNDBERG; *Co-chairman:* J. W. F. BEKS

Closing Comments

List of Senior-Authors

AKIOKA, T.: Department of Neurological Surgery, 2-5-1 Shikato-cho, Okayama City, 700 (Japan)

ASANO, T.: 2-11-7, Kajino-cho, Koganei-City, Tokyo (Japan)

AVEZAAT, C.J.J.: Dijkzigt Ziekenhuis, Dr. Molewaterplein 40, Rotterdam-3002 (The Netherlands)

BECKER, D.P.: Medical College of Virginia, Division of Neurosurgery, 1200 East Broad Street, Richmond, VA 23298 (USA)

BEKS, J.W.F.: University Hospital of Groningen, Department of Neurosurgery, Oostersingel 59, Groningen (The Netherlands)

BROCK, M.: Medizinische Hochschule Hannover, Neurochirurgische Klinik, Karl-Wiechert-Allee 9, D-3000 Hannover (Federal Republic of Germany)

BRUCE, D.A.: Department of Neurosurgery, The Children's Hospital of Philadelphia, Philadelphia, PA 19104 (USA)

CASTEL, J.P.: Neurochirurgien des Hôpitaux, Place Amélie Raba Leon, F-33076 Bordeaux Cedex (France)

COLD, G.E.: Neurokirurgisk Afdeling, Århus Kommenehospital, DK-8000 Århus (Denmark)

COLLICE, M.: Ospedale Maggiore "Ca' Granada", Piazza Ospedale Maggiore 3, I-20162 Milano-Niquarda (Italy)

CROCKARD, H.A.: The Royal Victorial Hospital, Belfast 12 (Northern Ireland)

DJORDJEVIC, M.: Branisevska 10, YU-1100 Beograd (Yugoslawia)

ECKSTEDT, J.: Department of Neurology, University of Umea, S-90185 Umeå (Sweden)

ENEVOLDSEN, E.M.: Department of Neurosurgery, Århus Kommenehospital, DK-8000 Århus (Denmark)

FURUSE, M.: Neurosurgical Department, Nagoya University, 65 Tsuruma-cho Showa-ku, Nagoya (Japan)

GJERRIS, F.: Neurosurgical Department, Rikshospitalet, DK-2100 Copenhagen (Denmark)

GO, K.G.: University Hospital of Groningen, Department of Neurosurgery, Oostersingel 59, Groningen (The Netherlands)

GOBIET, W.: Universitätsklinikum der Gesamthochschule Essen, Neurochirurgische Klinik, Hufelandstraße 55, D-4300 Essen 1 (Federal Republic of Germany)

GRANHOLM, L.: Karolinska Sjukhuset, S-10401 Stockholm (Sweden)

GREENBERG, R.P.: Medical College of Virginia, Division of Neurosurgery, 1200 East Broad Street, Richmond, VA 23298 (USA)

HAMER, J.: Neurochirurgische Abteilung des Chirurgischen Zentrums der Universität Heidelberg, Kirschnerstraße 1, D-6900 Heidelberg (Federal Republic of Germany)

HAYASHI, M.: Department of Neurosurgery, Kanazawa University, School of Medicine, 13–1 Takaramachi, Kanazawa 920 (Japan)
HOCHWALD, G.M.: New York University Medical Center, 550 First Avenue, New York, NY 10016 (USA)
HORTA, M.: Unidade de Neurocirurgia, 1° Hopital Distrital, Brasilia D.F. (Brasil)
HULME, A.: Frenchay Hospital, Bristol BS 16 1 LE (United Kingdom)

KASSELL, N.F.: The University of Western Ontario, Faculty of Medicine, Division of Neurosurgery, London, Ontario (Canada)
KINDT, G.W.: The University of Michigan, Department of Neurosurgery, Ann Arbor, MI 48109 (USA)
KULLBERG, G.: University Hospital of Lund, Department of Neurosurgery, S-22185 Lund (Sweden)

LAMAS, E.: Service of Neurosurgery, Ciudad Sanitaria "1° de Octubre", Madrid (Spain)
LANGFITT, T.W.: Univ. of Pennsylvania, Division of Neurosurgery, Philadelphia, PA 19104 (USA)
LEWELT, W.: Ul Zachnodnia 1/42, PL-20-620 Lublin (Poland)
LÖFGREN, J.: Neurokirurgiska Kliniken, Sahlgrenska Sjukhuset, S-41345 Göteborg (Sweden)
LORENZ, R.: Neurochirurgische Universitätsklinik, Klinikstraße 29, D-6300 Gießen (Federal Republik of Germany)

MARMAROU, A.: Albert Einstein College of Medicine, Yeshiva University, 1300 Morris Park Avenue, Bronx, NY 10461 (USA)
MARTIN, G.: Wellington Hospital, Riddiford Street, Newtown, Wellington 2 (New Zealand)
McGRAW, C.P.: The Bowman Gray School of Medicine, Wake Forest University, Winston-Salem, NC 27103 (USA)
MELLO, P.: Unidade de Neurocirurgia, 1° Hopital Distrital, Brasilia D.F. (Brasil)

NORTH, J.B.: Royal Adelaide Hospital, Neurosurgical Clinic, S.A.-5000 Adelaide (South Australia)

PAPO, I.: Ospedale Civile "Umberto 10", I-60100 Ancona (Italy)
PHILIPPON, J.: Clinique Neurochirurgicale, Hôpital de la Pitié, 83, Boulevard de l'Hôpital, F-75634 Paris 13 (France)
PRICE, D.J.: Wakefield Area Health Authority, Western District (Wakefield), Aberford Road, West Yorkshire WF1 4DG (United Kingdom)

DE ROUGEMONT, J.: Hospitalier Reg. et Université de Grenoble, Service de Neurochirurgie, F-30843 Grenoble Cedex, La Tronche (France)

STEVENAERT, A.: Hôpital de Bavière, Clinique Neuro-Chirurgicale, B-4020 Liège (Belgie)
SUNDBÄRG, G.: University of Lund, Department of Neurosurgery, S-22185 Lund (Sweden)
SYMON, L.: The National Hospital, Department of Neurological Sciences, Queen Square, London WC 1N 3BG (United Kingdom)
SZEWCZYKOWSKI, J.: Polish Academy of Science, Medical Research Centre, Bialobrzezeska 58, Warsaw (Poland)

TAKAGI, H.: Kitasato University, 1, Asamizodai, Sagamihara, Kanagawa, 228 (Japan)
TANAKA, K.: Department of Neurosurgery, Osaka City University, 1–5–7 Asahi-machi, Abeno-ku, Osaka (Japan)
TURNER, J.M.: The Midland Centre for Neurosurgery and Neurology, Holly Lane, Smethwick, Warley Worcs B67 7JX (United Kingdom)

VAPALAHTI, M.: University Central Hospital, SF-70100 Kuopio (Finland)

Session A

Basic Concepts I

Chairman: N. N. Zwetnow
Co-chairman: F. Isamat

Studies of Kinetics of Fluid Movements Within Brain Tissue[1]

A. Marmarou, K. Shapiro, W. Pöll, and K. Shulman

Introduction

Elevation of brain tissue pressure (BTP) and the development of BTP gradients have been implicated as factors affecting the continued formation and spread of edema (1, 3, 5). In a parallel study we found that the magnitude of tissue pressure gradients developed after cold-induced edema are less than 10 mm Hg (3). The objective of this study was to determine the rate of increase in local tissue fluid associated with BTP gradients of this magnitude and thus establish by an indirect means, whether these small BTP gradients can support bulk flow of fluid within brain parenchyma.

Methods

Adult cats were anesthetized with sodium pentobarbital (30 mg/kg), paralyzed with gallamine (4 mg/kg) and artificially ventilated. Catheters were introduced into femoral artery and vein for measurement of blood pressure and routine administration of drugs. Ventricular (VFP) and cisternal (CMP) CSF pressures were monitored using low compliance strain gauges referenced to the interaural line. Fluid was infused into the brain through a 23-gauge needle stereotaxically positioned in deep white matter and connected to an infusion pump. A T-connector and valve, positioned at the midpoint between needle and pump, was inserted for measurement of the needle pressure by a low compliance strain gauge. Stiff plastic tubing of ID .58 mm and OD . 97 mm was used throughout. The entire system was prefilled with saline tagged with Evans blue. Specified volumes of fluid were added to the tissue with the rate of infusion adjusted so that the needle pressure did not exceed VFP by a level established for each experiment (5 or 10 mm Hg).

This was preceded by a slower rate of inflow until the net volume accumulation reached 50 μl so as to minimize tissue destruction at the needle tip. At selected intervals, estimates of regional tissue compliance and resistance were made by superimposing 1-5 ml volumes upon the steady inflow rate. Tissue compliance was calculated by dividing the change in volume (ΔV) by the observed increase in pressure (ΔP) and correcting for gauge conpliance. Effective tissue resistance was obtained by dividing the change in steady-state needle tissue pressure (NTP) by the change in inflow rate (ΔQ). These parameters were expressed in percentage decrease from control.

At the end of the study, brains were removed, and water content was determined by gravimetric technique in selected animals.

[1] This work was supported in part by Training Grant §5 TO1 NSO5511-10.

Results

With prestabilisation of the infusion system at a low rate of inflow ($75 - 10^{-6}$ ml/min), lowering of the needle into deep white matter produces an initial transient elevation of in-line pressure which equilibrates with CSFP within 3-4 min. Control values of the NTP measured by this technique fall within the respiratory excursions of the CSFP. The pulsatile components of NTP encountered during this initial phase are similar to those observed using wick tissue pressure catheters (3). Respiratory fluctuations of NTP were synchronous with the CSFP but had a smaller peak to peak magnitude. No arterial pulsations were observed.

The rates of inflow necessary to maintain a NTP-VFP gradient of 10 mm Hg during the first 2 h of infusion ranged from .045 ml/h to .090 ml/h. As time progressed it was necessary to increase the rate of inflow (.225 - .300 ml/h) in order to maintain the NTP-VFP gradient at a constant value.

Initial tissue resistance ranged from $1.0 - 1.8 \times 10^4$ mm Hg/ml/min and decreased from 40 to 80% during the first 2 h followed by an additional 10% decrease during the next 4 h (Fig. 1). Initial tissue compliance ranged from 1.0 to 10×10^{-4} ml/mm Hg and increased by 15 to 30% over the course of the infusion with the greatest change occurring during the first 2 h.

There was no uniform pattern in the time course of the CSFP. in 50% of the experiments, the rise in CSFP was less than 10 mm Hg. In the remaining studies, CSFP rose gradually, reached a plateau ranging from 20-25 mm Hg within 3 h, then slowly returned toward preinfusion levels. The VFP and CMP remained equal over the entire time course and could be classified according to the types described elsewhere (3). As long as the inflow was maintained and adjusted as necessary, the NTP remained above the VFP by an amount equal to the preadjusted gradient (5, 10 mm Hg). When the infusion was stopped, the NTP equilibrated with the VFP within a 10-min period.

During the early phase of infusion the magnitude of respiratory variation of the NTP was considerably less than the respiratory fluctuations of the VFP. As time progressed, the pulsations of NTP increased, remaining synchronous with those of the VFP and gradually approaching their value (Fig. 2).

Upon sacrifice, examination of the brain slices revealed that EBA staining was confined to the white matter of the infused hemisphere. Staining was greatest in the vicinity of the infusion site with a graded reduction extending radially for a distance of 8 mm.

For a typical experiment, maximum white matter water content in the vicinity of the needle tip equaled 78 ml H_2O/100 g tissue, decreasing gradually to normal values (68%) 9 mm from the site of infusion. The spread of water per mm from the infusion site was similar to the distribution found in the cryogenic lesion (3). Gray matter water content of the infused hemisphere was normal (81 ml H_2O/100 g). Contralateral white and gray matter were normal and equaled 68 and 81%, respectively. The total volume infused equaled .250 ml. Analysis of gravimetric data showed that the increase in brain water at 5 h was equal to .228 ml.

Discussion

Our findings show that in edematous tissue the needle pressure (NTP) is equivalent to the tissue pressure (2) measured by the wick method (3, 4). When care is taken to eliminate mechanical artifact, it is possible to infuse fluid through a needle which simultaneously measures the local brain-tissue pressure. This technique, then serves as a generator for interstitial edema while allowing control of the volume and rate of edema flow. The migration of fluid under these conditions is confined to the white matter of the infused hemisphere. The distribution of edema measured gravimetrically is similar to results obtained in the cold injury model of vasogenic edema (3).

With the start of infusion, local tissue pressure increases above the local compartmental CSFP. This increase in BTP (25 mm Hg) is transient and gradually decreases toward the CSFP within 2-3 h. The magnitude of BTP gradients associated with the rates of inflow used was in the range of 5-10 mm Hg. This suggests that the spread of fluid through brain parenchyma can indeed take place with relatively small tissue-pressure gradients acting as the propelling force for bulk flow. The concomitant reduction of tissue resistance observed as inflow of fluid distends the ECF space facilitates this process.

The reduction of tissue resistance (R_t) and increase in local compliance (C_t) must be viewed qualitatively since it was not possible to determine the amount of tissue involved in this process. Values obtained by this point source infusion ($R_t = 1.0-1.8 \times 10^4$ mm Hg/ml/min and $C_t = 1.0-10. \times 10^{-3}$ ml/mm Hg) are conservative and more significant reductions of tissue resistance would be expected in other models of brain injury, where local tissue distortion is proportionally greater.

The gradual increase of the pulsatile component of the local BTP in the infusion model was also found in the wick pressure catheters following cryogenic injury. This phenomenon may reflect increased fluid coupling secondary to the breakdown of tissue resistance. In a viscoelastic substance such as brain tissue, where reaction forces may be rate sensitive, the development of a pulsatile driving pressure may accelerate the widening of tissue space and enhance the further spread of edema.

Summary

1. Significant increases in white matter water content can take place in the presence of relatively small tissue pressure gradients (10 mm Hg).
2. The increase in white matter edema is accomplished by a concomitant decrease in tissue resistance and increase in local tissue compliance.
3. The biomechanical properties of tissue and the time course of events associated with brain edema support the concept of edema spread by bulk flow.

Key Words

Tissue resistance, Tissue compliance, Tissue pressure, Cerebral edema.

References

1. BROCK, M., FURUSE, M., WEBER, R., HASUO, M., DIETZ, H.: Brain tissue pressure gradients. In: Intracranial Pressure II (N. LUNDBERG, U. PONTEN, M. BROCK, eds.) pp. 215-220.

2. GUYTON, A.C., GRANGER, H.J., TAYLOR, A.E.: Interstitial fluid pressure. Physiol. Rev., 51, 527-563 (1971).

3. MARMAROU, A., SHULMAN, K., SHAPIRO, K., PÖLL, W.: The time course of brain tissue pressure and local CBF in vasogenic edema, Workshop on Dynamic Aspects of Cerebral Edema. Montreal, May 25-29, 1976.

4. PÖLL, W., BROCK, M., MARKAKIS, E., WINKELMÜLLER, W., DIETZ, H.: Brain tissue pressure. In: Intracranial Pressure (M. BROCK, H. DIETZ, eds.) pp. 188-194. Berlin-Heidelberg-New York: Springer 1972.

4. REULEN, H.J., KREYSCH, H.G.: Measurement of brain tissue pressure in cold-induced cerebral oedema. Acta Neurochir., 29, 29-49 (1973).

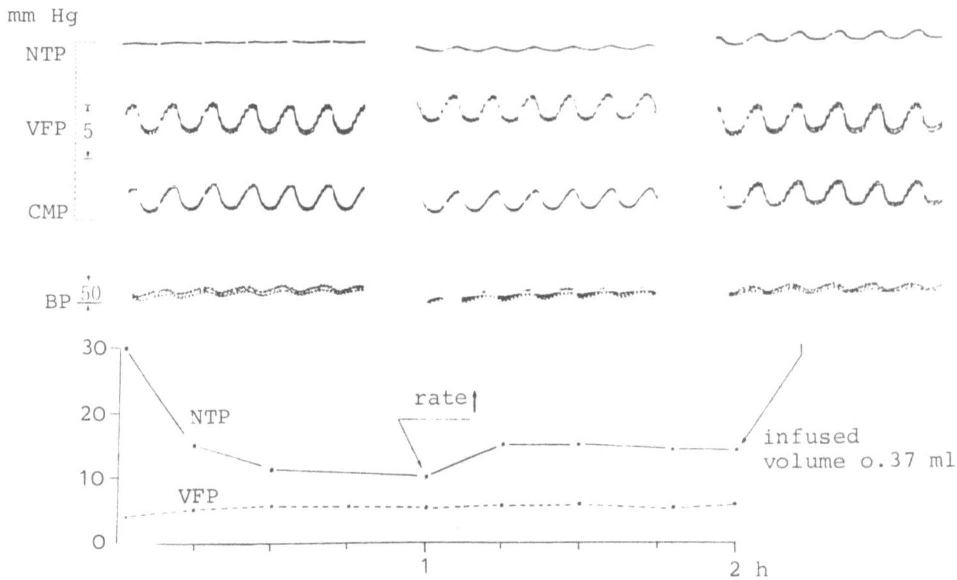

Fig. 1. Pulse waveforms for NTP, VFP, and CMP shown at hourly intervals during intraparenchymal fluid infusion. Amplitude of NTP increases as infusion progresses, and gradually approaches peak to peak magnitude of CSFP pulsations

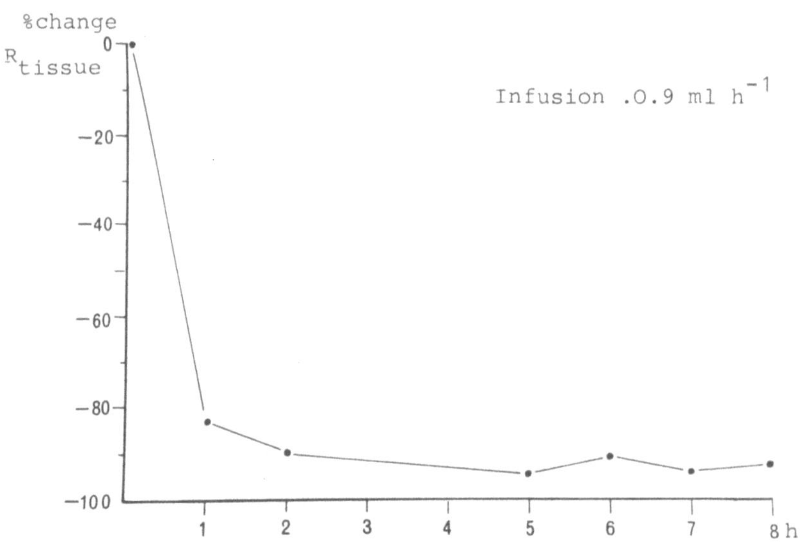

Fig. 2. Tissue resistance (R_t) decreases over duration of intraparenchymal infusion. This may account for dissipation of brain tissue pressure gradients observed in experimental animals following cryogenic injury

Responses of Cortical Vein Wedge Pressure, Ventricular Fluid Pressure, and Brain Tissue Pressure to Elevation of Arterial Blood Pressure Under Conditions of Hyperventilation and Freezing Injury to the Brain

K.G. Go, F. Zuiderveen, and T.I. Kuipers- de Jager

Introduction

As observed in a previous study (1), rises of cortical vein wedge pressure and ventricular fluid pressure concomitant to elevation of arterial blood pressure are increased after infliction of a freezing injury to the brain due to impairment of vasomotor autoregulation and consequent increased propagation of arterial blood pressure into the capillary bed of the cold-injured region. Since the impairment of vasomotor autoregulation seems to enhance the deleterious effect of the arterial blood pressure upon the development of vasogenic brain edema, it was the aim of this study to investigate whether hyperventilation might influence vasomotor activity under the conditions of brain injury.

Methods

Cats under endotracheal anesthesia (induced with pentobarbital and maintained with nitrous oxide-oxygen) were artificially ventilated after muscular relaxation with tubocurarine. Arterial blood pressure (P_a) was recorded through a cannula in the left femoral artery; cortical vein wedge pressure (P_{cvw}) was monitored through a thin polyethylene catheter with its tip inserted into the orifice of a cortical vein via the superior sagittal sinus; ventricular fluid pressure (P_{vf}) was measured through a needle stereotaxically introduced into a lateral ventricle, and brain tissue pressure (P_{if}) was recorded by a wick[1] catheter introduced into the white matter underlying the cortical area studied (via a craniotomy exposing the dura).

During spontaneous respiration the average arterial P_{CO_2} was 26.9 ± 4.3 mm Hg. After muscular relaxation the P_{CO_2} was maintained either at 26.1 ± 1.6 mm Hg (normal ventilation) or at 15.0 ± 1.5 mm Hg (hyperventilation), while the responses of P_{cvw}, P_{vf}, and P_{if} to elevation of P_a (by infusion of metaraminol during 5 min were recorded. After infliction of the freezing injury (5 min at -40°C) to the cortical area drained by the cannulated cortical vein, the responses of the various pressures to elevation of P_a were again recorded while P_{CO_2} was maintained either at 25.9 ± 1.6 mm Hg (normal ventilation) or at 14.3 ± 1.4 mm Hg (hyperventilation).

Results and Discussion

1. The Effect of Cold Injury

Prior to cold injury the mean arterial pressure P_a (taken as the sum of systolic and diastolic pressures divided by two) was on the average (i.e., comprising all values during normal ventilation and hyperventi-

[1] Kindly provided by Dr. W. Pöll.

Table 1. Average pressures (comprising observations during normal ventilation and during hyperventilation) before and after cold injury; with standard deviations

	Mean arterial pressure P_a (mm Hg)	Cortical vein wedge pressure P_{cvw} (mm H_2O)	Ventricular fluid pressure P_{vf} (mm H_2O)	Brain tissue pressure P_{if} (mm H_2O)
Before cold injury	142.34 ± 24.79	53.00 ± 51.59	24.54 ± 54.21	27.67 ± 44.65
After cold injury	132.99 ± 27.37	108.58 ± 66.44	146.22 ± 152.85	140.33 ± 153.26
P	> 0.05	< 0.001	< 0.001	< 0.001

lation) the same as after the cold injury.

Following cold injury, however, the cortical vein wedge pressure P_{cvw}, the ventricular fluid pressure P_{vf}, and the brain tissue pressure P_{if} were significantly increased ($P < 0.001$) with respect to the observations prior to the injury (both during normal ventilation and hyperventilation), see Table 1.[2]

The increase of P_{cvw}, P_{vf}, and P_{if} obviously indicate the development of cerebral edema after the cold injury; while the absence of any response of P_a point to the lack of a Cushing reaction. The relations between the various pressures are schematized in Figure 1.

With regard to vasomotor autoregulation, which was tested by studying the rises of P_{cvw}, P_{vf}, and P_{if} upon elevation of P_a, it appears that after cold injury the changes of P_{cvw}, P_{vf}, and P_{if} concomitant to elevation of P_a were all significantly greater than before cold injury, indicating that what has been called by LANGFITT (3) the vasomotor autoregulation for pressure, generally was disturbed after the cold injury (Table 2).

As to metabolic autoregulation, its state will be indicated by the responses to hyperventilation.

Table 2. Average increase of cortical vein wedge pressure ΔP_{cvw}, ventricular fluid pressure ΔP_{vf}, and brain tissue pressure ΔP_{if} concomitant to elevation of mean arterial pressure ΔP_a before and after cold injury (observations both during normal ventilation and hyperventilation)

	ΔP_a (mm Hg)	ΔP_{cvw} (mm H_2O)	ΔP_{vf} (mm H_2O)	ΔP_{if} (mm H_2O)
Before cold injury	65.10 ± 33.27	43.93 ± 55.81	27.61 ± 39.49	14.74 ± 23.02
After cold injury	66.88 ± 29.98	92.38 ± 66.13	106.88 ± 90.10	65.73 ± 76.76
P	> 0.05	< 0.001	< 0.001	< 0.001

[2] It is interesting to note that after cold injury P_{vf} exceeds P_{cvw}, which, however, as in vitro experiments demonstrated, does not imply collapse of cortical veins (2).

2. *The Influence of Hyperventilation*

It should be remarked that in this experiment hyperventilation induced a higher elevation (80.71 ± 26.26 mm Hg before and 81.30 ± 30.76 mm Hg after cold injury) of P_a during the infusion of metaraminol than occurred with normal ventilation (here the elevation of P_a being 52.96 ± 33.48 mm Hg before, and 55.24 ± 24.04 mm Hg after the injury), the difference between hyperventilation and normal ventilation being significant ($P < 0.001$). It may be explained by the occurrence of general vasoconstriction during hyperventilation.

Therefore, in comparing the changes of P_{cvw}, P_{vf}, and P_{if} upon elevation of P_a during hyperventilation with those during normal ventilation, the change of P_a due to the change of ventilation was corrected for by comparing the ratios of the respective pressure changes in relation to the elevation of P_a, i.e., $\Delta P_{cvw}/\Delta P_a$, $\Delta P_{vf}/\Delta P_a$, and $\Delta P_{if}/\Delta P_a$ (Table 3). Before cold injury, hyperventilation mostly (Fig. 2) resulted in a reduction of these pressure increase ratios, especially those of cortical vein wedge pressure and brain tissue pressure. After cold injury hyperventilation in many cases still resulted in a reduction of the pressure increase ratios, but in the other cases an augmentation of the pressure increase ratios occurred. These observations seem to be similar to the clinical findings of OVERGAARD (4), who observed an increase instead of a decrease of cerebral blood flow during hyperventilation in a number of patients with brain injury.

Table 3. Effect of hyperventilation on vectorial average ratios of increase of cortical vein wedge pressure, ventricular fluid pressure, and brain tissue pressure with respect to the elevation of main arterial pressure

	Before cold injury		
	$\frac{\Delta P_{cvw}}{\Delta P_a}$	$\frac{\Delta P_{vf}}{\Delta P_a}$	$\frac{\Delta P_{if}}{\Delta P_a}$
No. of animals with reduced pressure increase ratio	12	12	13
No. of animals with elevated pressure increase ratio	1	2	2
Total No. of animals	13	14	15
P	< 0.05	= 0.05	< 0.05

	After cold injury		
	$\frac{\Delta P_{cvw}}{\Delta P_a}$	$\frac{\Delta P_{vf}}{\Delta P_a}$	$\frac{\Delta P_{if}}{\Delta P_a}$
No. of animals with reduced pressure increase ratio	9	9	8
No. of animals with unchanged or elevated pressure increase ratio	6	5	5
Total No. of animals	15	14	13
P	> 0.05	> 0.05	> 0.05

It may be concluded that, following a cold injury to the brain, pressure autoregulation generally was disturbed, whereas metabolic autoregulation was impaired far less frequently.

References

1. GO, K.G., ZIJLSTRA, W.G., FLANDERIJN, H., ZUIDERVEEN, F.: Circulatory factors influencing exudation in cold-induced cerebral edema. Exptl. Neurol. 42, 332-338 (1974).
2. LANGFITT, T.W.: Personal communication.
3. LANGFITT, T.W.: Cerebral circulation and metabolism. Summary of international symposium June 6-10, 1973. J. Neurosurg. 40, 561-576 (1974).
4. OVERGAARD, J.: Personal communication.

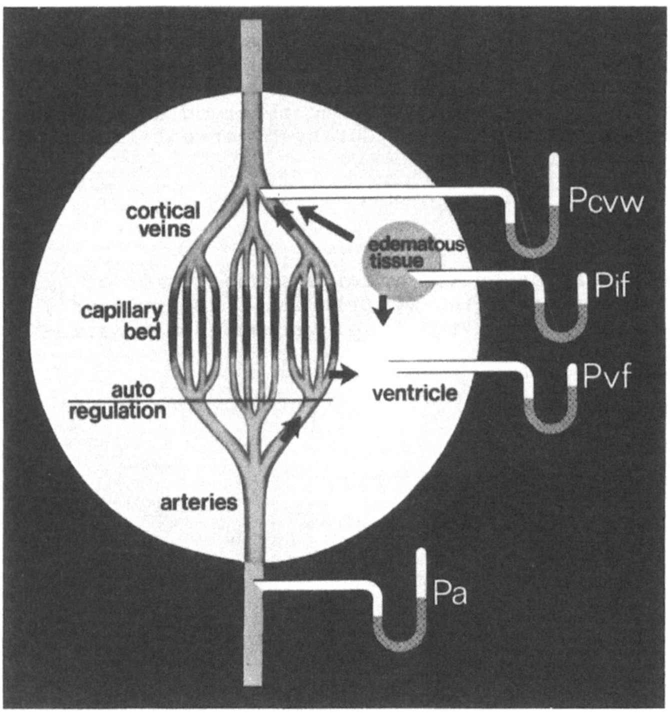

Fig. 1. Diagram representing relations between various pressures. P_a, arterial pressure, when not checked by vasomotor autoregulation, may come through into capillary bed, distending it and raisng ventricular fluid pressure P_{vf} and brain tissue pressure P_{if}; furthermore, the pressure wave will be apparent in P_{cvw}: cortical vein wedge pressure. Edema in the brain tissue elevates P_{if}, and by increase of volume, also elevates P_{vf} and P_{if} according to pressure-volume relationship

▷

Fig. 2. Recordings of P_{cvw}, P_{vf}, and P_{if} upon elevation of P_a. Upper part of figure shows that before cold injury, hyperventilation reduces rise of P_{cvw}, P_{vf}, and P_{if} with respect to normal ventilation. Lower half of figure shows recordings after cold injury, but rather an increase of changes of P_{cvw}, P_{vf}, and P_{if} upon elevation of P_a occur

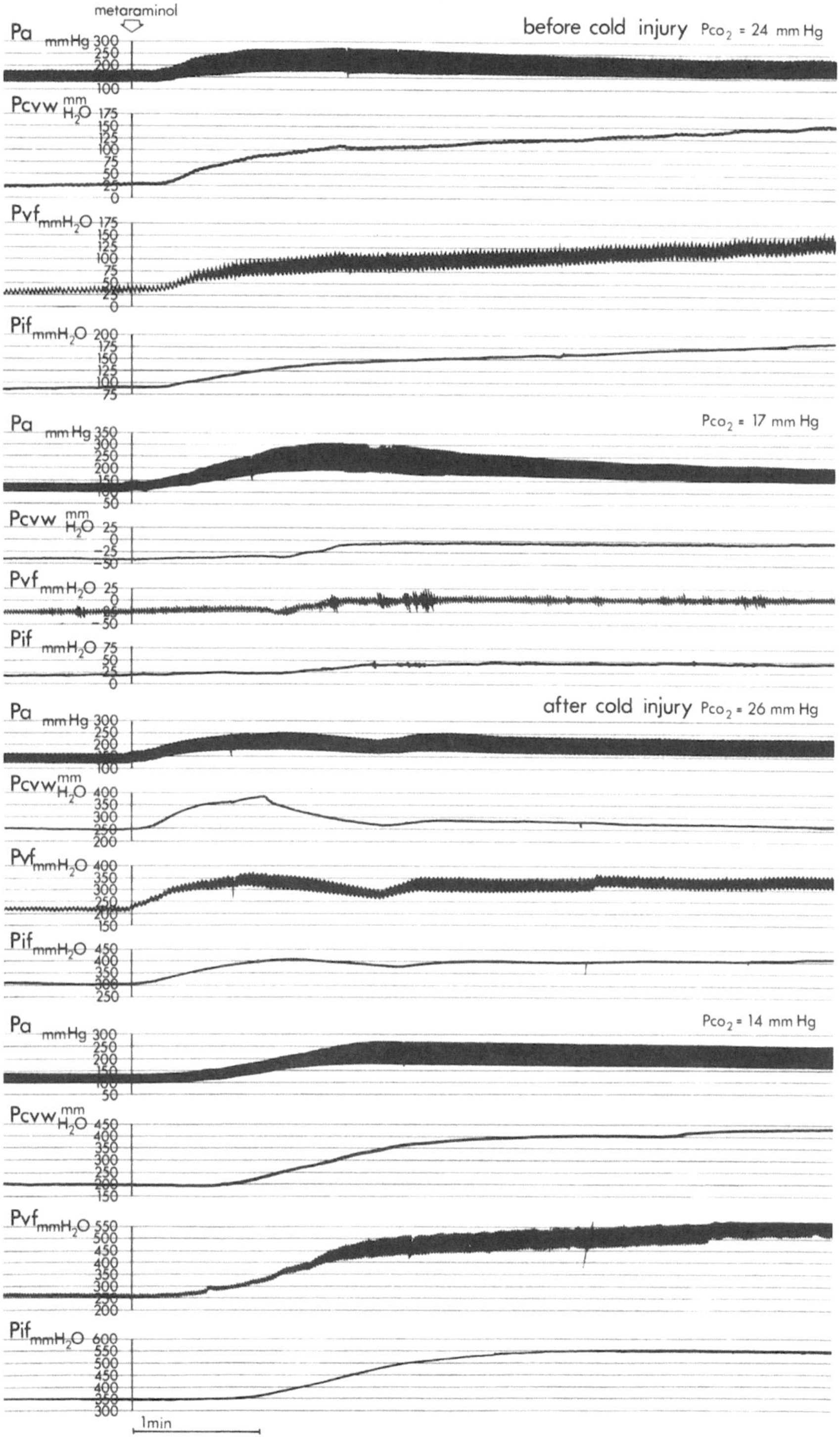

metaraminol
before cold injury Pco2 = 24 mm Hg
Pa mmHg
Pcvw mm H2O
Pvf mmH2O
Pif mmH2O
Pco2 = 17 mm Hg
after cold injury Pco2 = 26 mm Hg
Pco2 = 14 mm Hg
1min

The Influence of Brain Tissue Pressure Upon Local Cerebral Blood Flow in Vasogenic Edema[1]

A. Marmarou, W. Pöll, K. Shapiro, and K. Shulman

Introduction

Although the time course of brain tissue pressure (BTP) in vasogenic edema has been documented (2, 5, 7), the effect of these pressure changes upon local cerebral blood flow (CBF) is unknown. The local CBF represents the generating source of the edema seen in this model. Our objective in the present study was to determine the temporal response of local white matter CBF to vasogenic edema and correlate these changes with parallel studies of local white matter BTP.

Methods

There were 13 adult cats under pentobarbital (30 mg/kg) anesthesia and paralyzed with gallamine (4 mg/kg) mechanically ventilated and placed in a stereotaxic frame. Ventricular (VFP) and cisternal (CMP) pressures were monitored continuously as was systemic blood pressure. Regional CBF (rCBF) was measured by polarographic technique using Teflon-coated platinum electrodes (254 μ) implanted in deep white matter of left and right hemispheres. The electrodes were placed symmetrically to correspond to the location of glass encapsulated wick tissue pressure probes inserted in a parallel study using the same protocol (Fig. 1) (5).

In nine animals three steady-state flows were measured prior to a cryogenic injury of the left frontal pole (duration 5 min probe area 0.5 cm^2). Four animals served as controls and were not subjected to the cold injury. Thereafter, rCBF was determined at 40-min intervals for 5 h, along with continuous monitoring of VFP, CMP, and BP. Blood gases were determined prior to hydrogen saturation, at the peak of saturation, and after washout was complete. Upon sacrifice, brains were removed and sectioned, and water content of both gray and white matter was determined by gravimetric technique.

Results

Average steady-state levels of rCBF ranged from 13.1 to 17.4 ml/min/100 gm. No significant differences were found between probe sites: rCBF1 = 17.42 ± 9.0SD; rCBF2 = 15.3 ± 5. 95SD; rCBF3 = 13.11 ± 3.0SD; rCBF4 = 16.3 ± 5.62SD. These values are in agreement with those reported by other investigators (1, 3). Studies of control animals showed that after steady state is achieved rCBF does not change significantly over the 5-h period. rCBF remains constant within a systemic blood pressure range of 50 to 140 mm Hg. At elevated arterial blood pressures, "breakthrough" occurs and flow becomes pressure passive. Following breakthrough the white matter cerebral vascular resistance given by the slope Δ(BP-ICP)/ΔCBF was equal at all probe sites and averaged

[1] This work was supported in part by Training Grant #5 T01 NS05511-10.

6.12 mm Hg/ml/min. False autoregulation (6) of white matter flow was demonstrated in the left hemisphere of one animal, while intact autoregulation was apparent in the contralateral hemisphere. We found that the CO_2 responsivity pf the falsely autoregulating hemisphere was low ($\Delta CBF/\Delta PCO_2$ = .36) compared to the hemisphere with intact autoregulation ($\Delta CBF/\Delta PCO_2$ = 3.13).

Following cryogenic injury, a uniform maximal reduction occurred in the vicinity of the lesion (rCBF1). Flow at this site decreased by 34% in the 1st hour with an additional decrease of 16% in the following 3 h. The CBF ipsilateral (rCBF3) and 20 mm distal to the lesion decreased by 10% in the first 2 h followed by a hyperemia which reached 130% of control in 4 h (Fig. 1).

Flows in the contralateral hemispheres (rCBF2, 4) decreased by 25% with the greatest change occurring within the first 2 h.

In four animals autoregulation was tested 5 h after the lesion by measuring ΔCBF after progressive exsanguination. Autoregulation was intact at all probe sites in two animals. In two animals autoregulation was impaired and CBF pressure passive.

Two pressure response profiles were apparent. In the first group of animals (n=4) mean steady-state CSFP = 8.4 mm Hg. The maximum pressure elevation in these animals was less than 10 mm Hg. In the second group, (n=5) mean CSFP rose to 24.2 mmHg 2 h after cryogenic injury. ICP plateau at this level and gradually fell over the next 3 h. VFP to CMP gradients were not observed.

In control animals, white matter water content (WWC) and gray matter water content (GWC) were normal: WWC = 68.49, GWC = 82.40% H_2O/100 g tissue. In animals with cryogenic injury, WWC was maximal in the lesion area (WWC = 78.02 ± 2.16SD) decreasing to 69.5%, 12 mm distal from the site of injury. WWC of the contralateral hemisphere showed a uniform elevation of 2%. GWC of both hemispheres was 1% above normal. These latter elevations were not significantly different from control animals.

Discussion

Our results show that under normal conditions the autoregulatory dynamics of white matter rCBF are similar to those of cortex (8). Following cryogenic injury, the most consistent finding was the gradual decrease of rCBF in the vicinity of the lesion to 50% of control at 5 h after injury.

In relating these changes of rCBF to the time course of tissue pressure observed in a parallel study (5), we found that with the exception of white matter adjacent to the lesion there is no clear association between these parameters. Our results from the BTP study show that the response of tissue pressure was not uniform and three types of pressure increase of ICP and BTP following cryogenic injury could be distinguished: Type I, low (<10 mm HG); Type II, moderate (<20 mm Hg); and Type III, high (>20 mm Hg). The Type III response, characterized by a progressive increase in both BTP and ICP was associated with impaction in which case the tissue pressure above the tentorium tended to follow the local compartmental CSF pressure and did not exceed the VFP. We concluded from these results that (a) the ventricular fluid pressure is a reasonable estimation (±10 mm Hg) of the maximum brain tissue pressure and (b) excluding impaction, the maximum BTP gradients developed are transient, less than 10 mm Hg and dissipate within 2 h.

In the flow studies, animals were similar to the Type I and II categories of the BTP investigation and VFP did not exceed 25 mm Hg. Correlating these results, reductions of rCBF occurred in regions where transient elevations of BTP were limited to an estimated maximum of 35 mm Hg.

We suspect that the alterations of flow observed at four different electrode sites were not caused by the same mechanism. The maximal reduction of flow in the vicinity of the lesion can be correlated with the increased regional water content found in that area. These results and interpretation are in agreement with studies by FREI (4). The results of the present study which show that brain water was not elevated in the contralateral hemisphere nor in the hyperemic region of the damaged hemisphere implicate a mechanism other than increased water. The absence of marked elevations of BTP in these regions suggest that either a metabolic or neural factor may be operative at these probe sites.

Summary

1. The autoregulatory dynamics of white matter of rCBF are similar to those reported for cortex.
2. Following cryogenic injury, a uniform maximal reduction of white matter rCBF occurs in the vicinity of the lesion decreasing to 50% of control at 5 h.
3. Significant alterations of flow can occur at low levels of BTP (<30 mm Hg) and in regions which are nonedematous.

Key Words

White matter, Brain edema, Tissue pressure.

References

1. BOZZAO, L., FIESCHI, C., AGNOLI, A., NARDINI, M.: Autoregulation of cerebral blood flow studied in the brain of cat. International Conference on Blood Flow through Organs and Tissues (W.H. BAIN, A.M. HAROER, eds.) pp. 253-256. Edinburgh: Livingstone 1968.

2. BROCK, M., FURUSE, M., WEBER, R., HASUO, M., DIETZ, H.: Brain tissue pressure gradients. In: Intracranial Pressure II (N. LUNDBERG, U. PONTEN, M. BROCK, eds.) pp. 215-220. New York-Heidelberg-Berlin: Springer 1975.

3. FIESCHI, C., BOZZAO, L., AGNOLI, A., NARDINI, M., BARTOLINI, A.: The hydrogen method of measuring local blood flow in subcortical structures of the brain: including a comparative study with the C^{14} antipyrine method. Exp. Brain Res. 7, 111-119 (1969).

4. FREI, H.J., WALLENFANG, T., PÖLL, W., REULEN, H.J., SCHUBERT, R.: Regional cerebral blood flow and regional metabolism in cold-induced oedema. Acta Neurochir. 29, 15-28 (1973).

5. MARMAROU, A., SHULMAN, K., SHAPIRO, K., PÖLL, W.: The time course of brain tissue pressure and local CBF in vasogenic edema. Workshop on Dynamic Aspects of Cerebral Edema. Montreal, May 25-29, 1976.

6. MILLER, J.D., GARIBI, J., NORTH, B., TEASDALE, G.M.: Effects of increased arterial pressure un blood flow in the damaged brain. J. Neurol. Neurosurg. Psychiat. 38, 657-665 (1975).

7. REULEN, H.J., KREYSCH, H.G.: Measurement of brain tissue pressure in cold-induced cerebral oedema. Acta Neurochir. 29, 29-49 (1973).

8. SYMON, L., PASZTOR, E., DORSCH, N.W.C., BRANSTON, N.M.: Physiological responses of local areas of the cerebral circulation in experimental primates determined by the method of hydrogen clearance. Stroke 4, 632-642 (1973).

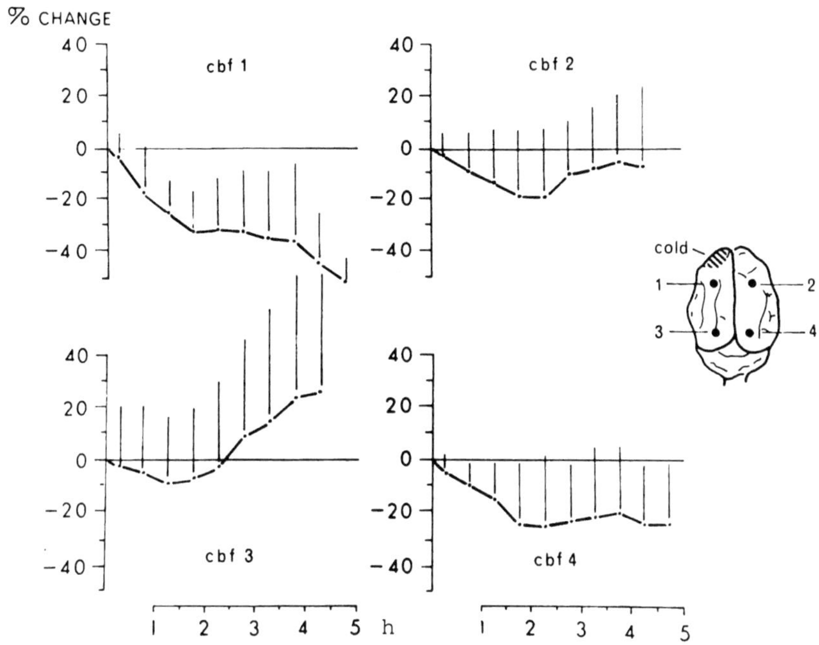

Fig. 1. Cerebral blood flow at each probe site is plotted as percent change from control versus time after freeze lesion. Limit of 150 is given for each rCBF value. The greatest reduction occurs at CBF1, with a delayed hyperemia at CBF3

Pathogenetic Role of the No-Reflow Phenomenon in an Experimental Subarachnoid Hemorrhage Model in the Dog

T. Asano, N. Basugi, I. Saito, and K. Sano

Introduction

Autopsies following death due to subarachnoid hemorrhage (SAH) showed that ischemia is undoubtedly the principal cause of brain damage in the acute stage of SAH (4). Since the result of SAH has been shown to depend on the mechanism of genesis of this anoxic-ischemic lesion of the brain is of great clinical importance. In the past, cerebral vasospasm has been regarded as a major factor in this respect (1, 8). However, most of the recent clinical and experimental studies have failed to show clear correlation between vasospasm and cerebral blood flow (CBF) (9, 10, 11). Obviously, more than one factor must be involved in the genesis of thos cerebral lesion, and an integrated investigation including all the possible parameters, such as intracranial pressure (ICP), CBF, cerebral function, and pathology, is definitely required to clarify this problem. Since such an extensive survey of SAH in humans is hardly possible from the clinical standpoint, we carried out the following experiment using an SAH-model in the dog.

Material and Methods

Various techniques were devised in the past to produce experimental SAH (5), but simulation of the pattern of ICP has been only rarely attempted. The influence of raised ICP has not been altogether neglected, however, and particular attention was paid to it in designing the present experimental model.

The intracranial portion of the internal carotid artery was approached by means of a craniectomy in the lateral base of the skull, after removing the zygomatic arch and the coronoid process of the mandibule.

Under an operating microscope, the dura was opened and the temporal lobe was gently retracted along the sphenoid ridge until the internal carotid artery could be seen. A 4-0 atraumatic needle was then inserted into the artery. There was no bleeding and only transient spasm of the artery was seen. The thread attached to the needle was then guided from the cranium. The dura was approximated by several stitches reinforced by pieces of Gelfoam. The bone defect was completely covered with a small silver plate which was fixed to the skull with tissue fixative. The wound was firmly closed in layers. SAH was induced by removing the needle 3 h later.

The experimental setup is shown in Figure 1. The dog was anesthetized with an intravenous injection of Nembutal and then immobilized by continuous infusion of Galamine. The normal level of blood gases was maintained by mechanical ventilation.

A double-needle type thermocouple (Shincorder, CTE-202) was inserted in the parietal region to a depth of 2-3 mm through small burr holes on the side in which SAH was induced. An epidural pressure transducer (ST lab. MH-AC) was inserted into the epidural space on the other side.

Cisterna magna pressure, systemic arterial pressure, and EEG were also monitored. The results of a preliminary experiment to evaluate the reliability of the thermocouple is reported elsewhere (3).

At 3 h after induction of SAH, the thoracic aorta was quickly cannulated and perfusion of the brain with an equal mixture of carbon black solution (biological ink, Pelikan) and 10% formalin was started at a pressure of 120 mm Hg. After fixation for 1 week, the status of cerebral microcirculation, as revealed by the filling defect, was checked macroscopically in coronal slices, together with microscopic examination using 100 μ sections.

Results

The ICP and CBF patterns in the 32 SAH thus induced were divided into two groups, Pattern I and Pattern II. Out of 32 SAH, 26 belonged to Pattern I, and the rest to Pattern II. In Pattern I (Fig. 2), there was an abrupt rise in ICP up to the level of the arterial diastolic pressure immediately after SAH. At the same time there was a drop in CBF accompanied by supression of EEG activity. After maintaining a plateau ranging from a few to 10 min, ICP fell gradually and smoothly to a level 10-30 mm Hg higher than normal. Together with the fall in ICP, there was a steep rise and overshooting in CBF. This appearance of reactive hyperemia is a characteristic feature of Pattern I, and it was invariably succeeded by complete or incomplete recovery of EEG activity.

In Pattern II (Fig. 3), the rise in ICP at the time of hemorrhage was even more severe. The secondary rise in ICP due to elevation of systemic arterial pressure was always observed. This tremendous elevation in ICP was accompanied by a marked drop in CBF and complete flattening of EEG activity, indicating almost complete cessation of CBF. Contrary to Pattern I, normalization of ICP did not take place in Pattern II. Extreme elevation of ICP in the range of 50-100 mm Hg persisted throughout. Accordingly, there was neither reactive hyperemia nor reappearance of EEG activity.

In 20 of the 26 dogs belonging to Pattern I, the filling defect was more or less recognized macroscopically as shown in Figure 4. Microscopic specimens taken from the poorly perfused area revealed extensive nonfilling of the capillary networks, while larger penetrating arterioles showed relative preservation.

It is characteristic that the filling defects were symmetrically distributed in both hemispheres.

The most frequently affected brain structures were the thalamus, basal ganglia, upper part of the midbrain, and the arterial boundary zone of the cerebral cortex, especially in the parieto-occipital region. The infratentorial portion of the brain and the hypothalamus were relatively well perfused in Pattern I.

In Pattern II, carbon black filled only the superficial pial arteries and the brain parenchyma was totally unperfused, while the infratentorial portion was relatively spared (Fig. 5).

Discussion

ICP elevation patterns in human SAH have been recently reported (7). The results of the present experiment are very similar to the clinical data, presented in these reports, such as to height and duration of the initial rise of ICP at the time of hemorrhage, as well as the basic patterns of subsequent changes in ICP. This similarity is considered as proof that the basic mechanism of ICP elevation due to rupture of an aneurysm was satisfactorily simulated in the present SAH model.

ICP elevation patterns, on the other hand, were found to have a close relationship with the status of cerebral microcirculation. In Pattern II, in which markedly raised ICP and depressed CBF persisted, the brain accordingly showed pronounced nonfilling. In Pattern I, the extent of nonfilling was far less and variable although its distribution was uniform in all the animals. The remarkable nonfilling of the cerebral hemispheres in Pattern II, together with its frequent occurrence in Pattern I, suggests that such microcirculatory disturbance takes place commonly also in the acute stage of human SAH.

As to the mechanism of genesis of nonfilling (no-reflow phenomenon) in the present experiment, the following speculations can be made.

In more than half of the animals belonging to Pattern I, the duration of the initial global ischemia due to maximal elevation of ICP ranged from several to 10 min. Since it is known that complete ischemia for more than 5 min can give rise to the no-reflow phenomenon (2), this initial global ischemia may well be a major initiating factor in the genesis of nonfilling. Besides the well-known occurrence of diffuse early spasm affecting the circle of Willis, possible constriction of pial arterioles and moderately or severely elevated ICP as in Pattern II, all contribute to lowering the perfusion pressure to the cerebral vascular bed and help persistence of no-reflow in the postischemic period. As all of the above-mentioned factors are present in the acute stage, the occurrence of the no-reflow phenomenon also in human SAH seems very likely.

There is still much debate about the pathogenic role of the no-reflow phenomenon (2), and in regard to this problem, the results of the present experiment are by no means conclusive. However, it should be stressed that the no-reflow phenomenon is quite likely to occur and its preference for areas in deep brain structures, such as thalamus and midbrain, may be the cause of sustained loss or lowering of the level of consciousness in the acute stage of SAH. Also it may be worthwhile to note that the location of cerebral infarction, as shown in many previous reports (4), corresponds to the sites of nonfilling demonstrated in the present SAH-model.

If the no-reflow phenomenon is a very common occurrence, the aim of therapy in the acute stage of SAH should be directed toward improvement of cerebral microcirculation, together with the definitive treatment of the ruptured aneurysm.

The results of the present experiment seem to indicate that this therapeutic approach to SAH in the acute stage is worthy of further investigation, and thus extends the hope of decreasing morbidity and mortality due to SAH.

Summary

In the present experiment which simulates SAH in dog, the frequent and pronounced occurrence of the no-reflow phenomenon (NRP) in the cerebral hemispheres was demonstrated. The initial elevation of ICP at the time of hemorrhage, which causes transient or sustained global ischemia, seemed to be the principal factor in the genesis of NRP in this model, although participation of other factors, such as early spasm. were also considered. This result suggests that NRP may play a significant pathogenetic role also in the acute stage of human SAH.

References

1. ALLCOCK, J.M., DRAKE, C.G.: Ruptured intracranial aneurysms: the role of arterial spasm. J. Neurosurg. 22, 21-29 (1965).

2. AMES, A.: Incidence and significance of vascular occlusion in focal and diffuse ischemia. In: Cerebral circulation and metabolism (LANGFITT, T.W., McHENRY, L.C., REIVICH, M., WOLLMAN, H., eds.) pp. 551-554. Berlin-Heidelberg-New York: Springer 1975.

3. ASANO, T., TAMURA, A., TAKU, Y., et al.: The influence of acutely raised intracranial pressure on cerebral microcirculation. Neurol. med. chir. 1976, in press.

4. CROMPTON, M.R.: Cerebral infarction following the rupture of cerebral berry aneurysms. Brain 87, 263-280 (1964).

5. ECHLIN, F.A.: Current concepts in the etiology and treatment of vasospasm. Clin. Neurosurg. 15, 133-159 (1968).

6. HUNT, W.E., HESS, R.M.: Surgical risks as related to timing of intervention in the repair of intracranial aneurysm. J. Neurosurg. 28, 14-20 (1968).

7. NORNES, H., MAGNES, B.: Intracranial pressure in patients with ruptured saccular aneurysm. J. Neurosurg. 36, 537-547 (1973).

8. ODOM, G.L.: Cerebral vasospasm. Clin. Neurosurg. 37, 316-324 (1972).

9. PETRUK, K.C., WEST, G.R., et al.: Cerebral blood flow following induced subarachnoid hemorrhage in the monkey. J. Neurosurg. 37, 316-324 (1972).

10. SIMEONE, F.A., TREPPER, P.J., BROWN, D.J.: Cerebral blood flow evaluation of prolonged experimental vasospasm. J. Neurosurg. 37, 302-311 (1972).

11. ZINGESSER, L.H., SCHECHTER, M.M., DEXTER, J., et al.: On the significance of spasm associated with rupture of a cerebral aneurysm; the relationship between spasm as noted angiographically and regional blood flow determinations. Arch. Neurol. 18, 520-528 (1968).

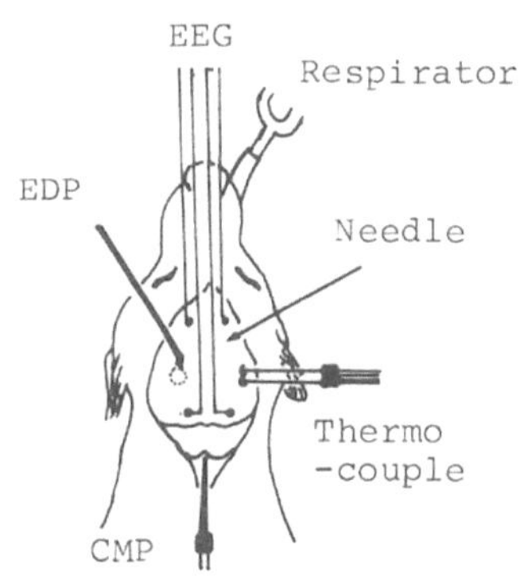

Fig. 1. Experimental setup. EDP (epidural pressure), CMP (cisterna magna pressure)

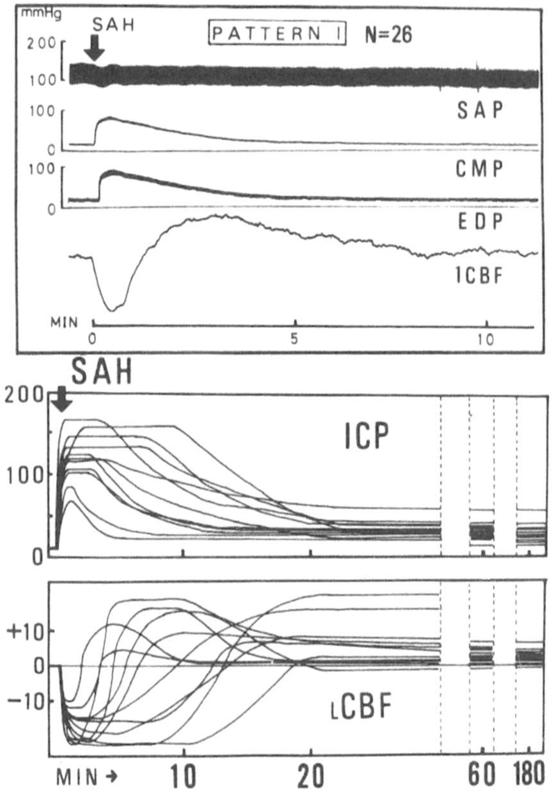

Fig. 2. Top: A representative polygraphic record in Pattern I. Below: ICP and CBF tracings of 11 dogs belonging to Pattern I.
1 CBF (local cerebral blood flow), SAP (systemic arterial pressure)

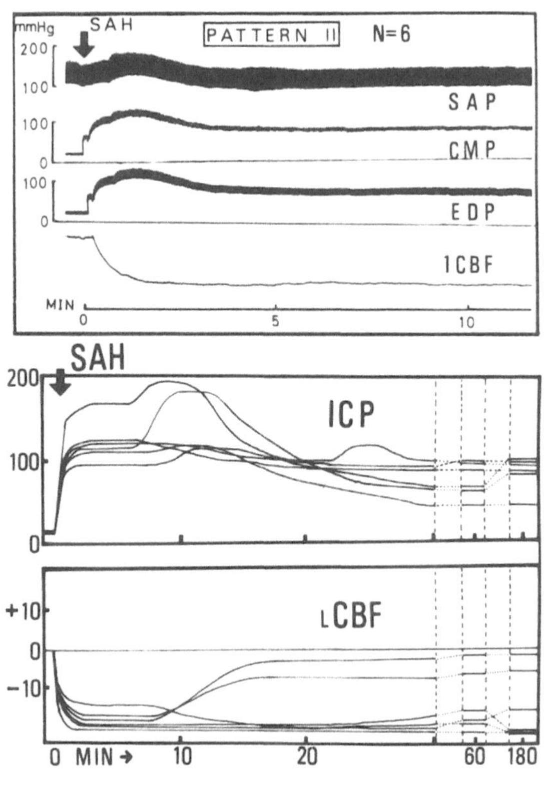

Fig. 3. Top: A representative polygraphic record in Pattern II. Below: ICP and CBF tracings of six dogs belonging to Pattern II

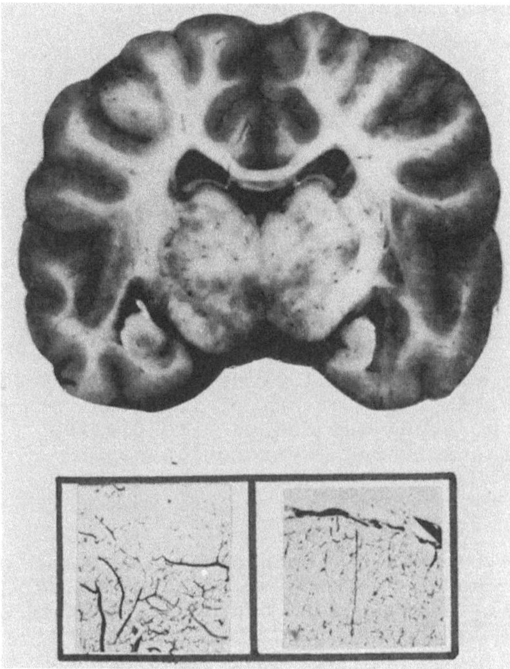

Fig. 4. Top: Coronal slices of brain in Pattern I, showing typical distribution of filling defect. Below: 100 μ-thick sections taken from thalamus (left) and cortex (right)

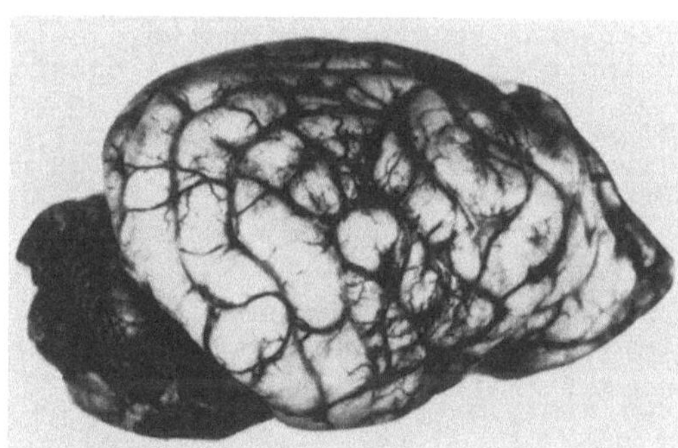

Fig. 5. External appearance of brain in Pattern II. Only relatively large pial arteries are filled with carbon black in both cerebral hemispheres. Infratentorial portion of brain was relatively well filled

The Role of CSF Resorption on the Intracranial Pressure/Volume Relationship

M. Furuse, M. Hasuo, M. Brock, and H. Dietz

Introduction

Despite several speculations on the mechanisms of pressure/volume (P/V) relationship, this matter of theroretical and practical importance remains unresolved to date. The present study was designed to clarify the role of CSF resorption on the intracranial P/V relationship.

Materials and Methods

There were 16 adults apparently healthy mongrel cats of both sexes weighing 2.3 to 3.6 kg were studied under Nembutal anesthesia (35 mg/kg body weight, intraperitoneal). All animals were tracheostomized, paralyzed, and artificially ventilated under normocapnic conditions ($PaCO_2$ 27-35 mm Hg) with a Starling pump. The femoral vessels on one side were catheterized for continuous recording of systemic arterial pressure (Statham P 23Db), blood sampling, and administration of drugs as needed.

Following fixation of the animal's head in a stereotactic frame, a thin polyethylene catheter (outer diameter: 1.0 mm) was inserted into each lateral ventricle through a small burr hole. One catheter was used to measure ventricular fluid pressure (Statham P 23Db), while the other was utilized for intraventricular administration of soot dispersion and for ventricular infusion of saline as described below.

Intracranial volume loadings were obtained (1) by intraventricular infusion of 2 ml of saline at a constant pump rate of 0.5 ml/min and (2) by intermittent inflation of an epidural balloon (0.5 ml increments in 30 s at intervals of 15 min). CSF malresorption was induced by slow intraventricular administration of 2 ml of a neutral soot dispersion (containing 10% soot, 9.5% gelatin, and 1.3% phenol). Changes in VFP and SAP were continuously recorded on a polygraph throughout the experiments.

At the end of the experiment the animals were sacrified by intravenous administration of saturated KCl solution, the brain and spinal cord were carefully removed and shiftings of intracranial structures as well as the distribution of soot particles were examined.

Results

Prior to intraventricular soot administration, the constant-rate infusion of saline lead to an average VFP increase from the control value of 7.8 (± O.) SE) mm Hg to 38.5 (± 6.2 SE) mm Hg at the end of the infusion period (4 min, i.e., 2 ml). When the saline infusion was discontinued, pressure promptly returned to levels slightly higher than control values within next 4 min (Fig. 1). There was no difference in pressure response curves observed after 1 and 3 h.

Intraventricular administration of a neutral soot dispersion altered intracranial capacitance as a function of time lapse. At the end of the 1st hour following soot administration, resting VFP rose to 18.0 (± 1.4 SE) mm Hg and the constant-rate infusion of saline revealed a steady and steep pressure increase to value of 89.6 (± 14.1 SE) mm Hg, significantly different from the controls ($P < 0.01$). At the end of the 3rd hour, the saline infusion lead to an even steeper increase of VFP from 32.1 (± 4.8 SE) mm Hg to 140.8 (± 21.7 SE) mm Hg. When the saline infusion was discontinued, pressures sharply decreased, remaining, however, significantly higher than the preinfusion values (Fig. 1).

The balloon inflation experiments also revealed that the soot administration causes a shifting to the left along the P/V curve. Graded inflation of an epidural balloon 1 h following intraventricular soot administration increases VFP proportionally to the balloon volume, showing an almost linear correlation. This apparently linear P/V relation in response to a localized ICP increase following obstruction of the CSF resorption pathways is shown in Figure 2.

A rapid increase in intracranial elastance (calculated from pressure difference between VFPs before and after each balloon inflation) was observed in the control animals simultaneously to the steepening of the P/V curve. Such changes were also noted - however, at smaller balloon volumes - in the soot administration group (Fig. 3). Pupillary dilatation and flatening of EEG corresponded to the sharp increase in intracranial elastance. Typical transtentorial and foraminal herniations were observed postmortem.

Comments

Intraventricular administration of a neutral soot dispersion causes an acute malresorptive hydrocephalus leading to an imbalance of the fluid dynamics within the craniospinal system. The gradual increase in resting VFP following soot administration is an expression of the CSF malresorption, since no localized obstruction of the subarachnoid cisterns or the aqueduct are observed under these conditions (1). The "infusion test" performed in the first group of animals 1 and 3 h after soot administration demonstrates, furthermore, a significant reduction in intracranial capacitance.

The balloon inflation experiments indicate that the compensatory shifting of fluid from CSF spaces in response to an expanding mass plays an important role in intracranial spatial buffering capacity.

Changes in intracranial blood volume can also account for part of the volumetric buffering capacity (3, 5, 9), and the observation has been made (2) that the "squeezing out" of intravascular blood is related to the levels of brain tissue pressure attained in the presence of brain swelling. Further studies are necessary to clarify to what extent CSF and/or blood displacement account for the intracranial volume-compensation. The influence of the time-factor also remains inclear and it is unknown to what proportion CSF and blood are respectively displaced by fast or slow volume increases.

It is striking that increases in intracranial elastance can develop rather abruptly. This suggests that the rapid decrease in intracranial spatial buffering capacity in the late stage of intracranial hypertension may be due to morphologic factors such as herniations of brain tissue leading to compartmentation of the craniospinal system. The lack of communication along the CSF system (4, 8, 9) thus accelerates the total exhaustion of its spatial buffering capacity.

Summary

The factors influencing intracranial P/V relationship were studied by constant-rate intraventricular infusion of saline and by graded inflation of an epidural balloon under the condition of CSF-malresorption caused by intraventricular administration of a neutral soot dispersion.

At 1 h following soot administration, pressure responses to saline infusion become significantly steeper, corresponding to a marked reduction in intracranial capacitance. Balloon inflation leads to an even steeper, almost linear P/V relation in the presence of CSF-malresorption. It thus appears that CSF displacement along the resorptive pathways plays an important role in intracranial space-buffering mechanism.

Marked and rapid increases in intracranial elastance suggest that shifting and herniation of parts of brain may lead to a "watertight" compartmentation of the craniospinal system and contribute toward steepening the P/V curve.

Key Words

Intracranial pressure, Pressure/volume relationship, CSF-malresorption, Intracranial elastance.

References

1. BROCK, M., FURUSE, M., HASUO, M., DIETZ, H.: Influences of CSF-resorption pathways on intracranial capacitance. In: Advances in Neurosurgery (H. PENZHOLZ, M. BROCK, M. HAMER, M. KLINGER, O. SPOERRI, eds.) Vol. 3, Brain Hypoxia. Pain, pp. 109-114. Berlin-Heidelberg-New York: Springer 1975.

2. FURUSE, M., BROCK, M., WEBER, R., HASUO, M., DIETZ, H.: Intracranial pressure/volume relationship in acute water intoxication. In: Intracranial Pressure II (N. LUNDBERG, U. PONTEN, M. BROCK, eds.) pp. 101-106. Berlin-Heidelberg-New York: Springer 1975.

3. LANGFITT, T.W., WEINSTEIN, J.D., KASSELL, N.F.: Cerebral vasomotor paralysis produced by intracranial hypertension. Neurology 15, 622-641 (1965).

4. LÖFGREN, J., ZWETNOW, N.N.: Cranial and spinal components of the cerebrospinal fluid pressure/volume curve. Acta Neurol. Scandinav. 49, 575-585 (1973).

5. LÖFGREN, J., VON ESSEN, C., ZWETNOW, N.N.: The pressure/volume curve of the cerebrospinal fluid space in dogs. Acta Neurol. Scandinav. 49, 557-574 (1973).

6. MARMAROU, A., SHULMAN, K., LaMORGESE, J.: Compartmental analysis of compliance and outflow resistance of the cerebrospinal fluid system. J. Neurosurg. 43, 523-534 (1975).

7. NAKATANI, S., OMMAYA, A.K.: Volume pressure curves and pial vascular pressure gradients in the rhesus monkey. In: Intracranial Pressure II (H. LUNDBERG, U. PONTEN, M. BROCK, eds.) pp. 89-96. Berlin-Heidelberg-New York: Springer 1975.

8. PÁSTOR, E., PÁSTOR, A., BODO, M., BOGSCH, S.: The role of spinal arachnoidal spaces in compensation of intracranial hypertension. In: Intracranial Pressure II (N. LUNDBERG, U. PONTEN, M. BROCK, eds) pp. 82-85. Berlin-Heidelberg-New York: Springer 1975.

9. SHULMAN, K., MARMAROU, A.: Pressure-volume considerations in infantile hydrocephalus. Develop. Med. Child Neurol. 13 (Suppl. 25), 90-95 (1971).

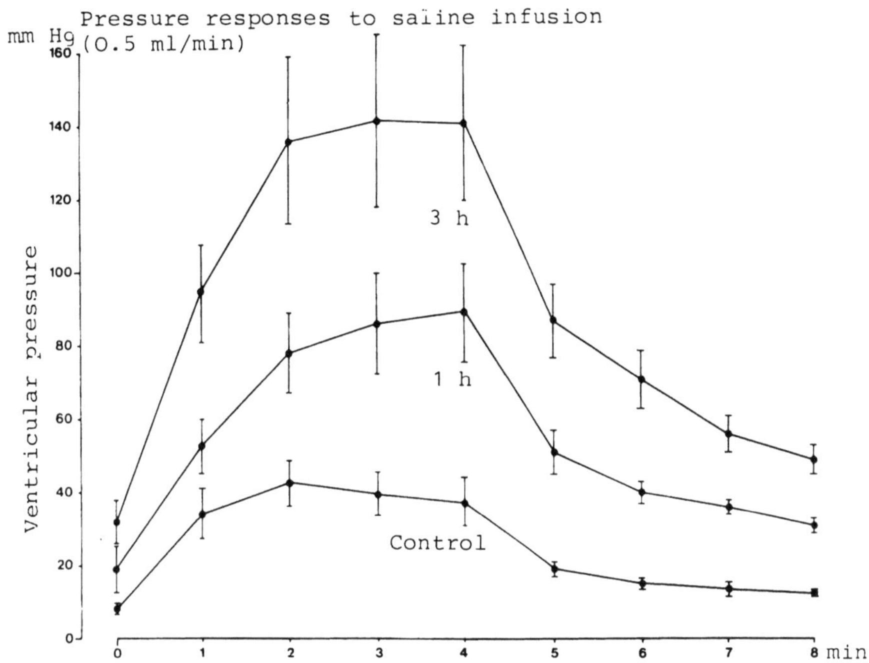

Fig. 1. Pressure-volume curves obtained by intraventricular infusion of 2 ml of physiologic saline (0.5 ml/min) before (control) as well as 1 and 3 h after intraventricular administration of a neutral soot dispersion

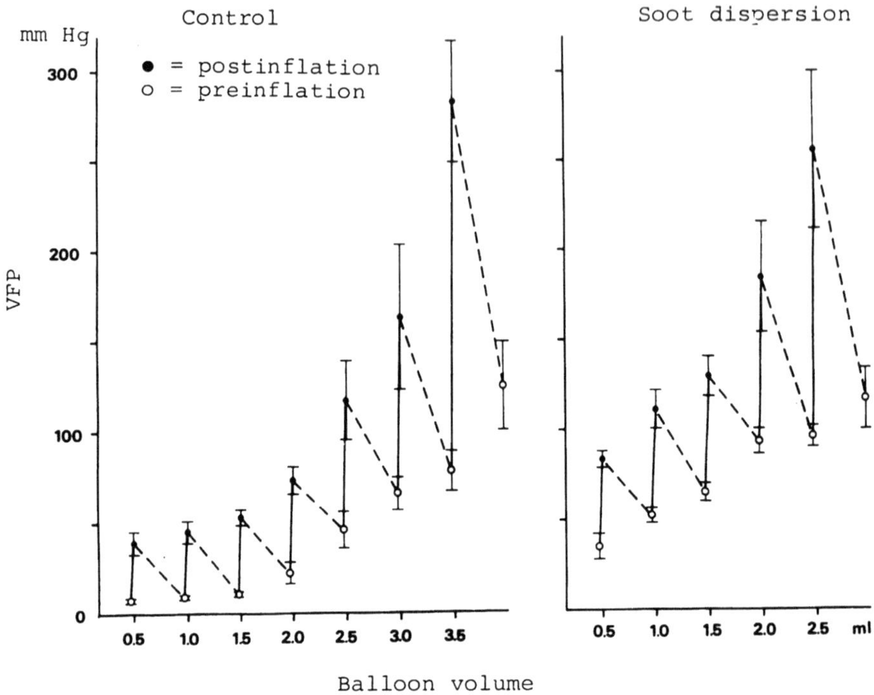

Fig. 2. Pressure response to intermittent inflation of epidural balloon. In soot dispersion, group volume buffering capacity is markedly reduced

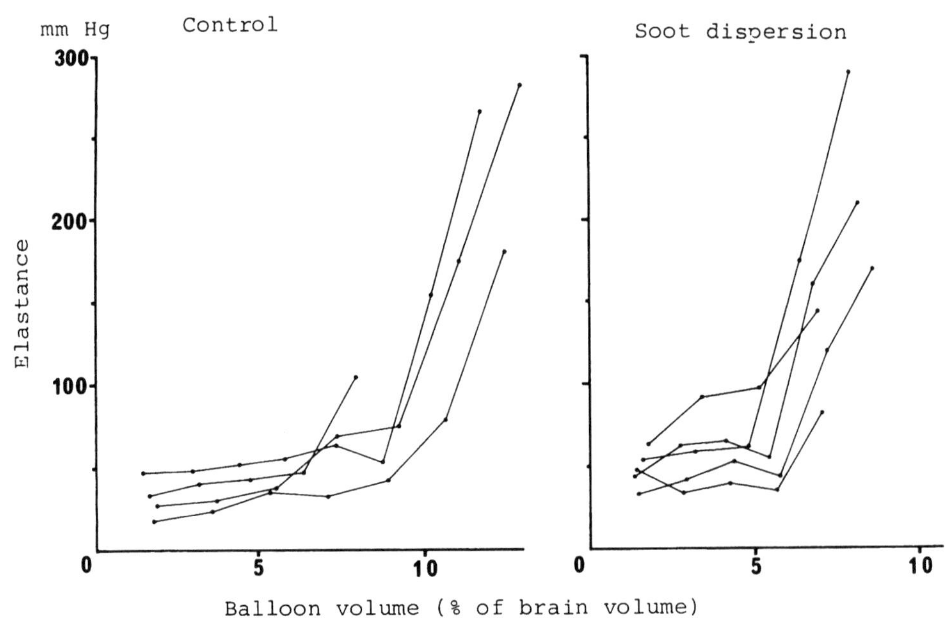

Fig. 3. Marked increase in intracranial elastance in response to balloon expansion in presence of CSF-malresorption

Intracranial Blood Volume and Its Variation with Changes in Intracranial Pressure

J. Löfgren and N.N. Zwetnow

Introduction

The intracranial blood volume (ICBV) may undergo rapid changes in connection with circulatory adjustments of the cerebral vascular bed. The effects of changes in the ICBV on intracranial pressure (ICP) are magnified by intracranial mass lesions and increased pressure. Under extreme conditions with cerebral vasoparalysis the vascular bed may assume excessive dimensions with adverse consequences (2). An accurate assessment of the mechanical effects of changes in the vascular volume demands a method for continuous, quantitative monitoring of the ICBV in different circumstances. The present paper is concerned with a description of such a method which has been worked out in dogs and applied to the problem of the effect on ICBV of increased cerebrospinal fluid (CSF) pressure.

Methods

Experiments were performed in dogs anesthetized with pentobarbital, intubated and ventilated mechanically on a respirator. The pressures were recorded in cisterna magna, femoral artery, and inferior caval vein. Technetium albumin was administered intravenously and the gamma emission measured extracranially by means of relatively widely collimated gamma-detector after stripping off skin and temporal muscle from the skull. In two experiments cerebral blood flow was recorded with the Xenon technique with injection into left vertebral artery. ICP was raised in steps by a pressurized bottle of saline connected to the subarachnoid space.

Calibration procedure (Fig. 1). In order to express ICBV in counts per minute (cpm) in ml blood, neck compression was performed with a sphygmometer cuff inflated to 50 mm Hg. This caused a partial obstruction of the venous outflow and distension of the cerebral vascular bed indicated by an increase in the gamma activity. The volume addition caused a parallel increase in CSF pressure (10-15 mm Hg). CSF was thereafter withdrawn until CSF pressure regained its initial steady state value. The aspirated volume of CSF, usually about 1.8 ml, corresponded to the increase in ICBV caused by the continuing compression of the neck. Thus changes in gamma activity could be evaluated directly in ml. The absolute quantity of the ICBV could be estimated by stopping the heart after the experiment with potassium chloride intravenously and raising the ICP to 200 mm Hg, presumably displacing most of the ICBV from the skull cavity. The decrease in cpm should correspond to total ICBV at the moment of cardiac arrest. By measuring brain weight

[1] This study has been supported by the Swedisch Research Council, Grant B77-17x-3500, which herewith is gratefully acknowledged.

and intracranial volume percentage expressions could be obtained of ICBV. The error in the method was estimated to be 15%.

Results

Maximum variation in ICBV during the course of the experiments was 2.5-6.0 ml or 3-8% of intracranial volume. Stepwise elevation of CSF pressure to the level of the diastolic arterial pressure, i.e., about 100 mm Hg, did not result in any significant change or alternatively in a slight progressive rise in ICBV (Fig. 2). Rapid normalization of the pressure after a period of high pressure caused a more or less prolonged overshoot of ICBV amounting to about 3 ml, i.e., ICBV increased to approximately twice its initial value. These changes in ICBV correlated well with the concomitant measurements of the cerebral blood flow.

Discussion

The values obtained of the ICBV and the range of variation are in agreement with those arrived at by other methods. The range of variation of up to 8% of the intracranial volume should be compared to the size of the intracranial CSF compartment which is about 10% under normal conditions. Thus there is normally a margin of safety in the process of spatial compensation involving reciprocal changes in CSF volume.

The finding of a constant or slightly increasing ICBV during intracranial hypertension may be interpreted as follows. Changes in the volume of a vascular bed are by definition related to the venous capacitance section. Increased CSF pressure compresses presumably the distal low pressure venous section of the intracranial vascular bed decreasing the venous volume in the system. The fact that ICBV is unaltered or even increased when the CSF pressure is raised implies that the volume reduction is balanced by a continuing dilation of some other "upstream" section of the vascular bed, the volume of which may be referred to as the "arterial" volume. The constancy of the blood flow during increasing ICP indicates a progressive dilation of the resistance vessels keeping total flow resistance approximately constant. Thus the dilation of the resistance vessels is associated with an increase in the arterial volume of the vascular bed. When CSF pressure is normalized after a period of high pressure there is an immediate overshoot in cerebral blood flow with the nature of a reactive hyperemia (1). The compressed venous section assumes its normal dimensions causing an increase in ICBV. The increase in the arterial volume during intracranial hypertension is consequently of the same order of magnitude as the decrease in venous volume. This a state of high ICP is characterized by a redistribution of CBV from distal venous to more proximal arterial sections of the vascular bed. This redistribution of blood volume may have important effects on intracranial spatial relations.

The quantitative data of these experiments are in agreement with previous measurements of the distribution of volume changes between the cranial and spinal compartments (3). It was shown that at CSF pressures higher than about 30 mm Hg, volume additions were distributed about equally, i.e., the elastance is approximately the same in the cranial and spinal compartments in this pressure range in the dog. An increase of CSF pressure to 100 mm Hg corresponds to a volume increment of about 5 ml starting from a normal pressure. Half this amount, 2.5 ml, is distributed to the cranial system, compressing the venous vascular bed, and the other half is displaced into the spinal compartment. These calculations conform precisely with the value of the venous vascular compression during similar increases in CSF pressure obtained in the present measurements of ICBV and support our earlier interpretation of the pressure-volume relations.

Summary

ICBV was measured in dogs with a continuous and quantitative method. The gamma activity was recorded extracranially after intravenous administration of technetium albumin. A calibration procedure was performed with neck compression causing an increase in ICBV and CSF pressure. A volume of CSF was aspirated which reduced the pressure to the control value. This volume corresponded to the increase in ICBV which henceforth could be expressed in ml. Increasing ICP apparently caused a redistribution of ICBV with a compression of the distal venous bed and a dilation of the upstream vascular bed, the total ICBV being unaffected or slightly increased.

References

1. HÄGGENDAL, E., LÖFGREN, J., NILSSON, N.J., ZWETNOW, N.N.: Prolonged cerebral hyperemia after periods of increased cerebrospinal fluid pressure in dogs. Acta physiol. scand. 79, 272-279 (1970).
2. LANGFITT, T.W.: Increased intracranial pressure. Clin. neurosurg. 16, 436-471 (1968).
3. LÖFGREN, J., ZWETNOW, N.N.: Cranial and spinal components of the cerebrospinal fluid pressure-volume curve. Acta neurol. scand. 49, 575-585 (1973).

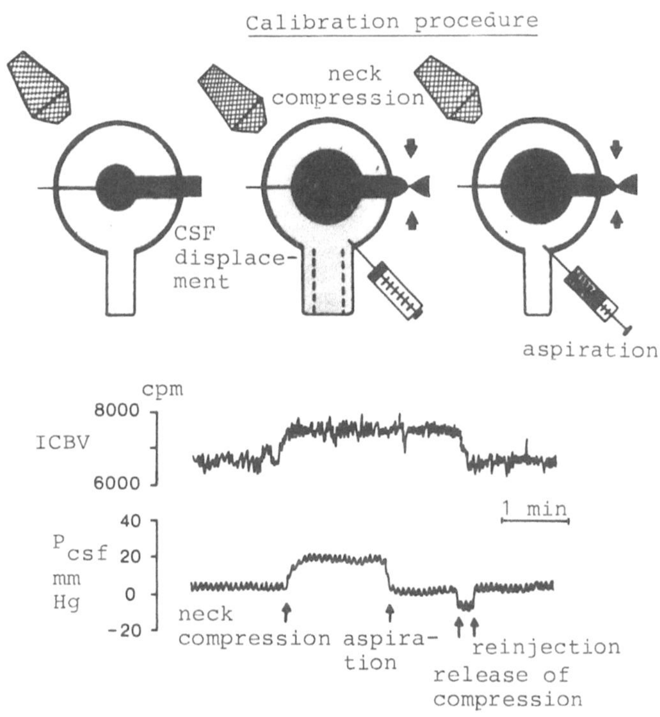

Fig. 1. Calibration procedure. Neck compression causes an increase in intracranial blood volume, resulting in increase in the γ-activity and an increase in the CSF pressure. CSF is aspirated to resettle the pressure to its initial value. Volume withdrawn corresponds to increase in cerebral blood volume

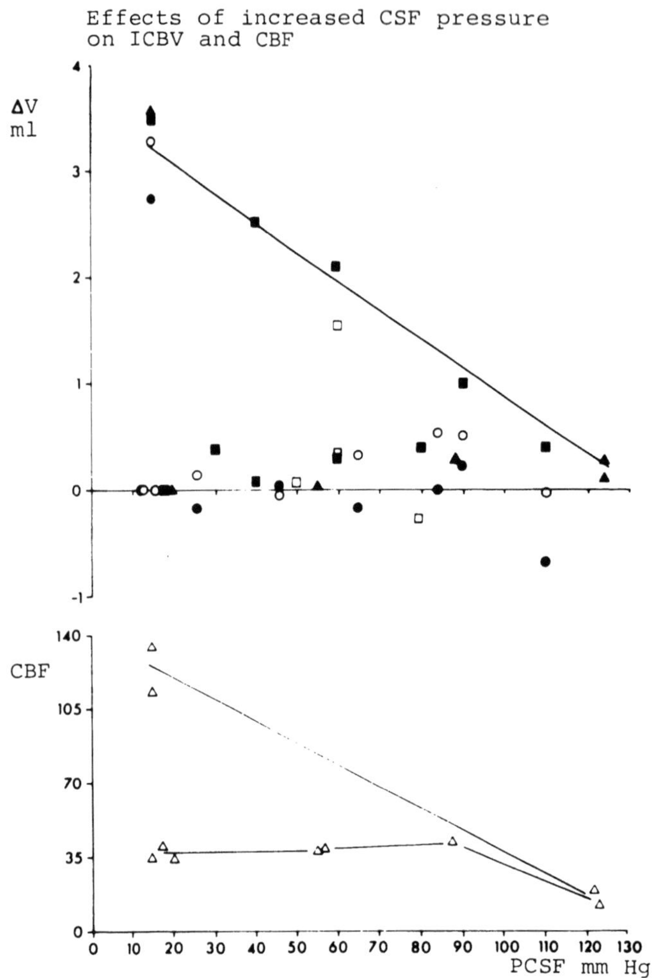

Fig. 2. Changes in blood volume and cerebral blood flow during increasing CSF pressure. Release of high pressure results in a reactive hyperemia and an increased intracranial blood volume

Summary

N. N. Zwetnow and F. Isamat

By measurements of cerebral tissue pressure gradients with wick catheters MARMAROU was able to show that fluid transport occurred within brain tissue in the presence of small pressure gradients of about 10 mm Hg. ROWAN discussed the accuracy of the pressure measurements and asked whether two or more wick catheters had been placed at equidistant points from the lesion to test the accuracy of measurement. MARMAROU answered that control experiments had shown the measuring error of the wick catheters to be less than 0.5 mm Hg. BRUCE asked MARMAROU which physical forces were supposed to contribute to the tissue water transport and specifically whether diffusion might be involved. MARMAROU answered that while diffusion might play a part the gradual decrease observed in tissue resistance would primarily point to a bulk flow as being most important.

GO's paper was discussed by LANGFITT, who wondered whether the difference between the intraventricular pressure and the cortical vein pressure was real or might be an artefact. GO admitted that an open head preparation might lead to errors in pressure measurements, but that possible errors did not affect the conclusions of his results. Answering SYMON's and SHULMAN's questions, GO stated that his preparation did not permit a closer analysis of tissue pressure being a possible autoregulatory stimulus.

Using cryogenic lesions to simulate intracranial expanding lesions MARMAROU et al. could demonstrate that significant reduction of regional CBF occurred close to the lesion, but also to a certain degree in the ipsilateral and the contralateral cerebral hemispheres at low tissue pressure. MILLER said MARMAROU's results were in good agreement with those presented at Aviemore 1975. The flow decrease seems to be caused by several factors (variation in local perfusion pressure, decrease in CMRO2, transhemispheric depression, etc.), the relative importance of which varies with each location. SYMON stressed the potential methodologic error in interpreting small variations in white substance flow, MARMAROU agreed, but said that even small flow differences in his study were found to be significant.

After experimental subarachnoid hemorrhage in dogs, ASANO et al. found no-reflow in cerebral tissue areas the extent of which depended on the increase in ICP. LANGFITT asked ASANO whether one might speak of a no-reflow phenomenon in the original sense of the term as long as the cerebral perfusion pressure had not been brought back to normal. ZWETNOW felt the two observed intracranial pressure patterns were directly related to the amount of bleeding in each experiment. Increased local pressure and a local vascular spasm might then be the factors responsible for the failing reperfusion in certain areas. The interesting results of the Japanese group await further confirmation and analysis, particularly with respect to their basal causative factors.

The paper of FURUSE et al. was another demonstration that an increase of the CSF outflow resistance may increase the intracranial pressure response to a volume increment. The increased pressure response in their experiments seems weel explained by the decrease in spatial compensation only. While the true form of the pressure-volume curve is less likely to be affected, the virtual increase in steepness of the apparent P/V curve after injection of sooth solution may thus be a phenomenon which appears only at relatively low injection rates of fluid.

The demonstration of a quantitative method for measuring changes in intracranial blood volume in experimental animals by LÖFGREN and ZWETNOW was the last paper of the session. Their results were confirmed by BENAMID, who measured intracranial blood volume semiquantitatively in terms of cerebral impedance. Other methods for measurement of intracranial blood volume were also discussed. BRUCE reported that intracranial blood volume measured with a positron-emitting tomograph in children with skull trauma showed a considerable increase many months after the trauma. If confirmed, these results would suggest the intracranial blood volume to consistute a parameter of certain clinical interest.

In conclusion, the papers of the session brought considerable new material and clarified concepts concerning intracranial tissue pressure gradients and the reciprocal relationships of CBF and ICP. There still is some controversy concerning the effects of arterial pressure and CBF autoregulation on the intracranial pressure-volume relationship. An agreement upon a common terminology seems justified.

The Chairmen felt greatly honored by the genuine interest in the work of the session showed by HER ROYAL HIGHNESS PRINCESS MARGRIET OF THE NETHERLANDS.

Session B

Basic Concepts II

Chairman: K. Shulman
Co-chairman: J. Hoff

Isolation of Factors Leading to Sustained Elevations of the ICP[1]

A. Marmarou, K. Shapiro, and K. Shulman

Introduction

Theoretical considerations suggest that the normal steady state level of the ICP is given by the product of CSF formation and outflow resistance ($I_f \times R_o$) added to the venous exit pressure Pv (4).

Equation (1): $ICP = (I_f \times R_o) + Pv$.

The objective of this investigation was to test: (1) the validity of this concept in clinical settings, and (2) to separate the contribution of CSF parameters (I_f, R_o) from venous exit pressure (Pv) in producing sustained elevations of the ICP.

Material and Methods

There were 13 patients selected from a large group of patients undergoing intraventricular ICP monitoring complemented by the Pressure Volume Index technique (6). The time course of ICP response to bolus CSF manipulation was recorded from transducers on fast speed strip chart recorders. All transducers were referenced to the patient's occiput with the patient flat in bed. As outlined in Table 1, bolus withdrawal (0.5 - 8 ml at 1 ml/s) was performed. Using the immediate fall in ICP from steady state, PVI and compliance (C) were calculated. The rate of ICP return to steady state permitted calculation of I_f. Using the PVI to predict the ICP response to bolus manipulation, appropriate increments were chosen for injection. PVI and R_o were calculated from the ICP response profile.

After a suitable control period, a Harvard pump was connected to the pressure line in eight of these patients and fluid was removed at the estimated rate of formation (I_f). The reduced steady-state pressure that resulted from this maneuver was considered a measure of venous exit pressure (P_v).

Results

The findings from the bolus withdrawal and injection sequence indicate a reduced volume buffering capacity (PVI = 13.9 ± 6 SD) for the group of patients undergoing continuous withdrawal. Average PVI was 56% of normal level (25 ml). When ICP was high, PVI was calculated only from bolus withdrawal data to prevent further increases in ICP. Steady-state ICP for this group was 29.2 mm Hg ± 11.2 SD. Mean arterial blood pressure (MABP) equalled 112 mm Hg ± 12.1 SD and was stable. CSF parameters derived from the test sequence are tabulated in Table 2.

[1] This work was supported in part by Training Grant No 5 T01 NS0511-10.

Table 1. Equations used to calculate CSF parameters (PVI, C, I_f, and R_o) are shown. These values are obtained by simple bolus manipulations of CSF. Evaluation of CSF system parameters from pressure response data

Record output	Known input	Extract parameters	Compute	Units	Restriction
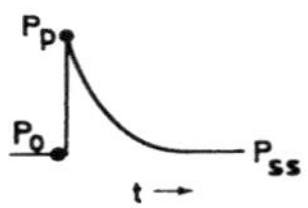	ΔV (ML)	P_o, P_p	$PVI=\frac{\Delta V}{\log_{10} P_p/P_o}$ $C=\frac{.4343 PVI}{P}$	ML ML/MMHg	$P > P_o$ $\frac{\Delta V}{\Delta T} \gg I_F$ $P_{ss} \approx P_o$
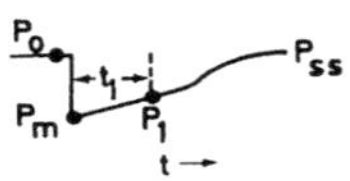	$-\Delta V$ (ML)	P_o, P_m, P_1, t_1	$PVI=\frac{\Delta V}{\log_{10} P_o/P_m}$ $I_{form}=\frac{PVI}{t_1}(\log\frac{P_1}{P_m})$	ML ML/MIN	$R_a \gg$ For $P < P_o$ $P_{ss} \approx P_o$
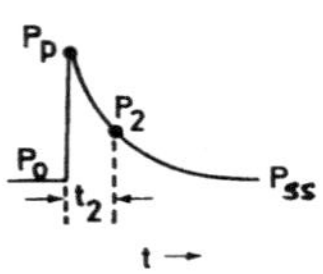	ΔV (ML)	P_o, P_p, P_2, t_2	$PVI=\frac{\Delta V}{\log_{10} P_p/P_o}$ $R=\frac{t_2 P_o}{(PVI)\log\left[\frac{P_2}{P_p}\cdot\frac{P_p-P_o}{P_2-P_o}\right]}$	ML MMHg/ML/MIN	$\Delta P_D = o$ $P_{ss} \approx P_o$

Table 2. Tabulation of CSF parameters used to characterize ICP dynamics in eight patients

	PVI ml	MABP mmhg	I_f ml/min	R_o mmhg/ml/min	$\overline{I_f R}$ mmhg	P_v mmhg	ICP mmhg
Mean	13.90	112.0	.49	14.63	5.27	22.63	29.2
SD	1.60	12.1	.20	20.71	5.91	8.67	11.2
SE	.56	4.1	.07	8.03	2.09	3.06	3.97

When fluid was removed at a rate equal to the patient's calculated formation (I_f = .49 ml/min ± .2 SD), ICP decreases and stabilized at a reduced steady-state level (P_v = 22.23 mm Hg ± 8.67 SD) within 5 min. When the withdrawal was stopped, ICP increased and returned to initial levels within 10 min.

The IxR product was computed for each patient using the estimated formation rate and resistance values obtained from the bolus withdrawal and injection tests. The average IxR component was 5.27 mm Hg. The sum of the IxR component and Pv value obtained by independent tests equalled 27.5 mm Hg, which compares well with the initial resting pressure (29.2 mm Hg). On a percentage basis, the contribution of the IxR pressure gradient was 18.1% of the ICP while 76.1% was accounted for by the Pv component.

These techniques were also applied in five patients with high ICP (range 26.5 mm Hg - 86.7 mm Hg). In three patients, the average IxR product was low (IxR = 2.50 mm Hg ± 1.05 SD) compared to the average ICP (35.8 ± 8.8 SD). The outflow resistance (R_o) of these patients was in the normal range. Results of withdrawal tests showed a high Pv (Pv = 29.7 mm Hg ± 7.00 SD), which accounted for 83% of the pressure rise. In the remaining two patients (Epidural hematoma, EDH: Subarachnoid hemorrhage, SAH) with ICP'd of 86.7 and 34.0 mm Hg, the resistance values were high (157.5 and 69.5 mm Hg/ml/min). The IxR products equalled 43.3 and 18.8 mm Hg and accounted for 49.8 and 55.6% of the elevated ICP, indicating impaired outflow resistance as a major factor in these ICP elevations (Table 3).

Table 3. Tabulation of CSF parameters used to characterize ICP dynamics in live patients with elevated ICP

Code	Po mmhg	R mmhg/ml/min	If ml/min	Pv mmhg	IxR mmhg	IR/P_o (%)	P_v/P_o (%)	TOTAL (%)
BT	26.5	1.95	.665	22.8	1.29	4.9	86.0	90.0
AVM	36.8	4.16	.719	29.4	2.99	8.1	79.9	88.0
CHI	44.0	9.05	.354	36.8	3.20	7.3	83.6	90.9
SAH	86.7	157.50	.275	-	43.3	49.9	-	-
EDH	34.0	69.50	.270	-	18.8	55.6	-	-

Comments

The theoretical basis of the steady-state relationship of ICP was first introduced by DAVSON (2) and PAPPENHEIMER (5). These workers assumed that normal flow out of the subarachnoid space should be proportional to the pressure difference between the CSF and venous compartment (ICP-Pv) divided by the resistance of the fluid pathway (R_O). At steady state, equation (1) is a restatement of this principle. Our laboratory as well as others have derived equations which reduce to this basic linear equation at equilibrium (1, 3, 4).

According to this principle, the ICP equals the sum of the ($I_f xR_O$) component, which is a measure of the pressure gradient that is developed across the absorption mechanism, added to tge sink pressure of the compartment absorbing fluid (Pv). The parameters ICP, I_f, and R_O can be measured or derived from the response data, leaving the pressure Pv to be determined. By withdrawing fluid at a constant rate equal to the rate of formation, the fluid that would normally be absorbed is diverted. This cancels the ($I_f xR_O$) component and the CSF compartment equilibrates to a reduced level of pressure which we believe is a measure of Pv.

Based on the data derived from patients, the sum of these components accounted for 94% of the measured ICP and supports the validity of the steady-state equation. We conclude that these simple dynamic tests, when coupled with standard ICP monitoring techniques, can be used to determine if the elevation of ICP is due to impairment of absorptive pathways. These patients are identified by an abnormally high ($I_f xR_O$) component (>25% of ICP).

It also suggests that the cause of sustained elevations of ICP with normal ($I_f xR_O$) is due to elevation of the effective venous sink pressure (Pv). We suspect that Pv may reflect both the venous exit pressure added to a valve opening pressure. The CSF dynamics examined thus far can only detect the combined effect of these mechanisms upon the ICP.

Although no extracerebral mass lesions were present in these patients, a mass effect of brain swelling could contribute to the initially high ICP and the decrease in buffering capacity (PVI). If so, the venous sink pressure (Pv), as we have determined it, would ne falsely high, i.e., effective venous sink pressure = actual P_V + mass pressure effect.

References

1. BENABID, A.L., de ROUGEMONT, J., BARGE, M.: CSF dynamics: a mathematical approach. In: Intracranial Pressure II (N. LUNDBERG, U. PONTEN, M. BROCK, eds.) pp. 54-60. New York-Heidelberg-Berlin: Springer 1975.
2. DAVSON, H., HOLLINGSWORTH, G., SEGAL, M.B.: The mechanism of drainage of the cerebrospinal fluid. Brain 93, 665-678 (1970).
3. GUINANE, J.E.: An equivalent circuit analysis of cerebrospinal fluid hydrodynamics. Amer. J. Physiol. 223, 425-430 (1972).
4. MARMAROU, A., SHULMAN, K., LA MORGESE, J.: Compartmental analysis of compliance and outflow resistance of the cerebrospinal fluid system. J. Neurosurg. 43, 523-534 (1975).
5. PAPPENHEIMER, J.R., HEISSEY, S.R., JORDAN, E.F., DORONER, J. deC.: Perfusion of the cerebral ventricular system in unanesthetized goats. Amer. J. Physiol. 203, 763-774 (1962).
6. SHAPIRO, K., SHULMAN, K., MARMAROU, A.: Clinical applications of the pressure volume index. Presented at the American Association of Neurological Surgeons Annual Meeting. San Francisco (1976).

Increases in ICP and Development of Plateau Waves in Decompensated Hydrocephalic Cats. A new Model[1]

G.M. Hochwald, A.E. Marlin, and A. Wald

Introduction

Since first described by LUNDBERG (7), intracranial pressure (ICP) plateau waves are a well-defined pathologic clinical entity. These waves generally occur, and are most clearly noted, as being concomitant with elevated ICP. The appearance of plateau waves is considered to be a harbinger of a continuing rise of ICP and decline of the patient's clinical status.

At any instant, the actual ICP is a net result of forces acting within the cranial vault. The reaction between the volume of the contents within the cranial vault and the rigidity of the vault determine the ICP level. The contents of the cranial vault can be described as consisting of several compartments (5). Arterial and venous blood, cerebrospinal fluid (CSF), extracellular fluid which may be in communication with the CSF, and brain parenchyma itself. Variation in the volume of any of these compartments without a compensatory change in another compartment will cause a corresponding change in ICP. Although, even under normal conditions, there are wide fluctuations of ICP, an average base line level can generally be defined. Plateau waves imply the existence of two stable states for intracranial volume contents. At either base line or plateau wave pressures the contents of the various intracranial compartments are in equilibrium with each other, and there is a relatively steady-state pressure.

In patients, the appearance of plateau waves demands immediate intervention, and precludes systematic study of this phenomenon. In animal models, it is difficult to maintain a reproducible model of elevated ICP, sufficient in time and magnitude to allow formation of plateau waves (4). Because of these limitations, the mechanisms by which plateau waves are created and their effects on brain function are still subject to investigation. We are presenting, in this report, a new model for the production of plateau waves, using experimentally obstructed hydrocephalic cats (5). In these animals the outlets of the fourth ventricle are occluded and communication between the ventricular system and the subarachnoid space is reestablished via the spinal cord central canal. Complete obstruction of the CSF circulation is then possible by placing a ligature around the lumbar spinal cord (1).

Materials and Methods

Experimental obstructive hydrocephalus was produced in cats by the intracisternal injection of kaolin. This technique has been previously described in detail (3). In short, 1 ml of CSF was withdrawn from the cisterna magna of adult, anesthetized cats (2.5 - 3.5 kg) and replaced

[1] This work was supported by NINCDS grants NS 05024, NS 06599, NS 07366 and the National Foundation-March of Dimes 1-416.

with 0.8 ml of kaolin (200 mg of hydrated aluminum silicate) suspended in saline. This causes a severe arachnoiditis which results in an obliteration of the cisterna magna and an obstruction to the outflow of fluid from the fourth ventricle. Subsequently, there is a rise in intraventricular pressure (IVP) which, in approximately 3 weeks, returns to within the normal range. The normalization of the IVP, or compensation of the hydrocephalic process, has been associated with the development of an alternate CSF absorption pathway which includes the enlarged central canal of the spinal canal.

At 3 or more weeks after intracisternal kaolin, five normal, adult, mongrel cats were anesthetized with pentobarbital sodium (20 mg/kg) and paralyzed with gallamine triethiodide (7 mg/kg). Supplemental doses were given as needed to maintain anesthesia and control ventilation. Some cats were anesthetized only, and were allowed to breathe unassisted.

The cats were put in a stereotaxic frame in the sphinx position. A saline-filled catheter was placed in a lateral ventricle and attached to a pressure transducer. The site of ventricular penetration was described previously in studies on ventricular perfusion (3). The intraventricular pressures were monitored and continuously recorded with a physiologic recorder. Arterial carbon dioxide pressure was kept between 25 and 30 torr by a respirator. End tidal CO_2 was monitored with a capnograph. Body temperature was maintained between 37 and 38°C by means of an automatically controlled heating pad. Arterial blood pressure was monitored through a catheter placed in a femoral artery.

After initial intraventricular pressures were recorded, an L_4-L_5 laminectomy was carried out in both normal and hydrocephalic cats. The central canal was obliterated with a ligature placed around the dura and spinal cord. The laminectomy site was closed by approximating the muscles and skin.

Results

Of 14 hydrocephalic cats studied, 12 developed plateau waves. Initial IVP ranged from 3 to 6 mm Hg. Shortly after the spinal cord was ligated, IVP increased gradually over a period of 4-8 h to an amplitude of 30-60 mm Hg. Figures 1 and 2 show, in a typical experiment, the development of plateau waves, as well as blood pressure and end tidal CO_2. Plateau waves developed in ventilated and spontaneous breathing cats, having amplitudes of up to 150 mm Hg. The waves were of 6-10 min duration, and occurred at intervals of 15-30 min. Precursor waves of lesser amplitude and duration, sometimes preceded the plateau waves. The plateau waves continued for anywhere from 12 to 36 h, ending when the cat died or the experiment was terminated.

The IVP of normal cats (n = 5) ranged between 0 and 3 mm Hg. As their spinal cords were ligated, an initial surge of pressure, up to 20 mm Hg, resulted. Within a few minutes, the pressure dropped to between 5 and 10 mm Hg. Over a subsequent period of 12-24 h IVP did not exceed 15 mm Hg and no plateau waves were noted.

There were no noticeable changes of end tidal CO_2 either at the start or end of a plateau wave on cats which were or were not being artificially ventilated. Typical end tidal CO_2 ranged from 3.5 to 4.5%. Arterial blood gases drawn prior to and during a plateau wave showed no significant difference in pO_2, pCO_2, or pH, which were all within normal limits.

Systolic blood pressure was generally higher than the peak of the plateau wave, typically in the range of 160-200 mm Hg. In the later portion of the plateau wave, systemic blood pressure often increased by about 10%. As the plateau wave terminated, systemic pressure decreased to below base line value, and then rose again after 5-7 min. It was not possible to discern whether the fall in systemic blood pressure was preceded or followed by the falling pressure portion of the plateau wave.

Discussion

The dilated central canal of the spinal cord playd an essential role as a conduit for the egress of CSF from the ventricular system of hydrocephalic cats (1, 2). Fluid flows into the spinal subarachnoid space and is absorbed there. A suture tied around the spinal cord occludes the central canal. Consequently, the IVP rises progressively, and will eventually result in the death of the cat.

The development of plateau waves appears to be a response to a persistent elevation of IVP. LANGFITT et al. (6), using a balloon in the extradural space, found that when the intracranial pressure of monkeys was elevated beyond the vasopressor threshold, there was an enormous increase in both arterial and intracranial pressures. This increase in arterial pressure was not confirmed in our experiments. This difference may be due to the methods used to increase intracranial pressure and to the rate at which this occurs. After the spinal cord is ligated, CSF accumulates, and a pressure develops within the ventricles which is transmitted uniformly throughout the entire cranial vault.

Plateau waves have been the subject of several clinical studies by LUNDBERG and his coworkers (7 - 10). From measurements of regional cerebral blood flow and volume, while monitoring ventricular pressure, these authors proposed a sequence of events to explain the appearance and disappearance of plateau waves (10). The appearance of the waves was based on the increases in both intracranial blood volume and intraventricular pressure and on the decreases in cerebral blood flow. The slow rise in ventricular pressure between plateau waves was due to reaccumulation of CSF. The precipitating event in the disappearance of the plateau waves is the compensatory outflow of CSF which, when combined with an increase in the tone of the vessels, causes a sudden fall in both ventricular and vascular pressures. Changes in arterial pCO_2 will also influence both the appearance and disappearance of these waves (11). It is not known with certainty, however, whether the sequence of events described above is the cause or the result of the plateau waves.

The monitoring of end tidal CO_2 and measuring of arterial blood pO_2, pCO_2, and pH, did not reveal any variation which could explain initiation or termination of the plateau waves. Small variations which are not detectable with our measuring techniques, or local tissue variations may, however, be significant. Changes in systemic blood pressure with respect to plateau waves were noted. The relevance of these changes to the pathophysiology of plateau waves is not known.

At the Second Intracranial Pressure meeting in 1974, the chairmen of the session on Pathophysiology of Rapid Variations of ICP stated that "there was no reliable experimental model for plateau waves" (12). It is hoped that the experimental model described above will be used to provide sufficient facts to formulate a comprehensive theory of plateau waves.

Summary

This report describes a means to produce an experimental model of plateau waves in the cat. Cats were first made hydrocephalic by the intracisternal injection of kaolin. Approx. 3 weeks later the spinal cord was ligated at a L4-L5 laminectomy site. IVP was continuously monitored for 8-30 h via a catheter in the lateral ventricle. The cats were artificially ventilated and arterial blood gases and pressure monitored. Gradually, plateau waves developed which had amplitudes up to 150 mm Hg, were of 6-10 min duration, and occurred at intervals of 15-30 min. Precursor waves of smaller amplitude and duration, typically noted with plateau waves, were also present. During the course of the plateau waves, blood pressure increased by a small amount; as the waves terminated, blood pressure decreased slightly. End tidal CO_2, arterial pCO_2, pO_2, and pH, during and between the waves were not different. In normal cats with similarly ligated spinal cords, IVP did not exceed 15 mm Hg and plateau waves did not develop.

Key Words

Plateau waves, Hydrocephalus, Intracranial pressure.

References

1. EISENBERG, H.M., McLENNAN, J.E., WELCH, K.: Ventricular perfusion in cats with kaolin-induced hydrocephalus. J. Neurosurg. 41, 20-28 (1974).

2. HOCHWALD, G.M., BOAL, R.D., MARLIN, A.E., KUMAR, A.J.: Changes in regional blood flow and water content of brain and spinal cord in acute and chronic experimental hydrocephalus. Proceedings of the Society for Research into Hydrocephalus and Spinal Bifida. Glasgow, June 25-28, 1975. Devel. Med. Child Neurol. Suppl. 35, 17, 42-50 (1975).

3. HOCHWALD, G.M., LUX, W.E., JR., SAHAR, A., RANSOHOFF, J.: Experimental hydrocephalus. Changes in cerebrospinal fluid dynamics as a function of time. Arch. Neurol. 26, 120-129 (1972).

4. JOHNSTON, I.H., ROWAN, J.O.: Raised intracranial pressure and cerebral blood flow. 3. Venous outflow tract pressures and vascular resistances in experimental intracranial hypertension. J. Neurol. Neurosurg. Psychiat. 37, 392-402 (1974).

5. LANGFITT, T.W.: Intracranial volume-pressure relationship. In: Intracranial Pressure II (N. LUNDBERG, U. PONTEN, M. BROCK, eds.) pp. 69-76. Berlin-Heidelberg-New York: Springer 1975.

6. LANGFITT, T.W., WEINSTEIN, J.D., KASSELL, N.F.: Cerebral vasomotor paralysis produced by intracranial hypertendion. Neurology 15, 622-641 (1965).

7. LUNDBERG, N.: Continuous recording and control of ventricular fluid pressure in neurosurgical practice. Acta Psychiat. Scand. Suppl. 149, 36, 1-193 (1960).

8. LUNDBERG, N., CRONQVIST, S., KJÄLLQUIST, A.: Clinical investigation on interrelation between intracranial pressure and intracranial hemodynamics. Progr. Brain Res. 30, 70-75 (1968).

9. LUNDBERG, N., TROUPP, H., LORIN, H.: Continuous recording of the ventricular-fluid pressure in patients with severe acute traumatic brain injury; a preliminary report. J. Neurosurg. 22, 581-590 (1965)

10. RISBERG, J., LUNDBERG, N., INGVAR, D.H.: Regional cerebral blood volume during acute transient rises of the intracranial pressure (plateau waves). J. Neurosurg. 31, 303-310 (1969)-

11. TINDALL. G.T., McGRAW, C.P., VANDERVEER, R.W., IWATA, K.: Cardiorespiratory chanfes associated with plateau waves in patients with head injury. In: Intracranial Pressure (M. BROCK, H. DIETZ, eds.) pp. 227.231. Berlin-Heidelberg-New York: Springer 1972.

12. TROUPP, H., de ROUGEMONT, J.: Chairmen's comments. In: Intracranial Pressure II (N. LUNDBERG, U. PONTEN, M. BROCK, eds.) p. 419. Berlin-Heidelberg-New York: Springer 1975.

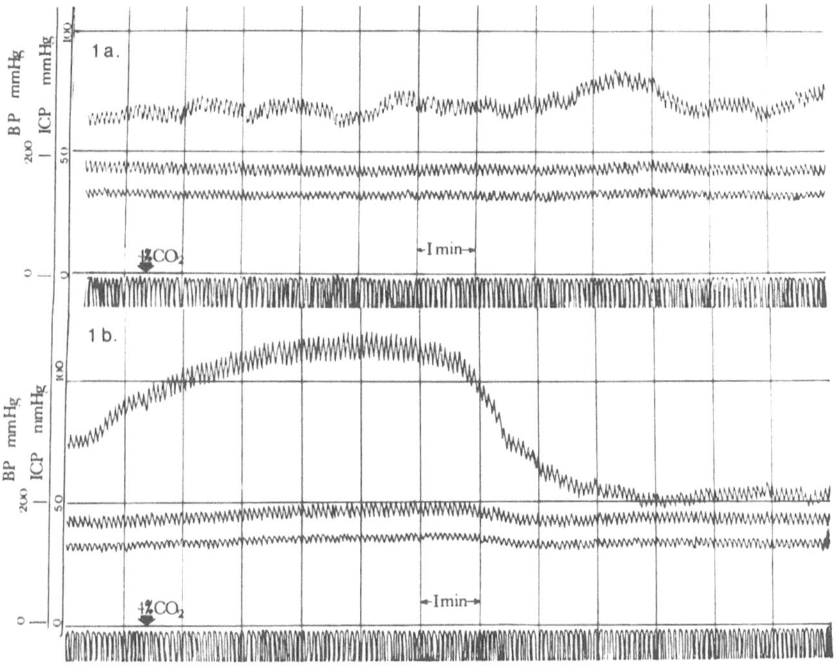

Fig. 1. Record from hydrocephalic cat showing appearance and disappearance of plateau wave. Systemic blood pressure (BP), and end tidal CO_2 also recorded. ICP is measured with cannula in lateral ventricle. Figure 1a shows events preceeding wave. Figure 1b shows complete wave

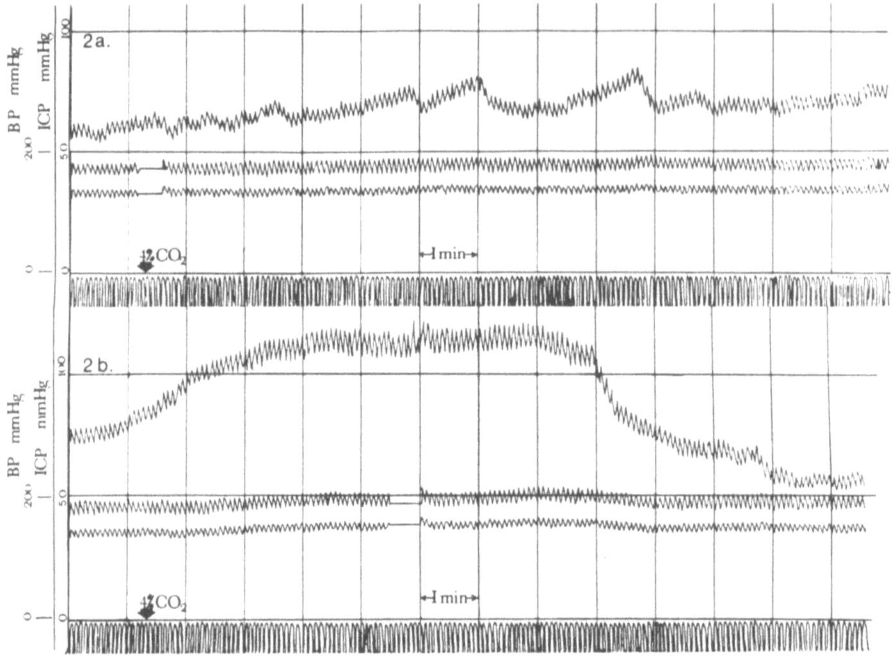

Fig. 2. Continuation of record from Figure 1. Figure 2a is record taken following previous plateau wave. Clearly seen are precursor waves of lesser duration and amplitude. Actual plateau wave is shown in Figure 2b. Also shown are blood pressure and end tidal CO_2

Increased Intracranial Pressure and Lung Water in Dogs

J. B. North and S. Jennett

Following head injury, hypoxemia is commonly observed and pulmonary edema sometimes occurs unpredictably. Whether this association is dependent on raised intracranial pressure (ICP) is not known, but there has been some experimental and clinical support for the hypothesis that there are neurally mediated effects on the lungs, which could cause an increase in venous admixture or in extravasation of fluid.

Attempts to reproduce hypoxia and neurogenic pulmonary edema in animals have produced variable results. We have raised ICP in spontaneously breathing cats and observed only a degree of hypoxemia which was compatible with the degree of hypoventilation due to central depression of breathing (3). HOFF (1) has found that lung water is increased in cats subjected to raised ICP, and suggested that such increases may represent an early stage of neurogenic pulmonary edema.

The purpose of this investigation was to make comparable observations in dogs by calculating lung water after raised ICP.

Eight beagle dogs (8-11 kg) were anesthetized with thiopentone, followed by intermittent pentobarbitone when necessary. They were paralyzed with suxamethonium and ventilated with room ain to maintain a constant arterial PCO, near to 40 mm Hg. ICP was recorded by a subdural catheter and external transducer; systemic arterial pressure (SAP), end-tidal CO_2, heart rate, and tidal volume were also recorded. Blood gases were sampled periodically.

With the animals in the prone position, cerebrospinal fluid (CSF) at $37^{o}C$ was injected into the cisterna magna to raise ICP by 1 mm Hg/s until ICP reached 100 mm Hg, and maintained at that level for 45 min.

During the rise in ICP, only small increases in SAP were observed such that cerebral perfusion pressure (CPP) was around 25 mm Hg. After 45 min, ICP was further raised to 150 mm Hg so that CPP was virtually zero; the total duration of raised ICP was just over 60 min. At the first sign of terminal hypotension, the animal was sacrified by an overdose of pentobarbitone. The lungs were removed immediately for gravimetric lung water analysis according to HOLCROFT's method (3). Three control animals were studied by the same method, but without raising ICP; an intravenous infusion of mock CSF was given, the volume of which was similar to that used to raise ICP.

Animals with raised ICP had no changes in total lung water (TLW) compared with the central group (Table 1). There were no significant differences in extravascular lung water relative to dry lung weight (EVLW/EVDW) or in lung blood weights in the raised ICP dogs when compared with the controls.

Table 2 shows that $PaCO_2$ did not change during 45 min of raised ICP. The absence of any degree of pulmonary edema in this preparation is in contrast to the findings in cats (1). This difference may be related to the relative absence of increase in SAP in the dogs; cats, despite

Table 1. Summary of total lung water and extravascular lung water (EVLM) results in control and raised ICP dogs; differences between groups are not significant

	Total lung water % lung water	$\frac{EVLM}{EVDW}$ ml/gm	$\frac{\text{Blood wt}}{EVDW}$ gm/gm
Control n = 3	76.1 ± 1.8	2.9 ± 0.5	2.3 ± 1.1
Raised ICP	77.8 ± 1.5	3.3 ± 0.3	1.9 ± 0.9

Table 2. Comparison of blood gas values before and after 45 min of raised ICP

	$PaCO_2$ mm Hg	$PaCO_2$ mm Hg	pH
Before ICP ↑	99.4 ± 8	40.5 ± 1.7	7.35 ± .02
After 45 min ICP ↑	99.5 ± 7	42.1 ± 3.5	7.33 ± .05

barbiturate anesthesia, consistently showed a marked increase. Therefore it is probable that a sympathetic discharge was not produced in our dogs by the degree of raised ICP, and may explain why increases in lung water were not observed.

References

1. HOFF, J.T., NISHIMURA, M.: A quantitative model of neurogenic pulmonary oedema. (R. McLAURIN, J. MULLAN, STRATTON, eds.) Chicago Conference on Neural Trauma (1976).

2. HOLCROFT, J.W., TRUNKEY, D.W.: Extravascular Lung Water following hemorrhagic shock in the baboon. Ann. Surg. 180, 408-417 (1974).

3. JENNETT, S., NORTH, J.B.: Effects of intermittently raised ICP on breathing pattern, ventilatory response to CO_2 and blood gases in anesthetized cats. J. Neurosurg. 44, 156-167 (1976).

Differences in the Behavior of Afferent Vessels in Autoregulation to Increased Intracranial Pressure and to Diminished Systemic Blood Pressure[1]

L. Symon, N.M. Branston, and A.J. Strong

Introduction

The cerebral circulation maintains constant blood flow in arterial hypotension (8) and raised intracranial pressure (ICP) (4) within the limits of its capacity. Both decrease the transmural pressure across the cerebral resistance vessels, and it has seemed reasonable to assume a probable identity of mechanisms for autoregulation in the two circumstances, at any rate as far as the intracranial vessels have been concerned.

There have been suggestions from our own and other laboratories that the autoregulatory process in relation to raised intracranial pressure appears more efficient than to hypotension. The present data results from a study of 14 animals in which the pressure drop between the aorta and the major branches of the middle cerebral artery was measured, while cerebral perfusion pressure was reduced in seven by raising the intracranial pressure, and in seven by lowering the systemic blood pressure.

Methods

There were 14 adult baboons (PAPIO CYNOCEPHALUS) in the weight range 8 - 16 kg used. Techniques of anesthesia (12), cannulation of pial arteries, and maintenance of intact catheter placement are described elsewhere (10, 11). Systemic blood pressure was measured from the aorta, end tidal CO_2 continuously, and arterial pH, pCO_2, and pO_2 episodically, monitored. As a rule, a posttemporal branch of the middle cerebral artery of a diameter of about 400 μ was chosen for pressure measurement.

Several of the animals which formed a portion of a study of autoregulation (12) had, in addition, a catheter placed in Labbé's vein. Following catheter placements, the integrity of the intracranial cavity was restored by closing the skull with acrylic, and this also greatly simplified maintenance of catheter position and patency during the course of the experiment. Systemic blood pressure was lowered by withdrawal of arterial blood. Intracranial pressure was raised by a continuous slow infusion of Ringer lactate solution through a needle in the cisterna magna, using a Palmer slow infusion pump.

[1] This study was supported by the Medical Research Council.

Results

Lowered Systemic Blood Pressure

The ratio of pial arterial pressure to systemic blood pressure under control circumstances in both groups of animals was between 70 and 90% depending on the size of pial artery used, and with lowering of the systemic blood pressure showed a progressive decline. This is illustrated in Figure 1. During exsanguination, attempts were made to stabilize the blood pressure at appropriate levels for measurement, but these levels were somewhat different for each individual animal. In the animals where ICP was raised, the relationship between pial arterial pressure and mean systemic blood pressure (PAP/MSBP) showed a progressive increase with rising ICP, beyond about 20 mm Hg (Fig. 2). Further ICP-rise produced a progressive rise in the ratio, which flattened off when the ICP rose above 70 mm Hg. Stepwise increments in ICP were achieved by varying the rate of the infusion pump, and measurements in the seven animals made at 10 mm Hg increments as the pressure rose. Over the whole range of tests from low intracranial pressure to pressures approaching 90 mm Hg, the relationship between PAP/MSBP ration and ICP was nonlinear, but over the range between 25 and 70 mm Hg there was approximately a linear relaxation of resistance determined by the pressure drop between systemic and pial artery.

Discussion

Autoregulation to lowered systemic blood pressure appears to involve two different processes in the cerebral circulation, and the body of current evidence suggests that constriction of the afferent vessels is in conflict with the efforts of the intracranial circulation itself. SYMON (12) showed that, assessed by transmission of pulse from artery to vein, the intrinsic portion of the cerebral circulation continued to dilate down to very low levels of PAP, much lower than the limit which in comparable preparations showed failure of autoregulation assessed by tissue blood flow, suggesting that the cerebral vascular resistance might not be a homogenous entity but that progressive vasoconstriction in the extravascular bed might compete with progressive dilatation within the resistance vessels in the tissue itself. Collateral work with DU BOULAY and SYMON (1) at the same time showed, by serial angiography in oligemic hypotension, constriction in the extracranial vasculature as high as the circle of Willis while intrinsic vessels dilated, indicating inhomogeneity of cerebral vascular resistance.

JAMES (6) and his colleagues suggested a modulating effect of the sympathetic nervous system on cerebral blood flow, which had its effect principally in the responses to hypocapnic vasodilatation - a sympathetic stimulation reducing the hypocapnic response and sympathetic paralysis increasing it. Similar findings were reported by HARPER and his colleagues (5), who elaborated the hypothesis of dual control of the nervous system, further supporting the concept of inhomogeneity of the cerebral vascular resistance. In studies of the relationship between pial arterial pressure and systemic pressure, JANSEN and KANZOW (7) working in the cat, have indicated a considerable influence of afferent vasculature on cerebral vascular resistance during a variety of pharmacologic tests, and have suggested that in this species approximately half the cerebral vascular resistance is localized in relatively large vessels. Pharmacologic modification of sympathetic activity (3) indicated that, during sympathetic paralysis, autoregulation to hypotension is more effective.

The suspicion has thus been clear for some years that the autonomic nervous system has an important part to play in autoregulation, and that the sympathetic portion of this system counteracts some of the autoregulatory capacity of the cerebral circulation in hypotension, while inhibition of the sympathetic nervous system enhances regulation. We know from the work of OWMAN and his colleagues in Scandinavia (2) that nerve endings on the intracranial vessels probably represent terminals both of the sympathetic and parasympathetic system.

The potential modification of vasoactivity in major afferent vessels therefore by these two major systems, would appear to be soundly anatomically based. HARPER and his colleagues (5) have presented the hypothesis that the autonomic nervous system controls the extracranial vessels, and the intracranial vessels largely perform independently. The present work and the succeeding paper from Japanese workers (15) suggest that inhibition of the sympathetic nervous system is important in the maintenance of autoregulation to raised ICP. It still seems likely that the ultimate mechanism of autoregulation - a reaction of the musculature of the cerebral vessels themselves to change in transmural pressure - is similar in the two types of autoregulation (9, 13, 14). Differences in detail, however, result from stimulation of the sympathetic nervous system during autoregulation to diminished perfusion pressure from hemorrhage, and inhibition of the sympathetic nervous system during autoregulation to diminished perfusion pressure from raised ICP.

References

1. DU BOULAY, G.H., SYMON, L.: The anaesthetist's effect upon the cerebral arteries. Proc. Roy. Soc. Med. 64, 77-80 (1971).
2. EDVINSSON, L., OWMAN, Ch.: Pharmacological characterization of amine receptor mechanisms in brain vessels. In: The Cerebral Vessel Wall. Erwin-Riesch Symp. Berlin, 1975 (in press).
3. FITCH, W., McKENZIE, T., HARPER, A.M.: Effects of decreasing arterial blood pressure on cerebral blood flow in the baboon: Influence of the sympathetic nervous system. Circ. Res. 37, 350-557 (1975).
4. HÄGGENDAL, E., LÖFGREN, J., NILSSON, N.J., ZWETNOW, N.N.: Die Gehirndurchblutung bei experimentalen Liquordruckänderungen. Verhandl. Int. Neurochirurgen Kongreß Bad Durkheim (1966).
5. HARPER, A.M., DESHMUKH, V.D., ROWAN, J.O., JENNETT, W.B.: The influence of sympathetic nervous activity on cerebral blood flow. Arch. Neurol. 27, 1-6 (1972).
6. JAMES, I.M., MILLAR, R.A., PURVES, M.J.: Observations on the extrinsic neural control of cerebral blood flow in the baboon. Circ. Res. 25, 77-93 (1969).
7. JANSEN, J., KANZOW, E.: Pressure drop and vascular resistance in cerebral circulation. In: Advances in Neurosurgery (W. KLUG, M. BROCK, M. KLINGER, O. SPOERRI, eds.), pp. 314-315. Berlin-Heidelberg-New York: Springer 1975.
8. LASSEN, N.A.: Autoregulation of cerebral blood flow. Circ. Res. 15 Suppl. 1, 201-204 (1964).
9. MILLER, J.D., STANEK, A.E., LANGFITT, T.W.: A comparison of autoregulation to changes in intracranial and arterial pressure in the same preparation. In: Cerebral Blood Flow and Intracranial Pressure (C. FIESCHI, ed.), pp. 34-38. Basel: Karger 1972.
10. SYMON, L.: Observations on the leptomeningeal collateral circulation in dogs. J. Physiol. 154, 1-14 (1960).
11. SYMON, L.: Leptomeningeal collateral circulation in macacus rhesus. J. Physiol. 159, 68-86 (1961).

12. SYMON, L.: Regional vascular reactivity in the middle cerebral arterial distribution: An experimental study in baboons. J. Neurosurg. 33, 532-541 (1970).

13. SYMON, L., DORSCH, N.W.C., HELD, K.: A study of regional autoregulation in the cerebral circulation to increased perfusion pressure in normocapnia and hypercapnia. Stroke 4, 139-147 (1973).

14. SYMON, L., PÁSZTOR, E., BRANSTON, N.M., DORSCH, N.W.C.: The effect of supratentorial space-occupying lesions on regional intracranial pressure and local cerebral blood flow: An experimental study in baboons. J. Neurol. Neurosurg. Psychiat. 37, 617-626 (1974).

15. SYMON, L., PÁSZTOR, E., DORSCH, N.W.C., BRANSTON, N.M.: Physiological responses of local areas of the cerebral circulation in experimental primates determined by the method of hydrogen clearance. Stroke 4, 632-642 (1973).

16. TANAKA, K., HASHI, K., NISHIMURA, S., MATSSURA, S.: Changes of the sympathetic vasomotor activity during increased ICP. This symposium - Session B(5).

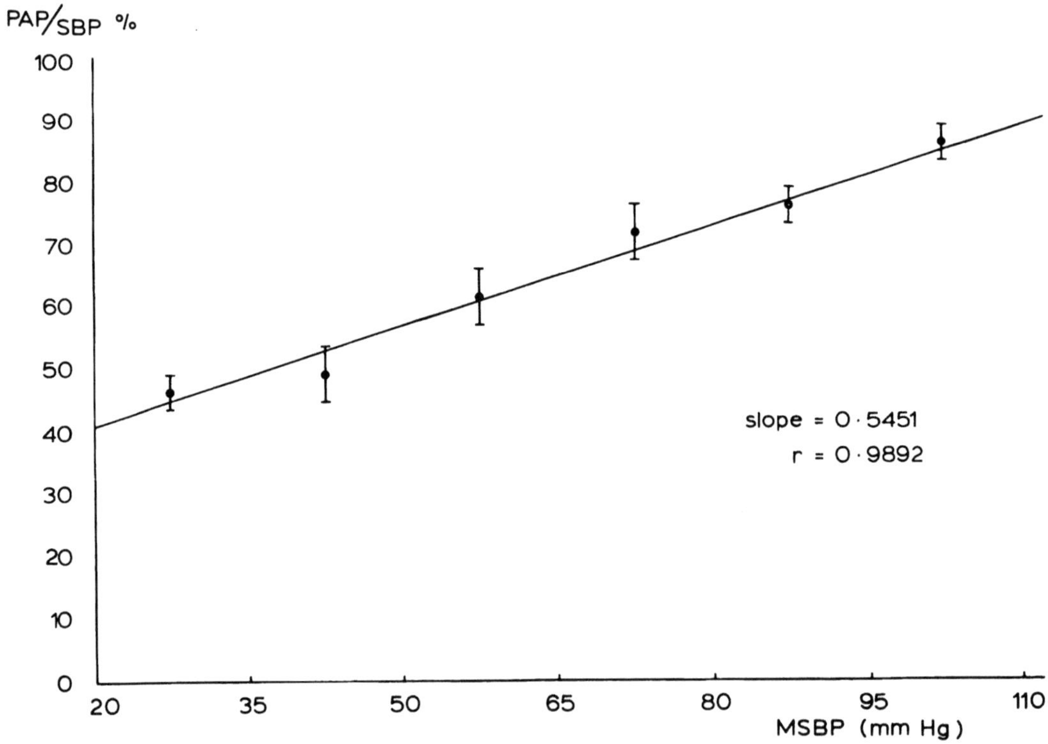

Fig. 1. Ratio of pial arterial systemic blood pressure in relation to falling systemic blood pressure. Relationship between percentage PAP/SBP and MSBP

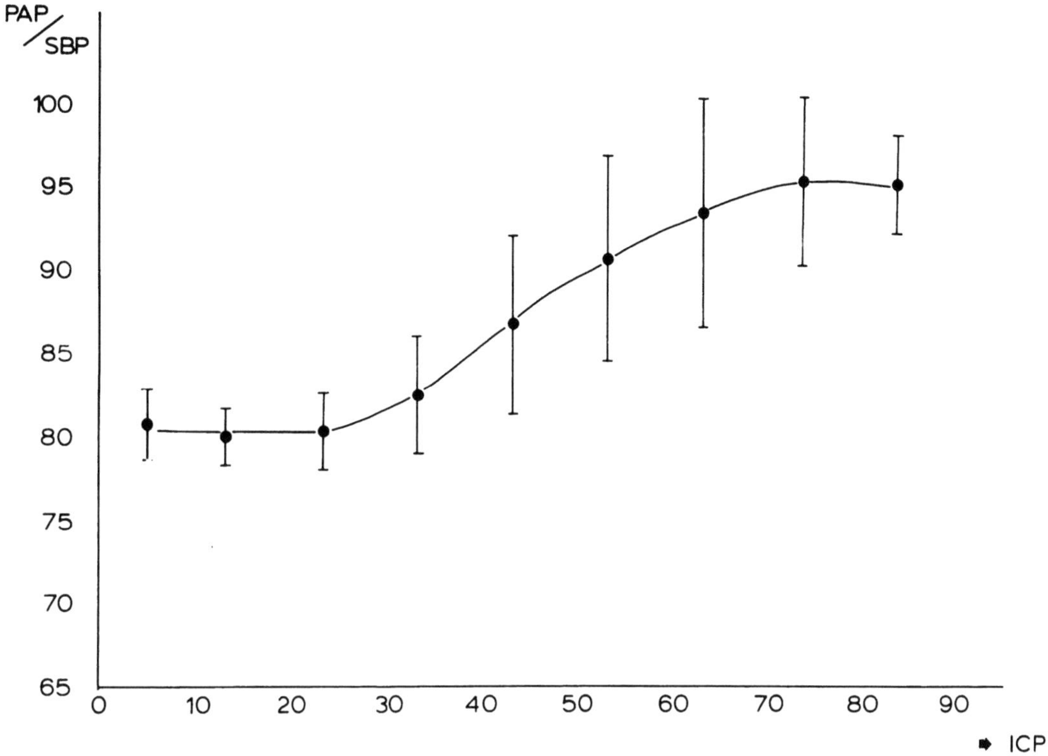

Fig. 2. Ratio between pial arterial pressure and mean systemic blood pressure in relation to rising intracranial pressure. Relationship between PAP/SBP ratio and ICP

Changes of the Sympathetic Vasomotor Activity During Increased Intracranial Pressure

K. Tanaka, K. Hashi, S. Nishimura, and S. Matsuura

Introduction

Although it has been suggested that the sympathetic nervous system participates in the development of the pressor response, vasoparalysis, or plateau waves during increases in intracranial pressure (ICP), the precise mechanisms remain unclear. Therefore, in the present study the direct observation of the sympathetic vasomotor activity during increases in ICP was attempted by measuring the efferent discharge from the renal nerve of the cat.

Materials and Methods

There were 18 adult cats anesthetized with intraperitonal injection of pentobarbital sodium (30-35 mg/kg). Cannulae were inserted into the femoral artery and vein for monitoring blood pressure (BP) and administering fluids and drugs. End-tidal CO_2 was monitored continuously by an infrared analyzer, and ventilation was controlled with a respirator after the animal was paralyzed with gallamine triethiodide (10 mg/kg). Body temperature was maintained (36-38°C) by a heating pad. Arterial pO_2, pCO_2, and pH were intermittently measured.

Two cannulae were inserted into the cisterna magna, one for monitoring ICP and one for raising ICP by infusion of saline at constant temperature.

The renal nerve was exposed retroperitoneally around the renal artery and the surrounding connective tissue was carefully stripped off under the operating microscope. The nerve was cut near to the renal hilus, and the proximal end was placed over a pair of silver electrodes and immersed in mineral oil. The postganglionic efferent discharge of the renal nerve was amplified with a high gain biological amplifier (Nihon Kohden, RB-5) and displayed on an oscilloscope. The output signals from the amplifier were also transfered to an integrator (Nihon Kohden, RFJ-5) in order to evaluate the renal nerve activity (RNA) quantitatively. All these parameters were continuously displayed on an inkwriting polygraph (Nihon Kohden, RBL-85).

In one animal an ascending nerve fiber from the superior cervical ganglion was exposed around the internal carotid artery, and the discharge of this nerve and of the renal nerve were recorded simultaneously.

In two animals the bilateral aortic and sinus nerves were cut at the neck in order to eliminate the effect of the baroreceptor reflex.

After the spontaneous activity of the renal nerve and the typical changes in the activity following alteration of BP were observed, ICP was increased by infusion of saline into the cisterna magna. In five animals, ICP was increased stepwise by 25 mm Hg until ICP reached the level of BP. In another five animals, a rapid increase of ICP beyond the level of BP was achieved by rapid infusion of saline.

Results

The efferent impulses from the renal nerve consisted of groups of action potentials of 50-100 μV in magnitude, and usually were synchronous with heart beats and respirations (Fig. 1-A). A branch of the superior cervical ganglion showed a similar pattern of activity (Fig. 1-B). A rise in BP by infusion of saline or a fall by rapid withdrawal of blood resulted in a decrease or increase, respectively, in the RNA (Fig. 1-C). Inhalation of 5% CO_2 increased the RNA, while hyperventilation decreased the activity (Fig. 1-D).

Stepwise Increment of ICP

During the initial increments of ICP, the RNA was progressively suppressed in all animals, except for the animal whose baroreceptor nerves were cut, in which this suppression of the RNA was no longer apparent. At a cerebral perfusion pressure (CPP) of 29 ± 5.9 mm Hg RNA began to increase, followed by a significant rise in BP (Fig. 2). It continued to increase as ICP was further increased to the level of BP. When ICP was then rapidly lowered to the initial level, the RNA which had been remarkably increased, decreased to the level less than the steady-state value within 5 min and remained depressed for several minutes, while BP returned to the initial value within 3 min. As the procedure of raising and lowering ICP was repeated, the value of CPP over which the RNA began to increase was progressively shifted higher. On the third trial of this procedure, in one animal out of five, a temporary disappearance of RNA for approximately 5 min was observed during the stage of moderately increased ICP, when the ICP was elevated from 95 to 110 mm Hg and BP rose from 125 to 150 mm Hg (Fig. 3). BP was unchanged despite the loss of RNA and there was no response to withdrawal of blood which usually causes RNA to increase.

Rapid Increment of ICP

In five cats, ICP was elevated beyond the level of BP and maintained for 5-7 min at that level. Then it was lowered rapidly. When this procedure was repeated several times, in three cats out of these five, it was observed that the increased RNA (Fig. 4-B) gradually declined despite a sustained increase in ICP above the level of BP. Thereafter, it finally reached to the point of complete disappearance of RNA (Fig. 4-C). The loss of RNA persisted for several minutes even after the ICP was lowered. The administration of 0.02 mg/kg of norepinephrine at this stage of loss of RNA resulted in a significant rise in ICP accompanied with a rise in BP (Fig. 4-D). Several minutes later, RNA had recovered spontaneously and showed an activity greater than that before the procedure. The administration of norepinephrine at this stage of reactivity resulted in only a slight rise in ICP, while the rise in BP was similar (Fig. 4-E).

Discussion

Since the sympathetic nerve firings are known to have a tendency to go into action as a whole and to be bilaterally synchronous (1, 7), changes of the renal nerve activity would represent changes of the sympathetic tone in the cerebral blood vessels. The finding that the activity of an ascending branch from the superior cervical ganglion showed synchronous discharge to that of the renal nerve may further substantiate the above concept.

The results of the present study agree with the idea that the pressor response following increased ICP was due to excitation of the sympathetic nervous system. Moreover, it was further indicated that the trigger stimulus for the pressor response may be the ischemia of the brain, because the value of CPP over which the RNA was increased was around 30 mm Hg, which corresponds to the point autoregulation becomes disturbed (6).

The suppression of the RNA in the period of slightly increased ICP may deserve considerations in relation to the earlier works. It has been known that CBF could be maintained at a lower level of CPP when it was decreased by increasing ICP than by decreasing systemic BP by withdrawal of blood (6). JOHNSTON et al. have reported that in the early stages of increased ICP, an increase in CBF may occur despite a falling CPP (3). It is possible, therefore, to presume that the autoregulation of CBF to changes in ICP may be augmented by the decrease of the sympathetic vasoconstrictor tone of the cerebral blood vessels. In addition, the participation of the reflex on this mechanism via the baroreceptor nerve may suggest a more complex sequence of events.

LANGFITT, et al. have shown that an extreme increase in ICP sufficient to disturb cerebral metabolism may result in the state of vasoparalysis and acute brain swelling (4). The results of the present study showed that the activity of the sympathetic vasoconstrictor nerve may also be paralyzed after repeated insults of severe intracranial hypertension. Interestingly, the transmission of BP to ICP was much greater in the state of depressed sympathetic activity. This phenomenon agrees with the report that the neurogenic mechanism may play a role on the production of acute brain swelling (2). A sudden temporary disappearance pf the sympathetic activity observed during the state of moderately increased ICP in this experiment is therefore of significant importance, because ICP will be significantly increased by the enhanced transmission of BP and the decreased compensatory capacity which may have been already exhausted as the result of existence of increased ICP. This situation may correspond to the phenomenon well known clinically as plateau wave (5) in many aspects.

Summary

Sympathetic vasoconstrictor nerve activity during increase in ICP was studied by monitoring the renal nerve activity in cats. In the stage of slightly increased ICP, the sympathetic activity was suppressed, but when CPP reached the level of 30 mm Hg, it began to increase accompanied by a significant rise in BP. After repeated insults of severe intracranial hypertension, the sympathetic activity could be paralyzed accompanied by the manifestation of cerebral vasoparalysis. Besides the paralysis of the nerve activity described above, a temporary disappearance of the sympathetic activity could occur in the stage of moderately increased intracranial pressure. This phenomenon was considered to be corresponding to the plateau waves clinically.

References

1. BARD, P.: Medical physiology. St. Louis: Mosby 1956.

2. ISHII, S.: Brain-swelling. Studies of structural, physiologic and biochemical alterations. In: Head injury (W.F. CAVENESS, A.E. WALKER, eds.), pp. 276-299. Philadelphia: Lippincott 1966.

3. JOHNSTON, I.H., ROWAN, J.O., HARPER, A.M., JENNETT, W.B.: Raised intracranial pressure and cerebral blood flow. I. Cisterna magna infusion in primates. J. Neurol. Neurosurg. Psychiat. 35, 285-296 (1972).

4. LANGFITT, T.W., WEISTEIN, J.D., KASSELL, N.F.: Cerebral vasomotor

paralysis produced by intracranial hypertension. Neurology 15, 622-641 (1965).

5. LUNDBERG, N.: Continuous recording and control of ventricular fluid pressure in neurosurgical practice. Acta Psychiat. Neurol. Scand., Suppl. 149, 1-193 (1960).

6. MILLER, J.D., STANEK, A., LANGFITT, T.W.: Concepts of cerebral perfusion pressure and vascular compression during intracranial hypertension. In: Cerebral Blood Flow (J.S. MEYER, J.P. SCHADÉ, eds.), pp. 411-432. Amsterdam: Elsevier 1972.

7. UVNÄS, B.: Central cardiovascular control. In: Handbook of physiology (J. FIELD, ed.), Section 1: Neurophysiology 2, pp. 1131-1162. Baltimore: Williams & Wilkins 1960.

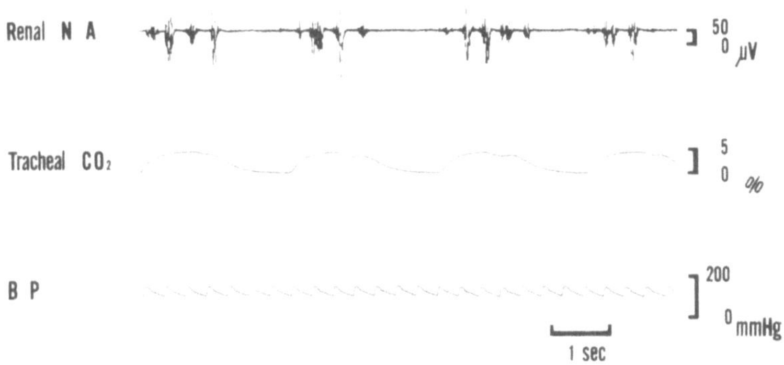

Fig. 1-A. Spontaneous activity of renal nerve. Activity was of 50-100 μV in amplitude showing groups of action potentials synchronous with the heart beats and respirations. Renal NA: renal nerve activity, RNA; BP: blood pressure

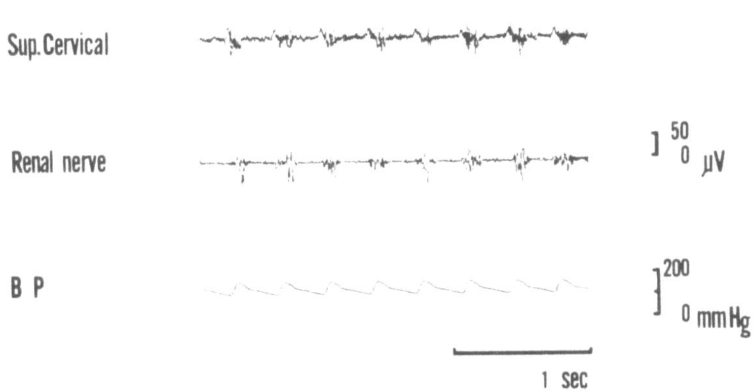

Fig. 1-B. Activities recorded simultaneously from renal nerve and branch of superior cervical ganglion. Note synchronicity of activities of both nerves

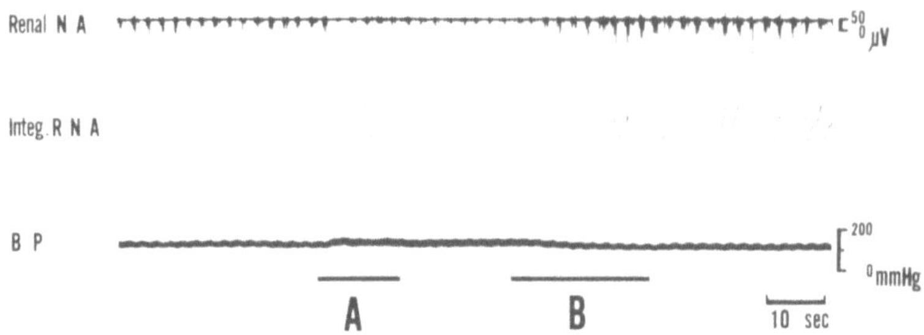

Fig. 1-C. Effect of raising and lowering of blood pressure on RNA. Raising of blood pressure by intravenous infusion of 10 ml of normal saline (bar A) caused suppression in RNA, while blood withdrawal (bar B) caused increase in RNA. <u>Integ. RNA</u>: Integration of renal nerve activity. Density of oblique lines means amount of RNA

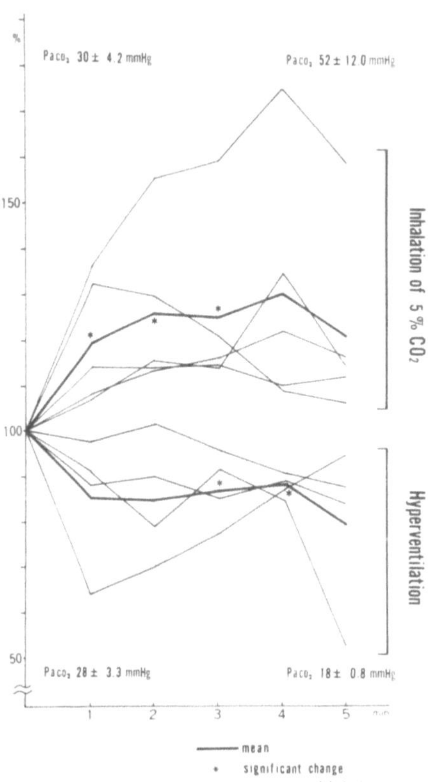

Fig. 1-D. Changes in RNA caused by 5% CO_2 inhalation and hyperventilation. Note increase in RNA by 5% CO_2 inhalation and suppression by hyperventilation. <u>Ordinate</u>: RNA integrated for every 1 min expressed in percentage (RNA before the study is expressed as 100%), <u>abscissa</u>: time duration following initiation of the procedure

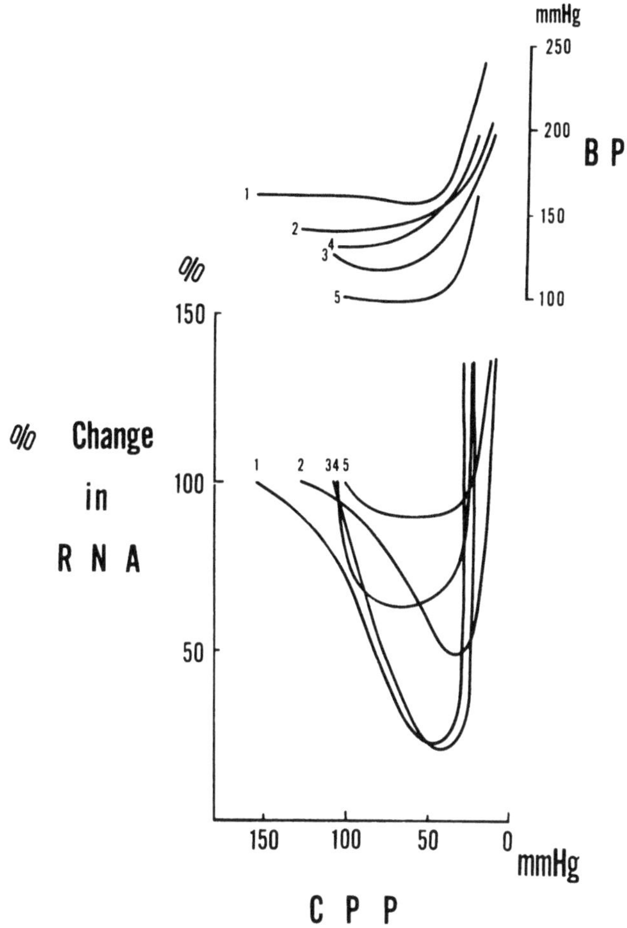

Fig. 2. Percent changes in RNA caused by increasing ICP. During initial period of increased ICP, RNA was progressively suppressed. When cerebral perfusion pressure became approximately 30 mm Hg, RNA began to increase followed by significant rise in BP. Ordinate: RNA change in percentage (RNA before study is expressed as 100%), abscissa: cerebral perfusion pressure, CPP

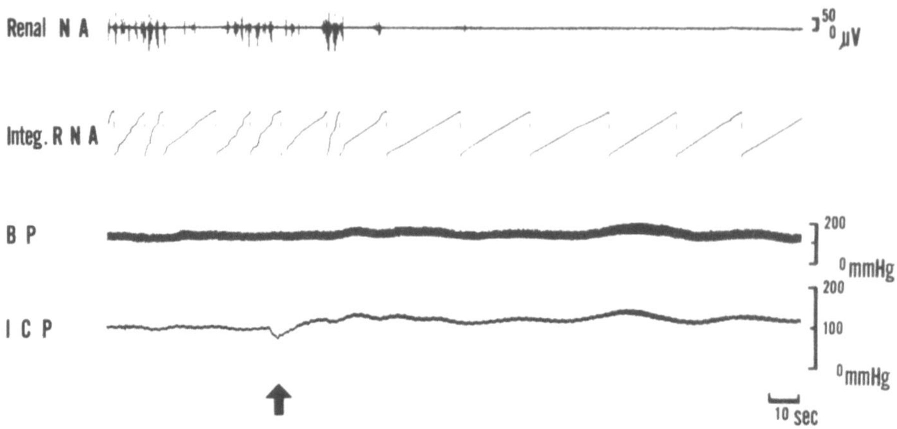

Fig. 3. Temporary disappearance of RNA during the stage of moderately increased ICP. At point of ↑, ICP was raised from 95 to 100 mm Hg. A sudden temporary disappearance of RNA was noted following a group of action potentials

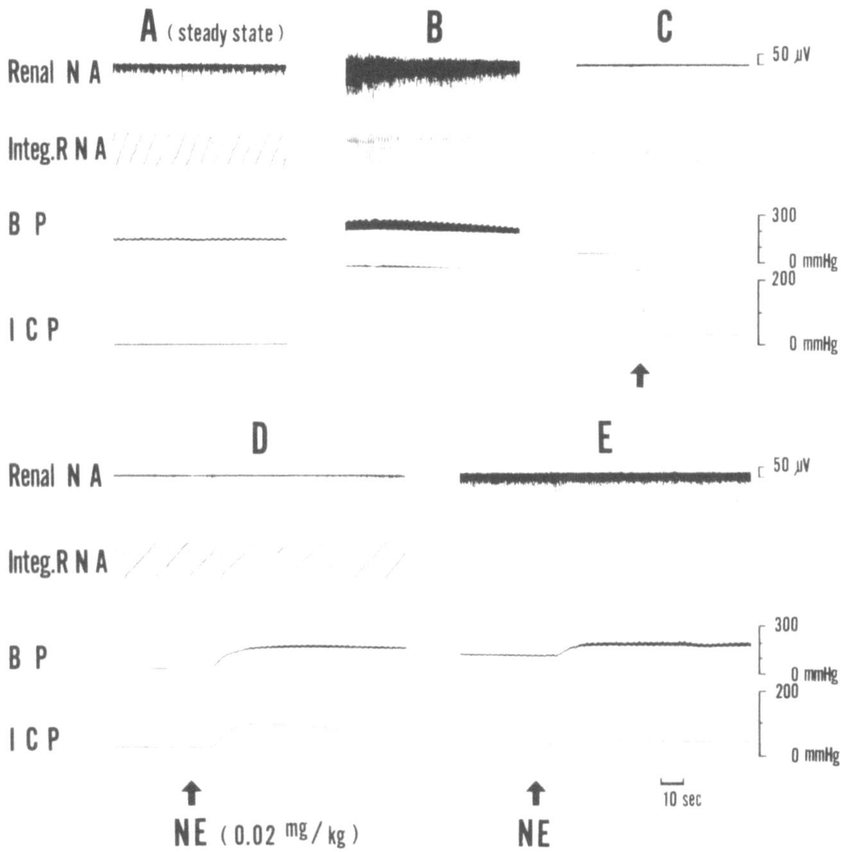

Fig. 4. Changes in RNA during a period of extremely elevated ICP and after decompression, and effect of norepinephrine during the stage of suppressed RNA and after RNA was reappeared.

A: Before procedure

B: When ICP was raised beyond level of mean BP, RNA increased markedly by 730% of state of A

C: 6 min after B. Increased RNA gradually decreased and finally disappeared. RNA remained absent even after ICP was decompressed at point of ↑

D: 2 min after C. RNA still disappeared. Administration of 0.02 mg/kg of norepinephrine (↑) resulted in rise in BP from 38 to 168 mm Hg followed by significant rise in ICP from 28 to 98 mm Hg

E: 3 min after D. RNA reappeared showing an activity of 218% of state A. Administration of 0.02 mg/kg of norepinephrine (↑) again resulted in a rise in BP from 114 to 187 mm Hg, while the rise in ICP was not striking, from 36 to 47 mm Hg

Correlation in Man of Intracranial Pressure and Neuroelectric Activity Determined by Multimodality Evoked Potentials[1]

R.P. Greenberg, D.J. Mayer, and D.P. Becker

Introduction

Intracranial pressure (ICP) measurements in man have not, by themselves, been well correlated with clinical findings or with final outcome. Perhaps ICP levels alone, like angiograms and pneumoencephalograms, etc., tend not to directly reflect neurophysiologic dysfunction, but rather mass alterations. In effect, elevated ICP may indicate only that a space-occupying lesion is present. It cannot indicate if the affected brain is physiologically compromised or normal. It is therefore difficult to assess the significance of ICP levels or when treatment aimed at lowering ICP should be started.

However, ICP, because of its effect on cerebral blood flow (CBF), $CMRO_2$, and ultimately on the metabolic vitality of cerebral neurons, has been convincingly related to brain electrical activity (5). Indeed, this association of ICP and neuroelectric activity suggests that ICP levels could be correlated with multimodality-evoked potentials (MEP) and clinical findings to uncover *an ICP level which alters normal cerebral metabolic function and therefore should be treated.* In a sense, we are utilizing multimodality-evoked potentials to evaluate the effective metabolic state produced by different ICP ranges and clinical situations, in our comatose head injury and brain tumor patients, in an effort to discover and correct neuronal metabolic dysfunction before it becomes irreversible. It would appear from our results that in an *acute* brain injured man, *an ICP of 40 mm Hg or greater can significantly compromise brain cell function and should be treated.*

Patients and Methods

In order to sample, quantitatively, the electrical activity of the largest possible population of cerebral neurons, we have recorded somatosensory, visual, auditory, brain stem-evoked potentials and MEP during every patient study and compared these results with simultaneously recorded intracranial pressure measurements. The ICP was continuously monitored either by the subarachnoid screw technique or by ventricular catheter and printed to obtain a permanent record for analysis by a brush recorder.

There were 20 patients from 11 to 62 years old, all unresponsive to verbal commands, with an ICP range from 2 to 80 mm Hg who were continuously monitored for periods of 2-14 days. There were 17 patients with severe head trauma and 3 with brain tumors studied by these methods. Also, 9 patients had serial MEP recordings performed bringing the total number of studies comparing ICP levels with MEP to 31.

[1] Supported by NIH Grant No. 1P01 NS-12587-01A1 NSP-A and by a Grant from the Southern Medical Association.

The evoked potentials were recorded from 16 scalp electrodes distributed symmetrically over both hemispheres according to the International 10-20 system. Electroretinograms, eighth nerve action potentials, and peripheral nerve action potentials were recorded when indicated to verify the integrity of peripheral receptors. A filter bandpass range of .1-1000 K.C. was used for all evoked potentials except those from the brain stem, which were recorded at 30-3000 K.C. A dedicated mini-computer was used to average out the background noise (E.E.G., muscle artifact, 60 cycle interference, etc.). The data was digitized for storage on IBM compatible tape and analyzed off-line as well as printed immediately by an X-Y plotter.

Multimodality-evoked potentials were analyzed for abnormalities by a grading system developed from our overall experience[2] and categorized for this particular study into normal or abnormal. When an evoked potential was flat line it was placed in the abnormal category.

The clinical status of these comatose patients was evaluated, at the time MEP and ICP were recorded, by the presence or absence of posturing (1). Oculocaloric responses were also examined and closely correlated with posturing as a criteria for determining a given patients clinical conditions. Final outcome classification follow those used by BECKER et al. (2).

In analyzing the data, all tables were collapsed to 2 x 2 tables and Fischer's exact test for 2 x 2 tables was then used to determine P values.

Results

Comparison of ICP Level and Multimodality-Evoked Potentials

A significant pattern emerged when the range of ICP (2-80 mm Hg) obtained from all patients in this study was compared with MEO categorized into normal or abnormal (Table 1). At an ICP level of 40 mm Hg or greater all MEP studies were abnormal. These were no normal MEP studies in this ICP range ($P \leq 0.025$). On the other hand, examination of MEP studies in the 0-40 mm Hg range revealed an equal distribution of 12 normal studies and 12 abnormal ones.

Table 1. Comparison of ICP and multimodality-evoked potentials

	Evoked potentials	
ICP	Normal	Abnormal
0-40 mm Hg	12	12
40+ mm Hg	0	7

Correlation of ICP and MEP Studies with Clinical Status

In this group we have compared both ICP and MEP to patients who were not posturing or better at the time of study and to patients who were posturing or worse (flaccid) (Table 2). A comparison was also done between ICP, MEP, and present or absent oculocaloric responses, which proved to be similar in outcome.

Patients who were posturing or worse had ICP levels equally distributed with 6 below 40 mm Hg and 6 above 40 mm Hg, indicating a lack of correlation of ICP with clinical status in this group. In these

[2] Manuscript in progress.

Table 2. Correlation of simultaneous ICP and MEP studies with clinical status

	ICP		MEP	
	0-40 mm Hg	40+ mm Hg	Normal	Abnormal
No Posturing or better	18	1	12	8
Posturing or worse	6	6	0	11

same patients there were no normal-evoked potentials; all 11 MEP were abnormal. The correlation between abnormal-evoked potentials and patients who were posturing or worse is significant at $P \leq 0.001$.

In the patient group who were not posturing or better there were 12 normal-evoked potential studies and 8 abnormal studies. No significant correlation between MEP and the group of patients not posturing at the time of the study was found. However, of the 8 abnormal studies 6 indicated focal deficit such as a hemiparesis but were otherwise normal.

Correlation of ICP, MEP, and Patient Outcome

We have collapsed the outcome categories into two groups: patients with good to excellent recoveries but who may have a focal residual deficit and patients with poor to dead outcomes. ICP and MEP were then compared to these two groups (Table 3).

Patients whose outcome was poor to dead had a 33% probability of having a mean ICP below 40 mm Hg. Of the ICP measurements in this group, 67% were above 40 mm Hg. The MEP results for this group indicated a highly significant correlation between abnormal MEP studies and poor outcomes or worse ($P \leq .001$).

In the outcome group good to excellent there were scattered ICP levels in the 0-40 mm Hg range but no ICP levels above 40 mm Hg. The evoked potentials were all normal in this group of good to excellent outcomes.

Table 3. Correlation of ICP, MEP, and patient outcome

	ICP		MEP	
	0-40 mm Hg	40+ mm Hg	Normal	Abnormal
Excellent to good	11	0	11	0
Poor to dead	3	6	0	9

Discussion

The value of continuous ICP monitoring to improve patient management and outcome would be greatly increased if correlations between elevated ICP and neurophysiologic compromise could be made in man. The level of ICP that should be treated could be determined according to physiologic criteria - perhaps before permanent brain dysfunction occurred.

Ultimately the neurophysiologic compromise caused by elevated ICP is probably secondary to decreased cerebral blood flow and decreased oxydative metabolism. One physiologic parameter that has been shown to quantitatively reflect depressions of neuronal metabolic function is the evoked potential (3). We have, therefore, correlated ICP levels with evoked potentials in man to determine at what level of ICP brain metabolic embarrassment occurs.

At ICP of 40 mm Hg or greater there was significant alteration of the evoked potentials in all cases leading us to believe that in acute brain injured man, treatment aimed at lowering the ICP should be instituted at this level.

The multimodality-evoked potential studies proved to be more sensitive than ICP in predicting patient outcome. Of the 20 patients studied, all 9, whose outcome was poor to dead, had abnormal or absent-evoked potentials while the 11 who recovered with little residual effects had normal-evoked potentials ($P \leq .001$). An important aspect of this result is that approx. 80% of the evoked potential studies were done within the first 9 days of hospitalization.

For evaluating each patient's clinical condition at the time of the ICP and evoked potential study, the ICP again was not as reliable as the multimodality-evoked potential, The evoked potential data, collapsed to normal versus abnormal categories for analysis, was not as good a predictor of clinical status as it was of final outcome (4).

Summary

Multimodality-evoked potentials were utilized to evaluate the neuronal metabolic state produced by different ICP ranges and clinical situations in comatose head injury and brain tumor patients. It would appear from this data that in acute brain injured man, an ICP of 40 mm Hg or greater can significantly compromise brain function and should be treated.

References

1. BECKER, D.P., VRIES, J.K., SAKALAS, R., YOUNG, H.F., WARD, J.: Early prognosis in head injury based on motor posturing, oculocephalic reflexed, and intracranial pressure. In: Head Injuries: Second Chicago Symposium on Neural Trauma (R.L. McLAURIN, ed.). New York: Grune and Stratton 1975 (in press).
2. BECKER, D.P., MILLER, J.D., YOUNG, H.F., WARD, J.D., ADAMS, W.E.: The critical importance of ICP monitoring in head injury. In: Intracranial Pressure III (J.W.F. BEKS, D.A. BOSCH, M. BROCK, eds.), pp. 97-100. Berlin-Heidelberg-New York: Springer 1976.
3. BRANSTON, N.M., SYMON, L., CROCKARD, H.A., PASZTOR, E.: Relationship between cortical evoked potential and local cortical blood flow following acute middle cerebral artery occlusion in the baboon. Experimental Neurology, 45, 195-208 (1974).
4. GREENBERG, R.P., BECKER, D.P.: Clinical applications of evoked potentials in severe head injury patients. Surgical Forum 26, 484-486 (1975).

5. GROSSMAN, R.G., TURNER, J.W., MILLER, J.D., ROWAN, J.O.: The relationship between cortical electrical activity, cerebral perfusion pressure, and cerebral blood flow during increased ICP. In: Cerebral Circulation and Metabolism (T.W. LANGFITT, ed.), pp. 232-234. Berlin-Heidelberg-New York: Springer 1975.

Summary

K. Shulmann and J. Hoff

MARMAROU et al. analyzed the factors leading to sustained elevations of ICP in 13 patients with various neurosurgical conditions. CSF formation rate, intracranial venous system pressure, and resistance of CSF outflow can be determined by the pressure volume curves using the PVI concept. The mean ICP of the patients was 29 mm Hg with the contributions of the various components as follows: 18% contributed by functional outflow resistance and 76% by the lumped venous component and/or mass lesion 6% remained unaccounted. In 3 of the 13 patients with subarachnoid hemorrhage the outflow resistance component comprised 49 to 55% of the increase in intracranial pressure.

The interesting observation of HOCHWALD's group that in no craniectomized kaolin hydrocephalic cats the central canal of the cord dilates with a terminal 5th ventricle has been confirmed by others. Ligation of the low cord preventing CSF escape from the central canal produces plateau waves and provides the first good model of this phenomenon for further study.

The work of NORTH calls attention to the problem of pulmonary edema after increased intracranial pressure. These authors did not demonstrate pulmonary edema in their cat model with cisternal elevations of ICP to 100 - 150 mm Hg for 45 min.

The papers of SYMON and TANAKA et al. were addressed to the role of the sympathetic nervous system on autoregulation and ICP. SYMON argues that autoregulation to a drop in blood pressure is associated with a delivery vessel vasoconstriction, while maintenance of CBF with increased intracranial pressure is in contrast associated with delivery vessel vasodilation, further suggesting the myogenic concept is the basis of autoregulation. TANAKA et al. demonstrated increased renal nerve sympathetic activity with increase intracranial pressure. Maximal renal nerve activity occurring at a cerebral perfusion pressure of 30 mm Hg.

Finally, in what promises to yield a good deal of data for future conferences, GREENBERG describes a beginning study of multimodal-evoked cortical potentials in patients undergoing ICP monitoring. Although the correlation with ICP and wave form of evoked potentials is only suggestive at this time. Patients with severe brain stem injuries and normal ICP can be clearly separated out.

In conclusion: all papers of this session have covered areas of considerable interest and potential for further investigation.

Session C

Trauma I

Chairman: T. W. Langfitt
Co-chairman: H. Nornes

The Incidence and Importance of Intracranial Hypertension in Head-Injured Patients

T. W. Langfitt

Introduction

The incidence and significance of intracranial hypertension in head injury has been a controversial issue. DANDY (6) among others believed that brain swelling and increased intracranial pressure (ICP) were the rule and were the most common causes of death in head-injured patients. In contrast, BROWDER and MEYERS (3), who measured lumbar subarachnoid pressure several times in the same patient, observed marked intracranial hypertension infrequently; and many patients who died did not have increased ICP any time during the course of their illness. Although these contradictory observations were made more than 40 years ago, and ICP has been measured directly and continuously in a large number of head-injured patients in the past decade, there is still disagreement among investigators on the frequency of intracranial hypertension and its contribution to morbidity and mortality.

There is general agreeement that increased ICP produces brain damage by a reduction in cerebral blood flow (CBF) below the critical level required to maintain cerebral metabolism and/or by brain herniation. The brain damage produced by herniation is also caused by a regional reduction in CBF. In CBF as in ICP studies there has been a large difference in mean values of CBF reported in series of head-injured patients, ranging from near normal to less than half the normal values.

The purpose of this "state of the art" presentation on ICP in head-injured patients is to report a survey of a number of clinical studies of ICP and CBF in which the data have been grouped together in order to attempt to determine:

1. The incidence and severity of increased ICP.
2. The contribution of increased ICP to morbidity and mortality.
3. The relationship of ICP to the presence of a mass lesion.
4. CBF values in head-injured patients.
5. The contribution of the hyperemic syndrome to large differences in mean CBF values among studies.
6. The relationship between ICP and CBF.

Many additional questions could be asked of the data available but, in fact, one of the disappointments of the review was the paucity of information published from some studies that were extensive and obviously performed carefully. The format also varied greatly; the data are not presented the same way in any two papers. This is particularly true of ranges of ICP from definitions of normal to markedly increased. Therefore, it has been necessary to exercise some editorial license in assembling the data in an understandable manner.

Analysis of Data

Incidence of Increased ICP

Table 1 illustrates ICP data from six reports totaling 280 patients. In one large series (15) the distribution of patients between normal/ mild and moderate/severe increases in ICP is nearly equal, whereas in another series of comparable size (5) only a few patients had a moderate and none of the patients a severe increase in ICP. In the series as a whole, 17% had severe and just over one third of the patients had either moderate or severe intracranial hypertension. However, the circumstances in which ICP was recorded (immediately following admission, with or without respiratory assistance, etc.) and the definitions of increased ICP (highest pressure throughout recording, plateau waves, base line between plateau waves, etc.) makes interpretation of the data difficult.

Table 1. ICP in head injury

	ICP (n = 280)			
Reference	Normal	Mild	Moderate	Severe
BECKER et al.	10	32	14	10
ROSSANDA et al.	13	6	6	5
TROUPP et al.	16	23	14	21
*KELLY et al.	11	12	9	9
BRUCE et al.	6	7	5	4
COLD et al.	14	28	5	0
Totals	70	108	53	49
% of total	25	39	19	17

Normal 0 to 10 torr,
Mild 10, 11 to 29, 30 torr,
Moderate 30, 31 to 50, 60 torr,
Severe >50, 60 torr.

*Data given as <30 and >30 torr.

ICP and Survival

Table 2 presents data on the relationship between ICP and survival, and the quality of survival, from reports with a total of 236 patients (2, 5, 15, 12, 10). The designation "recovered" includes patients with a neurologic status ranging from normal to severely impaired. Two-third of patients with a normal or mild increase in ICP recovered, whereas half of the patients with moderate or severe intracranial hypertension died. The number of vegetative patients in both groups is small.

Table 2. ICP and survival

	ICP (n = 236)			
	Normal/mild	%	Moderate/severe	%
"Recovered"	89	66	39	38
Vegetative	20	15	12	12
Dead	25	19	51	50

Moderate/severe >30, 40 torr
Data from one report <11 (Normal/mild) and >11 (Moderate/severe) torr.

Table 3. ICP and survival

	Recovered	Vegetative/dead
Normal	50	22
Increased (>11, 15, 20, 30 torr)	78	86
Normal	50	22
Severe increase (>60 torr)	2	19

Table 3 presents the same data in a different format. The purpose is to demonstrate that when the patients are divided into only two groups (normal and increased ICP) and into two categories of survival (recovered and vegetative/dead), the presence or absence of increased ICP has little influence on the clinical results. However, when the patients with normal and severe increased ICP are compared, it is clear that very few head-injured patients with an increase in ICP over 60 torr survive. Of equal importance is the observation that many patients with a normal ICP vegetate or die.

The latter observation helps clarify some disagreements among investigators; the fact that many patients who die following head injury do not have intracranial hypertension does not mean that intracranial hypertension is unimportant in head injuries; in fact, severe intracranial hypertension carries with it a very poor prognosis; nevertheless, approximately one-third of the mortality and severe morbidity is in patients with little or no intracranial hypertension (Table 2).

ICP and Mass Lesion

Table 4 illustrates clearly that when a mass lesion is present there is a strong likelihood that ICP is increased moderately or severely, and few patients without a mass lesion have significant intracranial hypertension. However, diffuse brain swelling is most common in the pediatric age group, and it appears that there were few children in these studies.

Table 4. ICP and mass lesion

	ICP (n = 88)			
	0-10	11-29	30-50	>50 torr
Mass	1	9	12	12
No mass	13	32	6	3
	0-29	%	>29 torr	%
Mass	10	18	24	73
No mass	45	82	9	27

Mean CBF

There are marked differences in mean CBF values in head-injured patients, the mean value among series of patients ranging from near normal to less than half the normal value (Table 5). Perhaps this should not be surprising when one considers the major variables that influence CBF and the fact that all of the variables pertain in head-injured patients (Table 6). Table 7 demonstrates the effect of a mass lesion on ipsilateral hemisphere CBF compared to mean values in patients without a mass lesion.

Table 5. Mean CBF in head-injured patients

(n = 180)

	n	Mean CBF (ml/100 g/min)
HASS et al.	45	43.4
ENEVOLDSEN et al.	23	30
OVERGAARD and TWEED	43	26
KELLY et al.	17	42.7
BALDY-MOULINIER and FREREBEAU	30	22.1
BRUCE et al.	22	39.5

Table 6. Major variables affecting CBF means

Neurologic status
Mass lesion
Hyperemic syndrome
Arrest of cerebral circulation
ICP, SAP > autoregulation
$PaCO_2$ - vasomotor reactivity
Cerebral metabolism

Table 7. Mass lesions and hemisphere CBF

	Mass		No mass	
	(1)	(2)	(1)	(2)
Mean CBF[a] (ml/100 g/min)	27.0	29.8	43.0	47.7
n	15	10	6	12

[a]Hemisphere ipsilateral to mass.
(1) BALDY-MOULINIER and FREREBEAU.
(2) BRUCE et al.

Table 8. Hyperemia

ENEVOLDSEN et al. (normal 50 ml/100 g/min)
2 of 23 patients > 50 - mean 53 ml/100 g/min

OVERGAARD and TWEED (CBF init. - normal 58.7 ml/100 g/min)
0-24 h - 2 of 15 > 58.7 - mean 64 ml/100 g/min
1-7 days - 10 of 20 > 58-7 - mean 68 ml/100 g/min

BRUCE et al. (normal 50 ml/100 g/min)
Patients with no mass lesion n = 12
4 of 12 > 50 - mean 74.7 ml/100 g/min
8 of 12 < 50 - mean 34.6 ml/100 g/min

KASOFF et al. (11) described hyperemic tissue peaks in regional cerebral blood flow (rCBF) studies in head-injured children, and several other investigators have noted that head-injured patients, particularly those without mass lesions, tend to fall into two categories, those with reduced and those with increased hemisphere CBF. The difference is most evident in the study of BRUCE et al. (4) (Table 8). When one also recalls that in a number of severely head-injured patients ICP equals the systemic arterial pressure, and CBF ceases (9 of 30 patients in the series of BALDY-MOULINIER and FREREBEAU), the differences in the mean values among series illustrated in Table 6 and the fact that mean CBF is nearly normal in some series are not so surprising observations.

ICP and CBF

Rarely have clinical data on the relationship of ICP to CBF been presented in detail. Therefore, it has not been possible to assemble data from several series as has been done here for ICP and CBF alone. Most investigators believe that there is no predictable relationship between ICP and CBF (7, 13, 4); in contrast, one group found an excellent inverse correlation between ICP and CBF (8).

Conclusions

1. Increased ICP is common in head-injured patients.
2. The mortality and severe morbidity rates are very high in patients with severe intracranial hypertension, but one-third of the patients die without significant increases in ICP.
3. ICP is higher in patients with mass lesions.
4. Mean CBF varies greatly among series of patients; two of the most important factors are hyperemia and cerebral circulatory arrest which skew the mean values even when the numbers of patients in these categories are small.
5. Probably there is no predictable relationship between ICP and CBF in head-injured patients.
6. Investigators in the field of ICP should adopt uniform methods for the collection and reporting of their data.

References

1. BALDY-MOULINIER, M., FREREBEAU, Ph.: Cerebral blood flow in cases of coma following severe head injury. In: Cerebral Blood Flow (M. BROCK, C. FIESCHI, D.H. INGVAR, N.A. LASSEN, K. SCHÜRMANN, eds.), pp. 216-218. Berlin-Heidelberg-New York: Springer 1969.

2. BECKER, D.P., VRIES, J.K., YOUNG, H.F., WARD, J.D.: Controlled cerebral perfusion pressure and ventilation in human mechanical brain injury: Prevention of progressive brain swelling. In: Intracranial Pressure II (N. LUNDBERG, U. PONTEN, M. BROCK, eds.), pp. 480-484. Berlin-Heidelberg-New York: Springer 1975.

3. BROWDER, J., MEYERS, R.: Observations on behavior of the systemic blood pressure, pulse, and spinal fluid pressure following craniocerebral injury. Amer. J. Surg. 3, 403-427 (1936).

4. BRUCE, D.A., LANGFITT, T.W., MILLER, J.D., SCHUTZ, H., VAPALAHTI, M.P., STANEK, A., GOLDBERG, H.I.: Regional metabolism in comatose patients. J. Neurosurg. 38, 131-144 (1973).

5. COLD, G., ENEVOLDSEN, E., MALMROS, R.: The prognostic value of continuous intraventricular pressure recording in unconscious braininjury patients under controlled ventilation. In: Intracranial Pressure II (N. LUNDBERG, U. PONTEN, M. BROCK, eds.), pp. 517-521. Berlin-Heidelberg-New York: Springer 1975.

6. DANDY, W.E.: Diagnosis and treatment of injuries of the head. JAMA 101, 772-775 (1933).

7. ENEVOLDSEN, E.M., COLD, G., JENSEN, F.T., MALMROS, R.: Dynamic changes in regional CBF, intraventricular pressure, CBF pH and lactate levels during the acute phase of head injury. J. Neurosurg. 44, 191-214 (1976).

8. GOBIET, W., BOCK, W.J., GROTE, W., BETTAG, M.: Cerebral blood flow in patients with traumatic cerebral edema. In: Intracranial Pressure II (N. LUNDBERG, U. PONTEN, M. BROCK, eds.), pp. 508-511. Berlin-Heidelberg-New York: Springer 1975.

9. HASS, W.K., KOBAYASHI, M., HOCHWALD, G.M., WALD, A., DOROGI, P., RANSOHOFF, J.: Relationship of cerebral metabolic rate to brain stem injury. In: Blood Flow and Metabolism in the Brain (A.M. HARPER, W.B. JENNETT, J.D. MILLER, J.O. ROWAN, eds.), p. 13-39-13.40. Edinburgh: Churchill Livingstone 1975.

10. JOHNSTON, I.H., JOHNSTON, J.A., JENNET, B.: Intracranial pressure changes following head injury. Lancet 1970 II, 433-436.

11. KASOFF, S.S., ZINGESSER, L.H., SHULMAN, K.: Compartmental abnormalities of regional cerebral blood flow in children with head trauma. J. Neurosurg. 36, 463-470 (1972).

12. KELLY, P.J., IWATA, K., McGRAW, C.P., TINDALL, G.T.: Intracranial pressure, cerebral blood flow, and prognosis in patients with severe head injuries. In: Cerebral Circulation & Metabolism (T.W. LANGFITT, L.C. McHENRY, M. REIVICH, H. WOLLMAN, eds.), pp. 241-244. Berlin-Heidelberg-New York: Springer 1975.

13. OVERGAARD, J., TWEED, W.A.: Cerebral circulation after head injury. Part I: Cerebral blood flow and its regulation after closed head injury with emphasis on clinical correlations. J. Neurosurg. 41, 531-541 (1974).

14. ROSSANDA, M., COLLICE, M., PORTA, M., BOSELLI, L.: Intracranial hypertension in head injury. Clinical significance and relation to respiration. In: Intracranial Pressure II (N. LUNDBERG, U. PONTEN, M. BROCK, eds.), pp. 475-479. Berlin-Heidelberg-New York: Springer 1975.

15. TROUPP, H., KUURNE, T., KASTE, M., VAPALAHTI, M., VALTONEN, S.: Intraventricular pressure after severe brain injuries: Prognostic value and correlation with blood pressure and jugular venous oxygen tension. In: Intracranial Pressure (M. BROCK, H. DIETZ, eds.), pp. 222-226. Berlin-Heidelberg-New York: Springer 1972.

ICP, CVR and Cerebral Metabolism Following Experimental Cerebral Missile Injury[1]

H.A. Crockard, F.D. Brown, A.B. Calica, and S. Mullan

Introduction

In an attempt to understand the cerebral gunshot injury, we have standardized an occipitofrontal missile injury in rhesus monkeys using an air rifle and recorded vital signs, cerebrovascular changes, and cerebral metabolism. Besides the conventional form of analysis of the data, we have used a multiple regression type of analysis in an attempt to predict accurately the survival time of each animal.

Materials and Methods

A Crossman 160 air rifle, firing a 3 mm diameter B.B. pellet weighing 0.31 g, was used. Missile velocity, calculated by using photoelectric cells, could be altered by varying the amount of compressed air used by the rifle. In this series, three velocities were used 56, 90, and 180 m/s. The air rifle was attached to a stereotaxic frame so that it could be adjusted very accurately in three planes allowing a similar injury in all animals.

There were 32 rhesus monkeys (Macaca mulatta), of either sex, weighing 5-9 kg used in this series. Surgical preparation of the animals is given in detail elsewhere (1). The animals were tranquilized with phencyclidine hydrochloride, 1-2 mg/kg; an endotracheal tube was passed and, for the surgical preparation, a small dose of barbiturate was given intravenously. No barbiturate was given 1 h before or immediately after the injury. Throughout the experiment the animals breathed spontaneously. The animal was placed in a stereotaxic head frame and the rifle adjusted so that the trajectory of the missile was 5° divergent from the sagittal plane through the occipital burr hole toward the upper outer quadrant of the right orbit. Immediately after injury the burr hole was sealed with nethyl methacrylate. $Xenon^{133}$ in saline was injected into the internal carotid arteries for the determination of hemispheric blood flow, using the flow initial technique. Control observations were made of MBP, heart rate, respiration, ICP, arterial and sagittal blood gases, hemispheric blood flow, $CMRO_2$ and CMR Lactate, and CVR. Following injury vital signs were continuously monitored, and the cerebrovascular measurements repeated at 1, 10, 30 min, and hourly until death or sacrifice.

The values of all the physiologic parameters were inserted into a computer program and, following initial analysis, six (MBP, ICP, CVR, CBF, CMRD, and CMR lactate) were identified as being most important. Single variables were compared with the length of survival following injury and generated (Fig. 1). Multiple linear regression analysis (2) was also performed and mathematical expressions evolved which could

[1]From Dept. of Neurosurgery, Univ. of Chicago Hospital. Supported by Grants No. F05-2144 and NS 7834-08.

predict individual animal's survival with considerable accuracy. Using only 30-min postinjury data, the following equation was evolved:
$2.4\ \text{MBP} + 4.7\ \text{CBF} - 31.4\ (r^2 = 0.46) = \text{Survival (min)}$.
With more data points, 76% of the variance could be explained ($r^2 = 0.76$).

Results

The results from the 32 animals will be presented in four groups. (a) There were 20 animals injured with a pellet travelling at 90 m/s releasing 1.26 joules of energy. This was designated a "standard" injury. Of these 14 died or were sacrified at 6 h. (b) A further 6 were allowed to live as long as possible - two survived 6 h and the other 14 lived 16, 21, and 28 h following injury. (c) Three animals were injured with a low energy injury, the pellet travelling at 17.1 m/s (0.05 joules of energy). (d) The fourth group has a high energy injury, missile velocity 180 m/s (5.02 joules). Two other animals were injured by passing a probe of the same diameter as the BB through the cerebral hemisphere. Vital signs were also monitored in them, and the brains used for comparative histopathology.
The changes in the standard injury group will be described, and the other groups compared to this.

(a) Standard Injury

At less than 1 s after the passage of the missile there were obvious changes in vital signs (Fig. 2). In several animals there was a brief period (2-5 s) of apnea, but the most noticeable change was that in tidal volume; there was no change in arterial pCO_2. At the same time there was a profound bradycardia which persisted for 10-20 min, and then the heart rate returned to control values at which it remained for the rest of the animal's life. There was a slight rise in MBP, which reached a peak at 10 min following injury, and then subsided to significantly lower levels from 30 min onward (77 mm Hg). Following injury there was also a marked increase in pulse pressure. ICP rose rapidly following injury, reaching a peak of 60-90 mm Hg 2-5 min following injury, and thereafter subsiding over the next 10-20 min to levels between 20 and 30 mm Hg. It remained at this level for the rest of the period of observation. CBF, which was 42.1 ml/100 g/min in the control period, fell to 26 ml/100 g/min at 1 min following injury, and it remained at this level for the rest of the animal's life, apart from a short period in each animal's life, between 10-40 min, when the flow was considerably reduced (11-15 ml/100 g/min). CBF from both hemispheres was involved, though the left side (the uninjured) usually had a faster flow. Control CVR, which was 2.2, fell at 1 min and was reduced further at 10 min, but at 30 min there was a reversal with an extremely high CVR, and this persisted for 2 h following injury (Fig. 3). Terminally the CVR fell again. $CMRO_2$ (control 3.12 ml/g), fell at 1 min and continued to fall until 30 min at which level it stayed for the rest of the observation period. CMR lactate (initially 0.25 mg/g), rose and remained high for 4 h after injury, and then fell.

There was a wide scatter in the results, some animals dying or becoming apneic within a few minutes after injury, and others surviving 28 h. Those who survived a short time had a more profound change in respiration, a marked bradycardia, a higher ICP, and a reduced perfusion pressure following injury. $CMRO_2$ was also much reduced at 10 and 30 min as compared to the others (Fig. 1).

(b) Long Survivors

The animals in this group showed fewer changes in vital signs. CBF rose to 30-50 ml/100 g/min 6 h after injury. CVR followed the same pattern early but after 12 h there was an increase in CVR. There were prominent episodes of B waves associated with MBP and respiratory changes.

(c) High Energy

The animals in this group showed much greater changes in vital signs and only two lived longer than 30 min without ventilatory support. There was a marked change in respiration resulting in hypocapnia, a profound bradycardia, a marked hypotension (50 mm Hg). ICP reached peak values up to 200 mm Hg at 1 min, and fell to 10-15 mm Hg at 10 min. There was an extremely high CBF at 1 min (66-135 ml/100 g/min), but by 30 min this flow was considerably reduced (11.6 ml/100 g/min).

(d) Low Energy

The three animals in this group showed very little change following injury. There was a slight change in respiration, but no change in PCO_2, a slight bradycardia at 1 min, but it had returned to control levels at 10 min and little or no change in MBP. There was a slight rise in ICP and it remained at 15-20 mm Hg for the rest of the period of observation. CBF was little affected.

The animals injured with the probe showed no change in ICP and no change in vital signs.

Discussion

The immediate brain stem signs illustrate the effects of the shock wave transmitted from the missile in this type of injury. The gradation in physiologic changes, with the amount of energy delivered to the brain, is in keeping with acceleration/deceleration experiments. Basically, we consider that this model delivers to the brain energy comparable to that released by the missile of a conventional hand gun after it has penetrated scalp and bone.

How may the physiologic changes be correlated? It is our opinion that immediately following injury there are direct brain stem effects as evidenced by the permanent hypotension. As well as this, there is loss of arteriolar tone shown by the immediate reduction in CVR, which produces a sudden increase in cerebral blood volume and hence a rise in ICP. Sudden transfer of arterial pressure to the capillary bed will cause disruption in the blood brain barrier, allow transudation of fluid, and thus effectively increasing brain volume. This increase in cerebral blood volume and brain volume occurring in a closed cavity will lead to the increase in CVR that is seen at 30 min. The CBF, reduced after injury, is dependent on the CPP, though in the first 30 min there is no linear correlation between them. At the time of maximum CVR, blood flow is severely compromised and, if the injury is severe, the downward trend will continue until the animal's death within a few minutes. In less severely injured animals, a new steady state will develop for the next 6-12 h. However, after that there is a further increase in CVR, perhaps due to the formation of cytotoxic edema and CBF is again compromised. With regard to cerebral metabolism, it is our belief that in the early stage, the reduction in $CMRO_2$ is primarily due to a reduction in flow, although in the longer surviving animals, we feel that this may also be due to a decreased oxygen extraction.

Conclusions

From this model we conclude that:

1. Following cerebral missile injury there are brain stem effects which can be related directly to the wounding energy.
2. There is a sudden increase in ICP, reduction in CPP and CVR, leading to an increase in cerebral blood volume.
3. There is a loss of autoregulation and, though there is no close correlation with CPP in the early stages, later CBF and CPP are linearly related.
4. There is a progressive reduction in oxidative metabolism, initially flow-dependent, but later due to decreased oxygen uptake by the brain.
5. Using multiple linear regression analysis it is possible to predict accurately an individual's survival time. On-line calculations may then allow each animal to be its own control when assessing therapy.

Summary

An experimental missile injury model in spontaneously breathing primates is described. The energy of wounding can be related directly to physiologic changes. The right cerebral injury produces generalized changes which may be conveniently divided into the brain stem effects and cerebral hemispheric effects. The former produces an hypotension which compromises CPP. The latter is responsible for loss of autoregulation, falling CBF, an increase in cerebral blood volume and, eventually, brain volume. CVR, which initially falls following injury, is increased due to these latter increases in volume, and this, in turn, compromises circulation. There is a reduction in $CMRO_2$ which is primarily flow-dependent.

References

1. CROCKARD, H.A., BROWN, F.D., JOHNS, L., et al.: An experimental cerebral missile injury in primates (in press).
2. CROCKARD, H.A., BROWN, F.D., CALICA, A.B., et al.: Physiological consequences of experimental missile injury and the use of data-analysis to predict survival (in press).

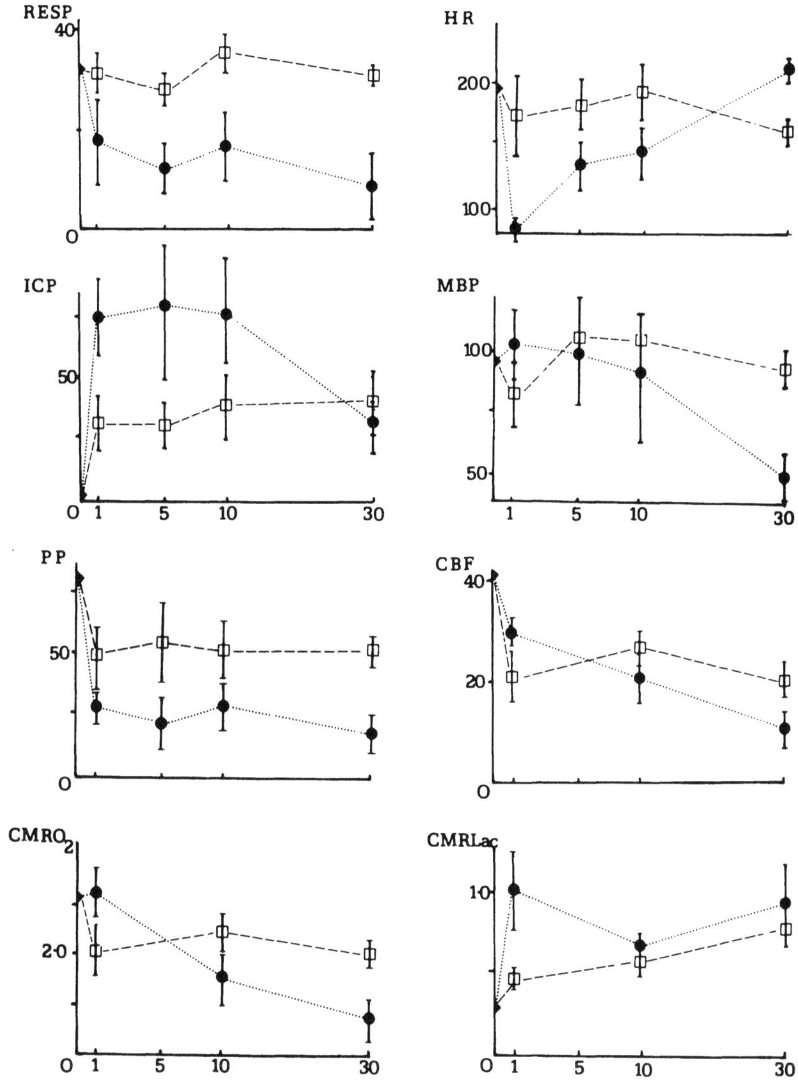

Fig. 1. Changes in eight parameters over first 30 min after injury. Open squares are from animals living 6 h after injury. Closed circles are values from animals which survived less than 1 h

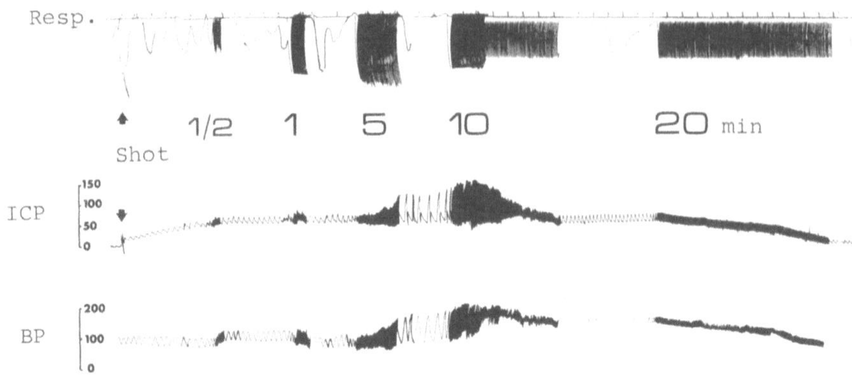

Fig. 2. Means and SE of three parameters over 6 h after injury. The marked reduction in CPP, associated with fall in CBF is seen. CVR initially falls, but at 30 min is significantly increased, perhaps due to increase in blood and brain volumes

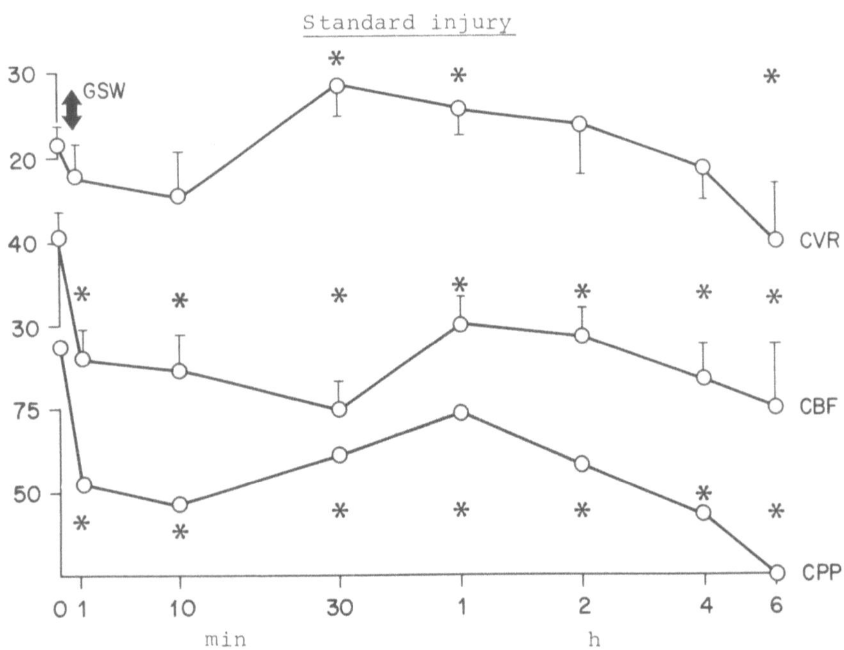

Fig. 3. Vital signs after injury. Note respiratory changes and immediate rise in ICP with a peak at 5-10 min. Cerebral perfusion pressure (CPP) is almost halved

Intracranial Pressure Effects of Missile Wounds[1]

M. Djordjevic[2], J. Löfgren, L. Steiner, and N. N. Zwetnow

Introduction

The passage of a missile through body tissues results in an explosive temporary cavitation and tissue destruction which is a function of the mass and probably the second power of the velocity of the missile (1). The aim of the present study was to evaluate the intracranial pressure (ICP) changes occurring after wounding with bullets of different velocities. In addition, there was an opportunity to study general neural responses to rapid energy loading. An advantage of the missile injury model is the ease with which input parameters can be precisely controlled over an extensive range.

Methods

Experiments were performed on dogs anesthetized with pentobarbital, intubated and usually ventilated mechanically in a respirator in order to eliminate secondary effects of disturbed respiration on ICP. Statham transducers were used for pressure measurements via catheters in the femoral artery, the inferior caval vein, and the lateral ventricle and a needle in cisterna magna. Considerable technical difficulties were encountered in preventing dislocation of the pressure recording devices during the firing. No attempts were made to record the dynamic pressure transients at the moment of injury. Cerebral blood flow was measured at intervals with injections into the left vertebral artery utilizing the xenon elimination method. EEG and ECG were monitored continuously.

The animals were shot transversely through the head in the posterior frontal region with an M-16 American carbine using jacketed lead spheres with a weight of 0.87 g and a caliber of 5.6 mm. Missile velocity was varied in stages between 122 and 785 m/s.

In some experiments blood pressure reactions were prevented by infusion of Arfonad. In another group of experiments vasodilation was induced prior to the wounding by means of administration of CO_2 or by producing a state of reactive hyperemia after a period of high ICP maintained artificially with a pressurized bottle of saline connected to the subarachnoid space (3).

[1]This study has been supported by the Swedish Research Institute of Defence. Invaluable technical help has been received from Senior Research Engineer Sven Sohlé, SRID, Stockholm, which herewith is gratefully acknowledged.

[2]On leave of absence from the Department of Neurosurgery, University of Belgrad (Yugoslavia), Recipient of the Doctoral Research Grant, Karolinska Institute, Stockholm.

Results

The degree of tissue destruction and fracturing of the skull was roughly proportional to missile velocity. Intracranial hematoma formation did not occur but post mortem examination showed thin layers of blood over the convexities and around the brain stem as well as small amounts of blood in the bullet tract. CSF was grossly blood-stained. After the shot the brain tissue rapidly herniated in the entry and exit wounds. Immediately after the wounding there was a rapid rise in the arterial pressure, sometimes to mean values exceeding 300 mm Hg (Fig. 1). The pressure leveled off and subsided thereafter gradually during the next 10 min, ultimately stabilizing on a slightly hypotensive level. Sometimes there was a continuing fall of the arterial pressure and the animal died. Concomitant with the arterial pressure response there were disturbances in cardiac action and ECG, especially ventricular extrasystoles.

The ICP showed corresponding changes increasing rapidly after the shot but to rather variable heights, from 30-40 mm Hg to values sometimes as high as 300 mm Hg. After a few minutes ICP decreased exponentially assuming finally a steady-state value of about 30-70 mm Hg. There was no apparent correlation between these changes in arterial and intracranial pressure and missile velocity. While the ICP reaction was modified by the arterial pressure it was basically independent thereof. Preventing the arterial pressor response by Arfonad did not abolish the ICP changes but decreased somewhat their amplitude (Fig. 2).

It has been suggested that an important mechanism in the ICP that changes after a mechanical head injury is cerebral vasodilation and an increased cerebral blood volume (4). Preinduced vasodilation prior to the wounding did not prevent or significantly modify the ICP reaction (Fig. 3). Further evidence against a vasodilation as a decisive factor was found in the blood flow measurements starting a few minutes after the wounding. Cerebral blood flow consistantly decreased by about 50% (Fig. 4). After low velocity injuries, there was some tendency toward a restitution of the blood flow with time. The decrease in the blood flow was not completely explainable on the basis of a reduced perfusion pressure. There was also an increase in cerebrovascular resistance, to some extent occurring progressively after the wounding, particularly in high velocity injuries. Autoregulation was abolished as indicated by linear pressure-flow relations after the wounding. During the first minutes after the wounding there were increasing EEG changes consisting of flattening and slowing of the baseline activity. After high velocity injuries the changes could progree to isoelectric recording. There was never an immediate extinction of the EEG activity after the wounding.

Discussion

The ICP changes produced by a missile wound of the severe type of these experiments seem related in part to primary events occurring intracranially and in part to modifying effects of a transient arterial pressor response. This pressor response is presumably due to a brief intense sympathetic discharge caused by the intracranial stress waves at the moment of injury. Cerebral vasodilation as the specific mechanism of the ICP effects seems unlikely. Missile injury in animals with a dilated cerebral vascular bed did not result in ICP changes different from the control. Furthermore, there was evidence of cerebral vasoconstriction and diminished cerebral blood flow a few minutes after the wounding. A transitory vasodilation may possibly contribute to the pressure changes during the first minutes (2). The increase in the cerebrovascular resistance may possibly at later stages also be dependent upon increasing tissue edema and pressure.

Consequently, it seems highly probable that the main reason for the ICP changes occurring after a missile injury is a transient bleeding in the skull cavity during the first minutes. This is in agreement with the somewhat variable responses as hemorrhage might be expected to occur as a random event to some degree independent of missile velocity. Actually the magnitude and time course of the pressure changes are practically identical to those seen in experimental intracranial bleedings (5, 6). The usual course of an intracranial hemorrhage is a phase pf rapid bleeding for about 30 s when the ICP rapidly rises counteracting the bleeding by a pressure tamponade. On the condition of intact hemostatic mechanisms, the bleeding may thereafter stop definitely within a few minutes and the dangerously high ICP is reduced by a compensatory increase in the outflow of CSF. The blocking of the CSF outflow passages, however, leads to an increase in the outflow resistance with a consequent elevation of the final steady-state pressure. Both arterial and venous hemorrhages follow similar courses in spite of different initial bleeding pressures. This is due to the mechanical fact that when a low-pressure venous bleeding starts and the ICP is built up, the venous pressure will successively rise, maintaining the bleeding until it ultimately reaches the level of the arterial pressure.

While no massive hematomas developed intracranially it was clear that a considerable amount of occult bleeding may have occurred. It should be remembered that the ICP effects are explainable by an intracranial hemorrhage of about 4-5 ml according to the existing pressure-volume relations.

It might be thought that the sometimes very extensive decompressions produced by the entry and exit wounds and fracturing of the skull should to some extent prevent an increase in ICP. This was not the case in any significant degree, evidently due to the rapid blocking of the openings by herniating brain tissue, taking up the internal stresses.

In conclusion, it is our contention that the ICP changes after a craniocerebral missile injury basically are dependent on intracranial accumulation of blood producing a transient pressure change due to a volume effect and an elevation of the steady-state pressure caused by an increased resistance to CSF outflow. It is tempting to speculate that the same basic mechanism of a brief period of intracranial bleeding immediately after the trauma also is operating in cases of severe blunt head injuries where the patients may arrive in a state of high ICP but without frank hematomas.

Summary

The time course and nature of the ICP changes occurring consequently to a missile injury were studied in dogs. There was a transient increase of ICP for a few minutes, whereafter it settled at a steady-state value usually in the range of 30-70 mm Hg. An arterial pressure response immediately after the wounding magnified the ICP change. Basically the alterations in ICP seem related to a short period after the wounding of intracranial bleeding, resulting in a transient pressure change related to the addition of volume and an increase in steady-state pressure secondary to an increase in CSF outflow resistance. Vasodilation was evidently not a factor as cerebrovascular resistance consistantly increased after the injury and vasodilation induced artificially prior to the wounding did not affect the ICP response.

References

1. deMUTH, W.E.Jr.: Bullet velocity and design as determinants of wounding capability: An experimental study. J. Trauma 6, 222-232 (1966).
2. GERBER, A.M., MOODY, R.A.: Craniocerebral missile injuries in the monkey: An experimental physiological model. J. Neurosurg. 36, 43-49 (1972).
3. HÄGGENDAL, E., LÖFGREN, J., NILSSON, N.J., ZWETNOW, N.N.: Prolonged cerebral hyperemia after periods of increased cerebrospinal fluid pressure in dogs. Acta physiol. scand. 79, 272-279 (1970).
4. LANGFITT, T.W., TANNENBAUM, H.M., KASSELL, N.F.: The etiology of acute brain swelling following experimental head injury. J. Neurosurg. 24, 47-56 (1966).
5. LÖFGREN, J., ZWETNOW, N.N.: Kinetics of arterial and venous hemorrhage in the skull cavity. In: Intracranial Pressure (M. BROCK, H. DIETZ, eds.), pp. 155-159. Berlin-Heidelberg-New York: Springer 1972.
6. STEINER, L., LÖFGREN, J., ZWETNOW, N.N.: Characteristics and limits of tolerance in repeated subarachnoid hemorrhage in dogs. Acta neurol. scand. 52, 241-267 (1975).

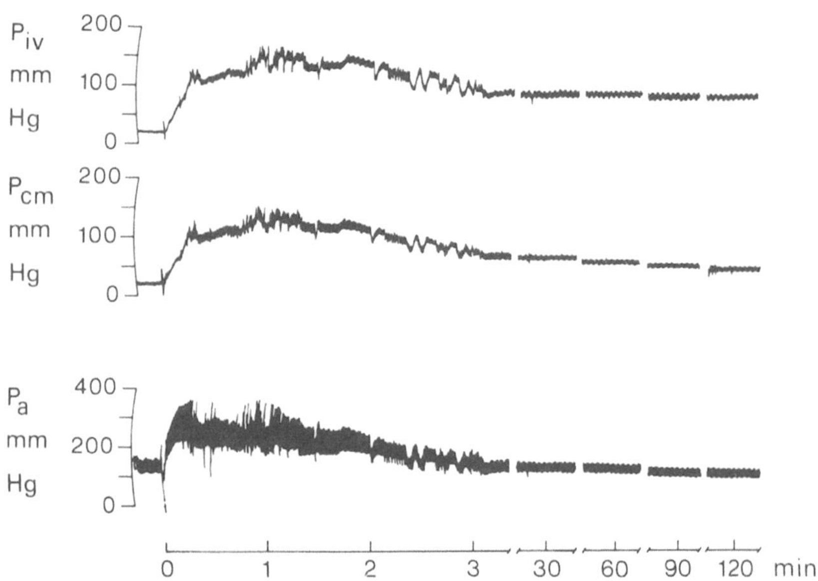

Fig. 1. Intraventricular (P_{iv}), cisterna magna (P_{cm}), and arterial (P_a) pressure courses after missile injury with missile velocity of 285.6 m/s. Intraventricular and cisterna magna pressures usually followed each other but sometimes a pressure differential developed indicating tentorial herniation

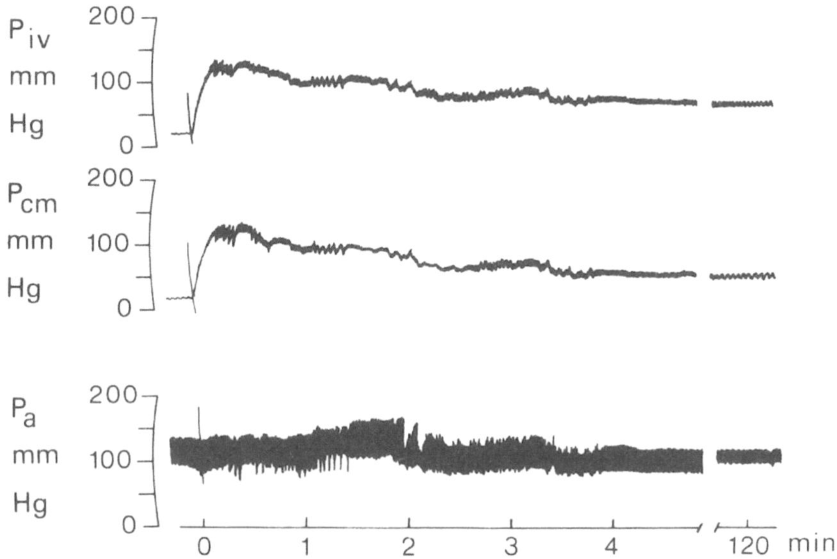

Fig. 2. Intraventricular (P_{iv}), cisterna magna (P_{cm}), and arterial (P_a) pressures following missile injury during continuing infusion of Arfonad to prevent a blood pressure response

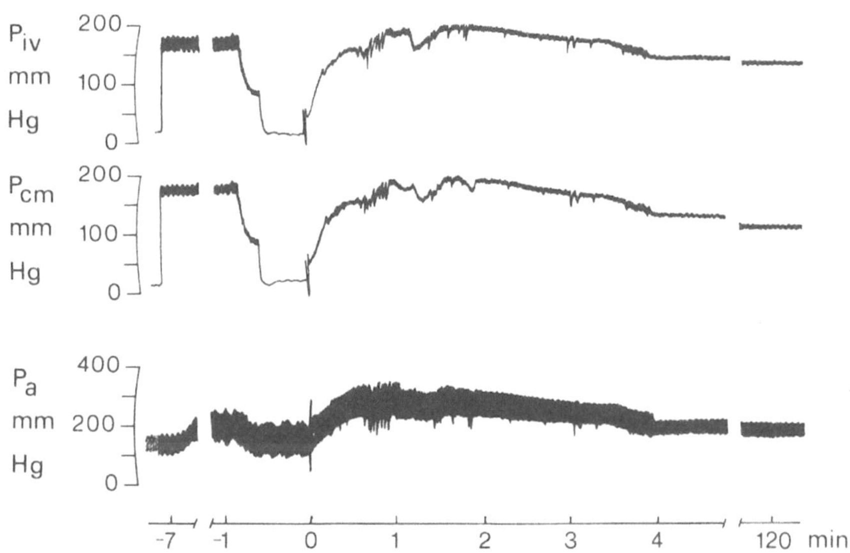

Fig. 3. Intraventricular (P_{iv}), cisterna magna (P_{cm}), and arterial (P_a) pressures following missile injury during state of reactive hyperemia produced by release of a high cerebrospinal fluid pressure maintained for a period of 8 min prior to wounding

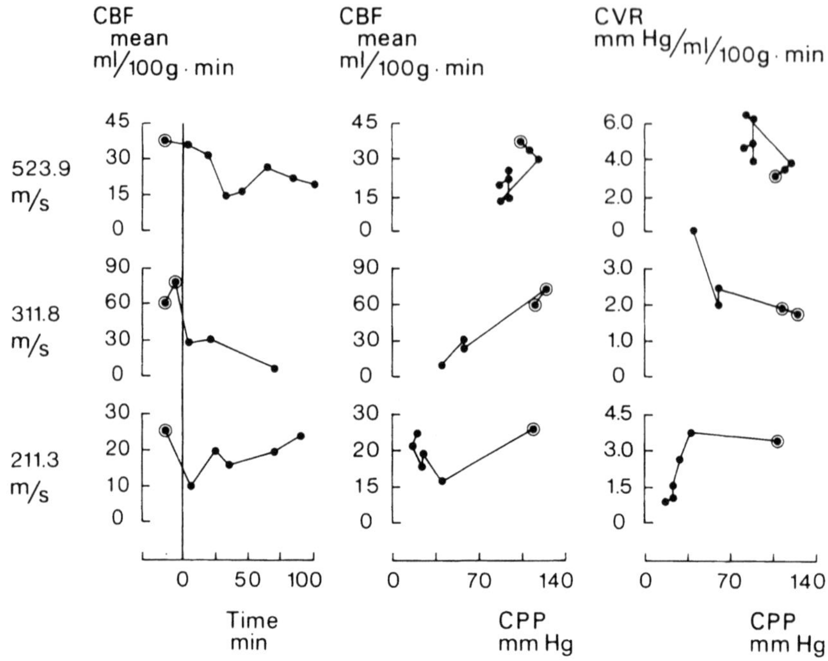

Fig. 4. Hemodynamic parameters after missile injury without different missile velocities. From right to left cerebral blood flow as a function of time, CBF as a function of perfusion pressure (CPP), and corresponding cerebrovascular resistance (CVR) as a function of CPP

Intraventricular Pressure in Patients with Chronic Subdural Hematomas Before and After Evacuation of the Hematoma

F. Gjerris

Introduction

Chronic subdural hematomas typically cause headache, dementia, and progressive neurologic signs such as hemiparesis and aphasia. Symptoms of increased intracranial pressure are uncommon. The incidence of papilloedema may vary between 25 and 90% (2), but in a large series of 216 patients with chronic subdural hematomas 22% had papilloedema (5). PLUM and POSNER (6) measured lumbar cerebrospinal fluid (CSF) pressure in conjunction with lumbar puncture and found it to be less than 150 mm of water in half of the patients and more than 150 mm of water in the other half. McKISSOCK et al. (5) measured lumbar CFS pressure on a single occasion in 86 patients with chronic subdural hematomas and found that 29% of the patients had a lumbar CSF pressure of more than 200 mm of water. These pressure measurements only reflect the pressure during a short period of time, but I am not aware of any studies where CSF pressure has been continuously recorded in this group of patients.

The purpose of the present study was to measure continuously the intraventricular pressure in patients with chronic subdural hematomas before and after evacuation of the hematoma in order to evaluate the effect of evacuation of the hematoma on the intraventricular pressure.

Material and Methods

Seven patients aged between 49 and 75 years with a one-sided subdural hematoma, angiographically verified, were studied. All patients had chronic subdural hematomas with membrane formation and more than 3 weeks had elapsed between a head trauma and operation. Six patients had severe preoperative hemiparesis or aphasia and all seven had alterations of consciousness (somnolence or confusion). One had papilloedema. All hematomas were evacuated through two burr holes and had a volume of 120 to 200 ml. At 24 to 48 h after surgery the symptoms had disappeared in six patients and all were awake. One patient with a very low intracranial pressure before operation (3-4 mm Hg) woke up during the evacuation under local anesthesia, but intraventricular pressure (IVP) remained very low and steady deterioration progressed, death occurring 3 weeks later.

In all patients IVP was measured continuously ad modum LUNDBERG (4) through a cannula in the anterior horn of the lateral ventricle contralateral to the hematoma. The transducer was placed at the level of foramen of Monro. The IVP was measured 8 to 24 h before and 1 to 24 h after evacuation using an ELEMA transducer and a SERVIGOR recorder.

No complications occurred. IVP was computed as diastolic pressure plus one-third pulse amplitude. The arterial blood pressure was measured repeatedly using a brachial cuff.

Results

The average values of IVP prior to operation in the six patients who recovered are shown in Table 1. The mean IVP was 22.6 mm Hg. IVP ranged from 0.5 to 19 mm Hg with a mean of 6.4 mm Hg, 1 h after operation. IVP increased to a mean of 20.2 mm Hg 8 h after operation. The IVP had increased further 24 h postoperatively attaining a mean of 23.4 mm Hg, which was similar to the pressure prior to surgery (Fig. 1). The patient with the highest IVP was the only one having papilloedema. In this patient IVP was still 25 mm Hg on the 3rd day after surgery, but all symptoms had disappeared excluding the papilloedema.

Table 1. Mean IVP before and after evacuation of chronic subdural hematoma

Patient No.		Mean intraventricular pressure (mm Hg) Before	1 h after	8 h after	24 h after
1	Average	19	11	15	17
	range	16 - 22.6	10 - 12.6	13.3 - 17.3	15.6 - 18.3
2	Average	20	3.5	18	19.5
	range	16.5 -24	2.3 - 4.6	17 - 19.3	17.3 - 21.6
3	Average	32	0.5	28.5	30
	range	27 - 37.6	0 - 1	21.6 - 35	23.3 - 37
4	Average	20	19	23	28.5
	range	18.3 - 22.6	16.3 - 21.3	15.6 - 29.8	23.3 - 34
5	Average	20	4	18.5	19
	range	17 - 23.3	2.3 - 6.3	17 - 20	17 - 20.6
6	Average	25	0.5	18	26.5
	range	20 - 30.3	0 - 1	15 - 21.6	23.3 - 30
Mean		22.7	6.4	20.2	23.4
SD		4.6	6.6	4.4	5.1
SEM		1.9	2.7	1.8	2.0

Discussion

Considering the six patients who presented a uniform pattern, this study shows that IVP returns to the preoperative levels about 8-10 h after the evacuation of the chronic subdural hematoma and remains there for at least the next 24 h. The fast normalization of the level of consciousness and the prompt improvement of hemiparesis following the evacuation of the hematoma indicate that raised ICP per se is not the cause of the clinical symptoms, but that the direct pressure of the hematoma on the underlying cortical area or the distortion of the brain stem causes the symptoms. In spite of an increased intracranial pressure, CSF formation remains constant (3) and the return of the IVP to the preoperative level after 8 h suggests that CSF, which is produced with a rate of 0.3 to 0.4 ml/min, then occupies the intracranial space previously taken by the hematoma (120 to 200 ml).

It is to be expected that IVP in patients operated upon for chronic subdural hematomas will normalize during the subsequent days in the same way as in patients undergoing surgery for brain tumors (1), but measurements have not been made.

In conclusion, it is not the raised IVP which causes the hemiparesis and somnolence, but the hematoma pressure on the underlying cortex and the distortion of the brain stem. The increased CSF pressure is caused by the blockage of CSF flow over the hemisphere and the demand for a constant bulk resorption of CSF.

Summary

Intraventricular pressure (IVP) was measured in seven patients, aged 49 to 75 years, before and after evacuation of a typical subdural hematoma. Before surgery mean IVP in six patients was 22.7 mm Hg (SEM = 1.9). At 8 h after surgery mean IVP was 20.2 mm Hg and 24 h postoperatively the mean IVP was again 23.4 mm Hg (SEM = 2.0) in the same six patients. One patient had an IVP of 3.5 mm Hg both before and after operation. He died 3 weeks later. At 24 h after evacuation, six patients presented good clinical improvement in spite of an intraventricular pressure at the preoperative level.

References

1. BECKER, D.P., YOUNG, H.F., VRIES, J.K., SAKALAS, R.: Monitoring in patients with brain tumors. Clin. Neurosurg. 22, 364-388 (1975).
2. LOEW, F., WÜSTNER, S.: Diagnose, Behandlung und Prognose der traumatischen Hämatome des Schädelinneren. Acta Neurochir. Suppl. 8 (1960).
3. LORENZO, A.V., PAGE, L.K., WATTERS, G.V.: Relationship between cerebrospinal fluid formation, absorption and pressure in human hydrocephalus. Brain 93, 679-692 (1970).
4. LUNDBERG, N.: Continuous recording and control of ventricular fluid pressure in neurosurgical pratice. Acta Psychiat. Neurol. Scand. Suppl. 149, 36 (1960).
5. McKISSOCK, W., RICHARDSON, A., BLOOM, W.H.: Subdural hematoma. A review of 389 cases. Lancet 1960 I, 1365-1370.
6. PLUM, F., POSNER, J.B.: Diagnosis of stupor and coma. Oxford: Blackwell Scientific Publications 1966.

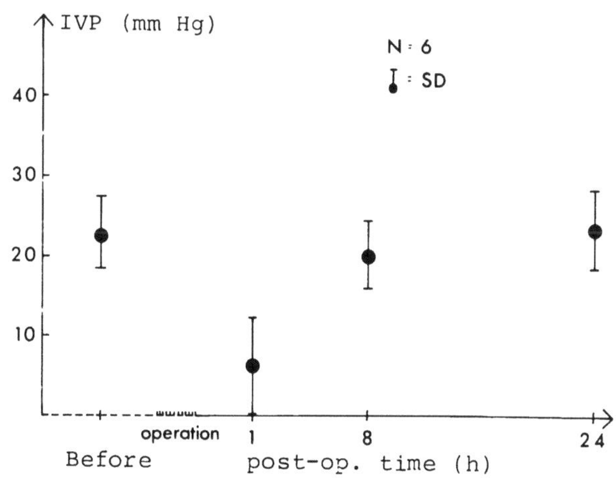

Fig. 1. Mean intraventricular pressure (mm Hg) in six patients before and after evacuation of chronic subdural hematoma

Intraventricular Isotope Encephalography and Continuous Intraventricular Pressure Recording in Patients Mentally Retarded Following Brain Injury

G. E. Cold and F. Jensen

Introduction

Since the first reports on normal pressure hydrocephalus (NPH) the interest in this treatable disease has resulted in many clinical studies. The difficulties in predicting the effect of a ventriculoatrial shunt on mental function by pneumoencephalography (PEG) or cisternography have led to the application of other diagnostic tools, including continuous intraventricular pressure (IVP) recording and the intralumbar infusion test. The value of these methods is still uncertain (2, 7, 11, 14). Since 1970, we have used intraventricular isotope encephalography (IIE) with ^{131}I albumin (5, 6). Simultaneously, we have recorded IVP continuously for a 24-h period and determined ventricular fluid Na^+, K^+, bicarbonate, lactate, pyruvate, protein, fractioned protein, pCO_2, pO_2, and pH.

The aim of the present investigation was to clarify the following questions: (1) Does IIE give valuable information concerning the effect of a ventriculoatrial shunt on mental function? (2) Does IVP on patients with abnormal IIE differ from that in patients with normal IIE, and is it possible to predict the effect of a shunt from the IVP recordings? (3) Will determination of electrolytes and metabolites in ventricular fluid give further information?

Material and Methods

A total of 29 mentallly retarded patients were examined 2-21 years after an acute brain injury. In 5 cases the primary brain injury was cerebral concussion; in the remaining 24 the diagnoses were cerebral contusion or laceration. Intraventricular isotope encephalography (IIE) was performed in all cases, applying 50 µCi ^{131}I albumin with an amount of albumin varying from 3 to 5 mg/ml. The isotope was injected through a frontal burr hole into the right lateral ventricle. Anteroposterior and lateral scintigrams were taken at 1, 3, 6, 24, and 48 h after the injection. The individual scintigrams were summed up to 15,000 counts and the time was recorded. The respective count rates were corrected for background radiation and physical decay. After the conclusion of the investigation, all count rates were calculated as percentages of the maximum count rate and plotted against time on semilogarithmic paper. IVP was continuously recorded by the method of LUNDBERG (8) with a STATHAM transducer P-37 or P-23 and a SERVIGOR recorder with a paper speed of 1-2 cm/min. The patients were in the straight supine position without a pillow. Mean pressure was recorded every hour and from this the mean pressure/day was calculated. In addition, the maximum pressure/min, peak pressure and maximum amplitude of 1-4 waves/min were determined every hour. The state of consciousnedd and periods of sleep were registered and so were involuntary movements and therapy. All patients had no premedication. Following the IVP recordings, but before IIE, about 10 ml ventricular fluid was withdrawn and its level of Na^+, K^+, bicarbonate, lactate, pyruvate, protein, frationd protein, pCO_2,

pO_2, and pH were determined. In all patients with whom intellectual contact was possible, psychologic tests by the method of WAIS were performed. Then, 6 months after the shunt operation the patients were retested.

Results

IIE revealed that 16 patients had communicating hydrocephalus and delayed albumin resorption. These patients received a ventriculoatrial shunt of the Pudenz type. A patient died 2 months after the operation, before psychologic re-testing was performed. Excellent improvement was noticed in 7 patients and some improvement in 2 while in 6 patients, including 2 with poorly functioning shunts, the condition was unchanged. Clinical improvement was thus seen in 9 of 13 patients with well-functioning shunts (69%).

The pressure levels in patients with or without prolonged resorption of ^{131}I albumin is shown on Table 1. Although the average pressure was higher in patients with prolonged resorption, the differences were not significant.

In comparison with patients without clinical improvement following the shunt operation, IVP levels in patients who improved were not significantly higher, but the differences in maximum amplitudes of 1-4 waves/min during periods of sleep and wakefulness were increased ($P<0.05$).

The results of ventricular fluid analysis are shown in Table 2. As indicated, Na^+ showed a significant difference ($P<0.05$). Ventricular fluid proteins, albumin, alpha, beta, and gamma fractions were significantly higher in patients with delayed resorption of ^{131}I albumin (Table 3).

Discussion

In a study od traumatic NPH from our clinic (1970) we found plateau-like waves in IVP during sleep (9). This observation was confirmed by SYMON et al. (14), while NORNES et al. did not find evidence suggesting that NPH patients have a higher-than-normal average IVP during sleep (11). In this study, transitory plateau waves were noticed in two patients during sleep. Both patients improved after shunt operation. Furthermore, a nonsignificant increase in the pressure level was found in patients with NPH, which is in accordance with the study of GRANHOLM & LÖFGREN (3).

The difference between maximum amplitudes during sleep and when awake was significantly increased in patients who improved clinically. This observation is consistent with the study of SYMON et al., who found episodic pressure waves in 9 of 16 patients during sleep (14). CHAWLA et al. also found that patients with rhythmical IVP oscillations discribed as B waves improved clinically after shunt operation (1). Recently MAIRA et al. have stated that pressure waves present during REM sleep and pulse synchronic oscillations in IVP are of importance in the pathogenesis of NPH (10).

While OJEMANN et al. found that the CSF protein was within the normal range (12), other investigators have reported increased CSF protein in NPH (4). In infants with communicating hydrocephalus. TVETEN found increased ventricular fluid protein (15). We found that total protein as well as fractionated protein were increased in patients with delayed resorption of ^{131}I albumin. It should be noted that precipitation of proteins in the drainage system can prevent CSF flow in the shunt (13). In two of our cases with poorly functioning shunts confirmed by IIE, CSF proteins were above 100 mg/100 ml. In one of these, transitory clinical improvement was observed after re-operation, but at the follow-up study 1 year later, the clinical state had deteriorated, and the shunt was not functioning. The average value of preoperative CSF proteins was 30.0 mg/100 ml in patients who improved mentally as against 35.8 mg/100 ml in patients who were unchanged. One reason for this could be precipitation of protein in the shunt system.

Table 1. IVP levels and maximum amplitudes of 1-4 waves/min in patients with or without delayed resorption of ^{131}I albumin

		Mean pressure/ day, mm Hg	Maximum pressure/ min mm Hg		Peak pressure mm Hg		Maximum amplitude, mm Hg	
			Sleep	Awake	Sleep	Awake	Sleep	Awake
Patients with normal resorption of ^{131}I albumin, 13 patients	Mean	8.8	16.7	12.8	24.3	17.2	10.7	4.9
	Range	4-17	7-25	5-20	13-40	9-25	3-27	3-13
	SD	3.3	5.1	3.6	8.1	4.1	6.8	2.6
Patients with prolonged resorption of ^{131}I albumin, 16 patients	Mean	10.1	17.3	14.5	24.8	19.8	9.1	5.6
	Range	4-20	9-44	8-25	12-55	11-30	4-25	2-17
	SD	4.2	8.8	4.9	10.9	6.2	5.5	4.3
Statistical analysis	Mann Whitney	P<0.2	P<0.2	P<0.2	P<0.2	P<0.2	P<0.2	P<0.2

Table 2. Ventricular fluid lacatate, pyruvate, L/P ratio, Na^+, K^+, bicarbonate, pO_2, pCO_2, and pH in patients with or without delayed resorption of intraventricular ^{131}I albumin

		Lactate, mmol/l	Pyruvate, mmol/l	L/P ratio	Na^+, Meg/l	K^+, Meg/l	Bicarbonate, Meg/l	pCO_2, mm Hg	pO_2, mm Hg	pH
Patients with normal resorption of ^{131}I albumin	Mean	2.3	0.15	16.1	148.8	2.55	21.6	49.5	56.5	7.302
	Range	1.7-3.6	0.11-0.21	10-29	146-156	2.2-2.9	19-24	37-63	40-67	7.23-7.39
	SD	0.85	0.039	5.26	2.86	0.197	1.43	8.4	10.5	0.053
Patients with prolonged resorption of ^{131}I albumin	Mean	3.1	0.14	24.3	145.4	2.46	21.1	46.1	53.9	7.299
	Range	1.8-7.4	0.06-0.42	10-40	139-150	2.2-2.8	18-29	35-65	28-81	7.25-7.34
	SD	1.98	0.127	13.7	3.32	0.219	4.31	10.9	17.0	0.033
Total number of observations		18	17	17	20	20	19	19	17	20
Statistical analysis	Mann Whitney	P>0.2	P>0.1	P>0.2	P<0.05	P>0.2	P>0.2	P>0.2	P>0.2	P>0.2

Table 3. Ventricular fluid proteins in patients with or without delayed resorption of intraventricular ^{131}I albumin

		Total protein mg/ 100 ml	Pre-albumin mg/ 100 ml	Al-bumin mg/ 100 ml	Alpha fraction mg/ 100 ml	Beta fraction mg/ 100 ml	Gamma fraction mg/ 100 ml
Patients with normal resorption of ^{131}I albumin	Mean	18.9	1.24	9.31	1.78	3.28	3.56
	Range	7-36	0.6-2.9	4.1-15.8	0.6-3.5	1.0-6.2	0.4-17.7
	SD	7.73	0.72	3.70	0.99	2.51	5.90
Patients with prolonged re-sorption of ^{131}I albumin	Mean	34.0	2.04	19.5	4.63	5.91	5.53
	Range	19-55	0-9-3.4	10.2-34.4	1.7-7.3	2.9-10.4	2.2-17.3
	SD	10.2	0.84	6.93	1.78	2.85	4.87
Total number of observations		27	16	16	16	16	16
Statistical analysis	Mann Whit-ney	P<0.002	P>0.1	P<0.002	P=0.002	P<0.05	P<0.05

References

1. CHAWLA, J.C., HULME, A., COOPER, R.: Intracranial pressure in patients with dementia and communicating hydrocephalus. J. Neurosurg. 40, 376-380 (1974).

2. COBLENZ, J.M., MATTIS, S., ZINGESSER, L.H., KASOFF, S.S., WISNIEWSKI, H.M., KATZMAN, R.: Presenile dementia. Arch. Neurol. 29, 299-308 (1973).

3. GRANHOLM, L., LÖFGREN, J.: A discussion on the intracranial pressure-volume relationship in normal pressure hydrocephalus. In: Intracranial Pressure II (N. LUNDBERG, U. PONTEN, M. BROCK, eds.), pp. 137-140. Berlin-Heidelberg- New York: Springer 1975.

4. HILL, M.E., LOUGHEED, W.M., BARNETT, H.J.M.: A treatable form of dementia due to normal-pressure, communicating hydrocephalus. Canad. Med. Ass. J. 97, 1309-1320 (1967).

5. JENSEN, F., MALMROS, R., HVID HANSEN, H.: Isotope encephalography in low pressure hydrocephalus. Proc. 19th Congress of Scand. Neurol. Acta Neurol. Scand. Suppl. 46, 93 (1970).

6. JENSEN, F., MALMROS, R., HVID HANSEN, H., COLD, G.E.: Intraventricular isotope encephalography. Dan. Med. Bull., in press.

7. KATZMAN, R., HUSSEY, F.: A simple constant-infusion manometric test for measurement of CSF absorption. Neurol. 20, 534-544 (1970).

8. LUNDBERG, N.: Continuous recording and control of ventricular fluid pressure in neurosurgical practive. Acta Psychiat. Scand. Suppl. 149 (1960).

9. MALMROS, R.: Commun. 19th Congr. Scand. Neurol., Aarhus 1970.

10. MAIRA, G., ROSSI, G.F., VIGNATI, A.: Intracranial pressure and pathogenesis of "normotensive" hydrocephalus. In: Intracranial Pressure II (N. LUNDBERG, U. PONTEN, M. BROCK, eds.), pp. 128-132. Berlin-Heidelberg-New York: Springer 1975.

11. NORNES, H., ROOTWELT, K., SJAASTAD, O.: Normal pressure hydrocephalus, long-term intracranial pressure recording. Europ. Neurol. 9, 261-274 (1973).

12. OJEMANN, R.G., FISHER, C.M., ADAMS, D., SWEET, W.H., NEW, P.F.J.: Further experience with the syndrome of "normal" pressure hydrocephalus. J. Neurosurg. 31, 279-294 (1969).

13. STEINKE, H.J.: Funktionstechnik und Komplikationsursachen bei ventrikulo-atrialen Shunts. Zbl. Neurochir. 29, 203-215 (1968).

14. SYMON, L., DORSCH, N.W.C., STEPHENS, R.J.: Long-term measurement of extradural pressure in "low pressure" hydrocephalus. In: Intracranial Pressure (M. BROCK, H. DIETZ, eds.), pp. 280-286. Berlin-Heidelberg-New York: Springer 1972.

15. TVETEN, L.: Cerebrospinal fluid proteins in obstructive lesions of the central nervous system. Acta Neurol. Scand. 41, 80-91 (1969).

Summary

T.W. Langfitt and H. Nornes

The principal differences in the findings of CROCKARD et al. and DJORDJEVIC et al. in animals subjected to missile injuries were a decrease in blood pressure in the former and a marked increase in blood pressure in the latter experiments, as well as a significant difference in the degree of intracranial hypertension observed. These differences appear to be explained by the amount of intracranial hemorrhage in the two experimental designs. In the studies of DJORDJEVIC et al., ICP rose to values of 300 torr or more, due apparently to immediate intracranial hemorrhage, and the arterial hypertension undoubtedly represented a vasopressor response. Little hemorrhage was seen along the missile track in the experiments of CROCKARD et al., but the ICP did increease to 60 torr or more. Cerebrovascular resistance was decreased initially; therefore, the rise in ICP probably was due to acute vascular dilatation. The immediate bradycardia observed in the experiments could be explained by brain stem distortion or displacement at the moment of the injury. Both arterial hypotension and hypertension have been observed in experimental closed-head injury, but the reason for the difference, according to the experimental model used, has not been adequately explained.

In the clinical studies of GJERRIS and of COLD and JENSEN, emphasis was placed on defective resorption of CSF in chronic head injury problems. GJERRIS demonstrated that the neurologic signs in a series of patients with chronic subdural hematomas were due to the hematoma and not to the mild intracranial hypertension that the patients had prior to surgery, since the patients remained improved following evacuation of their hematomas even though ICP returned to preoperative levels. In mentally retarded patients examined several years after acute brain injury, COLD and JENSEN found that those patients with pressure waves had a better clinical response to ventriculoatrial shunt than those patients who did not demonstrate pressure waves during the preoperative evaluation. These studies add to the ever increasing evidence that disturbances in CSF circulation are very common in head-injured patients. Serial computerized axial tomograms will provide more information on the time course of the alterations in CSF dynamics and, therefore, a better understanding of the clinical significance of posttraumatic hydrocephalus.

Session D

Trauma II

Chairman: M. Brock
Co-chairman: D. P. Becker

The Critical Importance of ICP Monitoring in Head Injury[1]

D. P. Becker, J. D. Miller, H. F. Young, J. D. Ward, and W. E. Adams

Introduction

The technical feasibility of continuous ICP monitoring is no longer in doubt and the risks are established. Guide lines for the clinical use of ICP monitoring have been laid down (2, 3) and several authors have cited their experience (1, 4, 5, 6). Despite this, many neurosurgeons still wish to know whether the yield of information from ICP measurement in patients with head injury is worth the expenditure in time, personnel, resources, and risk. It has been the policy at the Medical College of Virginia to incorporate early and continuous ICP measurement into the management of all patients with severe brain trauma. This paper is an endeavor to answer the question "Is ICP monitoring worth while as part of routine head injury management?".

Patients and Methods

Data is based on records of 150 comatose patients with blunt head injury seen at MCV Hospital between January 1973 and March 1976, who on admission were unable to obey commands, or worse. A rigid protocol has been followed. A right frontal twist drill hole was made in the hospital emergency room and intraventricular pressure measured as soon as stable airway and hemodynamic conditions had been obtained. Limited air ventriculography was then performed and all patients with 5 mm or more midline shift were taken directly to the operating room for wide craniotomy and removal of mass. Patients without shift but who had high ICP were directed to EMI Scan or angiography to seek bilateral lesions. Patients with no shift and normal pressure were admitted directly to the intensive care unit to be joined by the patients who had had surgical decompression. All patients in the ICU were ventilated at moderate hypocapnia (25-30 mm Hg) with further treatment of raised ICP by ventricular drainage and intravenous mannitol as required. In the early neurologic assessment two features have been emphasized, the oculocephalic response, classified as intact or impaired (including absent) and the motor response to painful stimuli, distinguishing as "posturing", "decerebrate", or "decorticate" responses. Outcome has been classified into five categories, ranging from excellent to dead.

Results

In the series of 150 patients, 59 had mass lesions requiring surgery (acute subdural and epidural hematomas and large temporal contusions often with intracerebral hematoma); all but one of these patients had increased ICP on admission and in most cases pressure was over 30 mm

[1] Supported by NHI Grant No. 1PO1 NS-12587-01A1 NSP-A.

Table 1. Admission ICP, mortality rate, and cause of death in patients in different diagnostic categories

	Admission ICP mm Hg			TOTAL No.	Cause of death		
	0-10	11-30	>30		Deaths (%)	Due to ↑ICP	Medical Cause
Acute subdural hematoma	0	6	20	26	13 (50%)	6	7
Acute epidural hematoma	0	4	6	10	1 (10%)	1	0
Cerebral mass contusion/ hematoma	1	16	6	23	9 (39%)	7	2
Diffuse injury shift < 4 mm	27	53	11	91	21 (23%)	8	13
Totals	28	79	43	150	44 (29%)	22	22

Hg (Table 1). Of the 91 patients without significant shift, 28 had normal ICP on admission. There was a significant association between mass lesions and increased ICP (X^2 18.45:P < 0.001).

There were 44 (29%) patients who died, half from raised ICP which could not be controlled and half from medical complications, e.g., pneumonia. The mortality rate in all patients with mass lesions (39%) was higher than the 23% mortality in patients with diffuse injury (X^2 4.37; P < 0.05), but there was no overall difference in outcome in the two groups; 54% of patients with mass lesions treated surgically ended in the "excellent" to "good" categories, versus 57% of those with diffuse injury. Of those patients with mass lesions who died, however, 61% did so because of uncontrolled intracranial hypertension compared with 38% of those who died from diffuse injuries.

In predicting the outcome of those patients with intracranial mass lesions, in whom ICP was almost invariably raised, the oculocephalic and motor responses were crucial. Thus 86% of patients with intact oculocephalic responses and no posturing ended up with excellent or good results while 80% of those with posturing and impaired oculocephalics finished as poor, vegetative, or dead (Table 2).

Table 2. Outcome related to motor and oculocephalic responses in groups of patients with mass lesions and with diffuse injuries with normal and with increased ICP. Knowledge of initial ICP, status of posturing, and integrity of OC reflexes provides strong predictive power

	Outcome from head injury					
	Excellent/good		Poor/vegetative		Dead	
Mass lesion (increased ICP)	19	2	1	1	2	3
	6	5	0	1	0	19
Diffuse injury with normal ICP	17	0	1	0	0	0
	4	0	0	3	0	2
Diffuse injury with increased ICP	28	3	0	0	1	0
	0	0	7	7	5	13

Key:		
	No posturing - OC intact	No posturing - OC impaired
	Posturing - OC intact	Posturing - OC impaired

In the 91 patients without shift, ICP was important in determining outcome - thus 78% of patients with low ICP ended up "excellent" and "good" while only 48% of those with elevated pressure at any level over 10 mm Hg finished in these categories ($X^2=6.67; P < 0.01$). Of those diffuse injuries with elevated ICP, all patients with posturing finished in the poor, vegetative, or dead categories and all but one with normal motor responses were "excellent" or "good". The oculocephalic response added little more information in this group. In the patients with diffuse injury and normal ICP, on the other hand, the oculocephalic response was important, impairment plus posturing indicating a uniformly bad outlook, while the four patients who had posturing but intact oculocephalics on admission all had excellent or good outcomes.

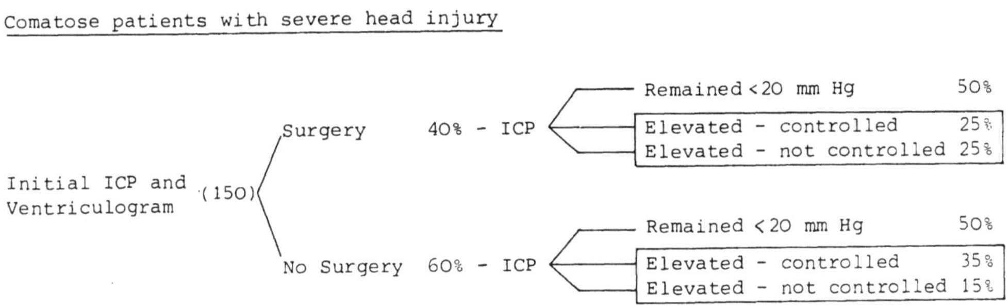

Fig. 1. Status of ICP during management of 150 patients with severe head injury

Increased ICP was also of considerable importance during the management of the 150 patients (Fig. 1). In only half of the 59 patients submitted to surgical decompression followed by artificial ventilation did ICP stay below 20 mm Hg; in the other half of the group ICP remained high or rose again and was controlled spontaneously or by ventricular drainage or mannitol in 25%; ICP was not controllable by these methods in a further 25%, progressing to death from intracranial hypertension. Intracranial hypertension was no less a problem in the patients with diffuse injury. In half of these patients also, artificial ventilation alone was insufficient to hold ICP below 20 mm Hg. The increased pressure was, however, controlled in most cases spontaneously or by further decrease in $PaCO_2$, ventricular drainage, or intravenous mannitol.

Discussion

The aim of the management protocol we have described is to detect and evacuate intracranial mass lesions before clinical signs of brain herniation and severe intracranial hypertension have appeared. ICP monitoring is used to detect brain swelling or other secondary processes prior to clinical deterioration and the results of treatment can be effectively monitored. How successful this regimen will be in improving the overall outcome of patients with severe head injury remains to be determined. What is already evident, however, is the frequency with which ICP monitoring provides important information which is unobtainable by other means.

The 75% incidence of increased ICP on admission, the relationship between intracranial hypertension and mortality, the value of ICP in prognosis, and the fact that 50% of the patients who die from severe head injury do so from uncontrollable intracranial hypertension all bear eloquent testimony to the value of ICP monitoring in head injury. Perhaps the most important finding to emerge, however, is that even after early and adequate decompression and correction of blood gas abnormalities, 50% of patients had recurrence or persistence of intracranial hypertension, which might not have been detected in some patients until brain herniation or cerebral ischemia had been produced.

We would submit, therefore, that the answer to this question "Is ICP monitoring in head injury worthwhile?" must be an emphatic "yes".

References

1. BECKER, D.P., VRIES, J.K., YOUNG, H.F., WARD, J.D.: Controlled cerebral perfusion pressure and ventilation in human mechanical brain injury: prevention of progressive brain swelling. In: Intracranial Pressure II (N. LUNDBERG, U. PONTEN, and M. BROCK, eds.), pp. 480-484. Berlin-Heidelberg-New York: Springer 1975.
2. JOHNSTON, I.H.: Intracranial pressure changes after head injury. In: Handbook of Neurology, Vol. 24, Part 1, Chapter 9 (R. BRAAKMAN, ed.), pp. 199-222. Amsterdam: North Holland 1975.
3. JOHNSTON, I.H., JENNETT, B.: The place of continuous intracranial pressure monitoring in neurosurgical practice. Acta Neurochir. (Wien) 29, 53-63 (1973).
4. LUNDBERG, N., TROUPP, H., LORIN, H.: Continuous recording of the ventricular fluid pressure in patients with severe acute traumatic brain injury. J. Neurosurg. 22, 581-590 (1965).
5. ROSSANDA, M., COLLICE, M., PORTA, M., BOSELLI, L.: Intracranial hypertension in head injury, clinical significance and relation to respiration. In: Intracranial Pressure II (N. LUNDBERG, U. PONTEN, and M. BROCK, eds.), pp. 475-479. Berlin-Heidelberg-New York: Springer 1975.
6. VAPALAHTI, M., TROUPP, H.: Prognosis for patients with severe brain injuries. Brit. Med. J. 3, 404-407 (1971).

Management of Head Injury by Means of Ventricular Fluid Pressure Monitoring

M. Collice, M. Rossanda, A. Beduschi, and M. Porta

Introduction

The aim of this paper is to summarize the most significant results of our experience with ventricular fluid pressure (VFP) monitoring in acute head injury.
The following has been analyzed: (1) intracranial pressure (ICP), clinical syndromes and outcome; (2) time of first appearance of intracranial hypertension; (3) plateau wave (PW) occurrence; (4) ICP and space-occupying lesions (SOL); (5) results of different treatments.

Materials and Methods

There were 73 patients aged 1 to 71 years with severe brain injuries studied. Out of 73 patients, 22 underwent surgery for different kinds of SOL. At the admission time or before surgery they were all unconscious: 48 did not show any sign of midbrain dysfunction (MBD), 25 showed some signs of MBD (usually bilateral decerebrate rigidity and/or disconjugate or absent oculocephalic reflex).
Using LUNDBERG's method (6) all were VFP monitored, most of them in the first 24-48 h from the onset of coma or after surgery. Recording was continued for 5-7 days when coma persisted. Out of 22 surgery patients, 18 were monitored in the postoperative period exclusively, 4 in both the preoperative and postoperative period.
Standard treatment (long-term hyperventilation (HV), intravenous Dexamethasone) and additional treatment (osmotics, barbiturates, CSF drainage) are reported in Table 1.

Results

ICP and Clinical Syndromes. Out of 73 patients, 32 developed high ICP (HICP). Table 2 shows the distribution of the patients in three pressure groups.
In the 51 nonoperated patients, HICP was not related to the clinical state on admission (HICP incidence between the two clinical syndromes is not significantly different).

In the 22 postoperative recordings, HICP appeared almost exclusively in the patients showing preoperative MBD signs.
A significant difference between the HICP incidence in the two clinical preoperative syndromes was disclosed (x : 602 P : < 0.001).
A correlation between the increasing pressure and a worsening condition was observed in 22 out of 32 patients. The remaining 10 cases did not show neurologic deterioration, not even after several hours or days of HICP.

Time of First Appearance of HICP. Out of 46 patients subjected to early and prolonged VFP monitoring, 26 showed HICP: 14 in the first 3 days, 12 after the 3rd day (usually on the fifth).

Table 1. Standard and additional treatment in the 73 cases studied

Standard treatment (73 cases)

- hyperoxic long-term hyperventilation ($paCO_2$-25-30 mm Hg)
- LV. dexamethasone (24 mg/day in adults) for the first 10 days. When coma persisted

Additional treatment (25 out of 32 cases with HICP)

- Osmotics (mannitol and/or Glycerol) 21 cases
  54 20% mannitol infusions (3.5-7 ml/kg) in
  15 cases (most cases 4 infusions (range 2-9)
  107 10% glycerol infusions (3.5-7 ml/kg) in
  14 cases (most cases 7 infusions (range 5-25)
- Thiopental (normal temperature) 9 of the above 21 cases
  43 injections (0.25-0.5 g) in 9 cases
  (most cases 4 injections (range 2-12)
- Repeated CSF withdrawals 8 of the above 21 cases
- Continuous CSF drainage
  (for 12, 20, 50, and 70 h respectively)
- (Moreover 2 patients of the osmotics group and 2 cases of the osmotic plus thiopental group were subjected to surgical decompression)

Table 2. Initial or pre-operative syndromes and VFP (highest value of base line) in 73 cases of severe brain injuries. For the 22 operated cases only post-operative recordings were considered

VFP mm Hg	Not operated Without MBD	With MBD	Operated Without MBD	With MBD	Total
0-15	19	7	12	3	41
16-45	10	3	1	3	17
> 45	6	6	0	3	15
Total	35	16	13	9	73

Plateau Wave Occurrence. Tracings obtained from 48 patients for a total of 215 days of recording were reviewed and 94 PW in 13 cases were found (one case showed 54 PW, most cases showed 2 PW). Out of these 13 cases 4 showed PW starting from a low base line (10-15 mm Hg). In two cases they appeared at the end of the HICP period. All but the last two cases developed actual HICP afterward. No relation between PW and clinical status was disclosed (7 out of 13 cases showed MBD signs when PW occurred).

ICP and SOL. Six recordings were obtained in the presence of a SOL. The following were the highest ICP values: 15-20-20-40-60 mm Hg. HICP appeared in two cases 1 and 5 days before focal signs, respectively.
In two cases PW preceded actual HICP. Four out of six cases were operated upon, and three recovered, the remaining two cases were treated without surgery and both recovered (patients with temporal edema and VFP 15-20 mm Hg).

ICP and Outcome. As shown in Figure 1, 29 of 73 patients (or 39%) died in coma; 21 of them showed HICP. Mortality rate in all patients with HICP (65%) was significantly higher than in the normal ICP group (19%) (x : 14.1 P : < 0.001). When clinical syndromes are considered separately, mortality rate in HICP groups is significantly higher only in the patients with MBD signs in comparison to that in the normal ICP group (x : 6.51 P : < 0.05).
When age was taken in consideration, a significant relationship between mortality rate and HICP was found only in the patients in the 16-46 years age group (see Table 3).

Table 3. Age groups, VFP (highest values of base line) and final outcome in 73 cases of severe brain injuries. Number of dead in brackets. (In 22 operated cases only post-operative recordings were considered

	VFP (mm Hg)			
Years	0-15	16-45	>45	Total
1-8	4 (0)	1 (0)	2 (0)	7 (0)
9-15	6 (3)	2 (1)	4 (4)	12 (8)
16-45	28 (5)	14 (7)	9 (9)	51 (21)
46-71	3 (0)	-	-	3 (0)
Total	41 (8)	17 (8)	15 (13)	73 (29)

Effect of Osmotics, Thiopental, and CSF Withdrawals on ICP. As shown in Figure 2, both mannitol and glycerol usually decreased ICP to 50% of the pretreatment level in 30 min. The decompressive action of the 3.5 ml/kg dose of both usually lasted from 2 to 3 h. The decompressive action of the 7 ml/kg dose of mannitol usually lasted from 5 to 6 h, while that of glycerol lasted from 3 to 4 h. A rebound effect following both osmotics was observed in a few cases.
Thiopental usually caused a sudden drop of ICP that promptly returned to approx. 70% of the pretreatment level within 30 min and usually did not rise again for 45 to 120 min.
HICP was controlled in 15 out of 21 cases that received osmotics or osmotics plus thiopental; 6 out of these 15 patients died in spite of the HICP control.
The duration of the decompressive action of different CSF volume withdrawals (1 to 14 ml) lasted from 15 min to 3 h (average 90 min).

The effect does not seem to be related to the pretreatment ICP level nor to the clinical picture. Figure 3 shows four examples of CSF withdrawals in four different cases.

Outcome of the Patients with HICP Related to Different Treatment. Figure 4 shows four treatment groups: osmotic, osmotic plus thiopental, CSF drainage, and HV with dexamethasone only. Recovery rate was 66%, 22%, 0%, and 14%, respectively. Recovery rate in the first, second, and fourth groups is significantly different according to RAYN's procedure for multiple comparisons.

Side Effects of Osmotic and Barbiturate Therapy. No side effects were observed in any patient. In two cases we had to interrupt osmotic therapy because of critically high serum osmolality.

Discussion

Usefulness of ICP Monitoring. Our data confirm the usefulness of ICP monitoring in both *diagnosis* and *treatment* (4, 6).

We would like to underline only two points: (1) PW as well as pre-PW (10) should be considered as extremely useful warning signs even though not very indicative as to the type of lesion that supports the future hypertensive state (2 of the 6 patients with SOL and 11 of the 42 without SOL showed PW); (2) the technique can sometimes avoid an unnecessary operation (twice in this series) in the sense that the compensatory reserve of the patient can be kept under continuous control (7).

As for the *prognostic value*, our data are not comparable to those of JOHNSTON (5) or those of VAPALAHTI (11), but seem to confirm de ROUGEMONT's (3) experience in the sence of a bad prognostic value of HICP in the presence of MBD signs. Moreover, children under 8 have tolerated HICP better than the other age groups, thus confirming the well-known age factor in prognosis.

Result of Treatment

Hyperventilation - Osmotics. The role of long-term HV in respect to ICP, as previously reported (2, 8) and also according to COLD (1) is confirmed by the relatively low incidence of HICP and especially of the severe HICP. Moreover, this may partially explain the good results obtained with the use of the osmotics. In fact, in the majority of cases, it has been sufficient to use moderate doses of mannitol or glycerol. The possible role of HV in delaying the appearance of HICP has not yet been clarified.
There is no doubt, however, that a final judgment about HV can only be reached by a comparison of the mortality rate, if it is taken as a criterion, in more numerous series. According to the clinical results, the absence of vegetative survival in this series seems particularly encouraging (only four patients had shown a "transition syndrome" before they died after 45 to 130 days from the injury).

The repeated *CSF withdrawals* have usually represented an emergency measure rather than chronic treatment. From the point of view of ICP the same observation should be made about thiopental. On the other hand, its action may not be exclusively on ICP (9). Anyhow, it has not improved the survival rate in this short series.

Continuous CSF drainage does not seem to be a useful method of treatment, at least in the head injury cases subjected to HV. Besides the final results (four dead out of four patients treated), all the patients showed during drainage a definite neurologic deterioration without any possibility of knowing the pressure level.

A conclusion about *surgical decompression* would be premature (two patients out of four treated died and none of them showed HICP after surgery). It is our impression that better results could be obtained if decompression were put into practice earlier, before other treatments had become completely ineffective, even though the clinical picture is still not dramatic.
In conclusion, the following lines of management arise from the use of VFP monitoring:

1. In patients needing surgery and showing MBD signs, VFP monitoring should be done after the removal of SOL, and bone decompression taken in consideration.
2. In patients without SOL, VFP monitoring should be done in all cases that remain unconscious after 24-48 h.
3. It should be continued for 5-7 days when coma persists.

4. New investigations for SOL should be performed when HICP or PW appear.
5. If the HICP is not maintained by SOL after having tested the effect of CSF withdrawals, these should be repeated or osmotic therapy should be applied.
6. In emergency situations, thiopental can be used.
7. In patients with MBD and HICP, the prognosis is so poor, except in children under 8, that any heroic measure could be considered.

Summary

A total of 73 patients with severe brain injuries, all unconscious and hyperventilated were studied by means of VFP monitoring. ICP and clinical syndromes, time of first appearance of HICP, PW occurrence, ICP clinical syndromes, and outcome were analyzed. For patients with HICP, final outcome was related to different treatments (osmotics, thiopental, CSF drainage, HV only). The data have been discussed from three points of view: usefulness of ICP monitoring, results of treatment, indications for a more correct management.

References

1. COLD, G., ENDEVOLDSEN, E., MALMROS, R.: The prognostic values of continuous intraventricular pressure recording in unconscious brain-injury patients under controlled ventilation. In: Intracranial Pressure II (N. LUNDBERG, U. PONTEN, M. BROCK, eds.), pp. 517-521. Berlin-Heidelberg-New York: Springer 1975.

2. COLLICE, M., PORTA, M., BOSELLI, L., ROSSANDA, M.: Enregistrements continus de la pression ventriculaire dans les traumatismes craniens graves. Neurochirurgie 7, 617-622 (1974).

3. de ROUGEMONT, J., BARGE, M., BENAIBID, A.L.: L'enregistrement de la pression intra-cranienne dans la surveillance des traumatismes craniens en période aigüe. Observation sur nos premiers résultats. Neurochirurgie 19, 125-134 (1973).

4. JENNETT, B., JOHNSTON, H.J.: The uses of intracranial pressure monitoring in clinical management. In: Intracranial Pressure (M. BROCK, H. DIETZ, eds.), pp. 365-368. Berlin-Heidelberg-New York: Springer 1972.

5. JOHNSTON, H.J., JOHNSTON, J.A., JENNETT, B.: Intracranial pressure changes following head injury. Lancet 1970 II, 433-436.

6. LUNDBERG, N.: Continuous recording and control of ventricular fluid pressure in neurosurgical practice. Acta Psych. Scand. 36, Suppl. 149 (1960).

7. MILLER, J.D.: Studies of intracranial pressure and volume in patients with head injury. J. Neurosurg. Sci. 17, 217-223 (1973).

8. ROSSANDA, M., COLLICE, M., PORTA, M., BOSELLI, L.: Intracranial hypertension in head injury. Clinical significance and relation to respiration. In: Intracranial Pressure II (N. LUNDBERG, U. PONTEN, M. BROCK, eds.), pp. 475-479. Berlin-Heidelberg-New York: Springer 1975.

9. SHAPIRO, H.M., WYTE, S.R., LOESER, J.: Barbiturate-augmented hypothermia for reduction of persistent intracranial hypertension. J. Neurosurg. 40, 90-100 (1974).

10. TINDALL, G.T., McGRAW, C.P., VANDERVEER, R.W., IWATA, K.: Cardio-respiratory changes associated with plateau waves in patients with head injury. In: Intracranial Pressure (M. BROCK, H. DIETZ, eds.), pp. 227-231. Berlin-Heidelberg-New York: Springer 1972.

11. VAPALAHTI, M., TROUPP, H. Prognosis for patients with severe brain injuries. Brit. med. J. 3, 404-407 (1971).

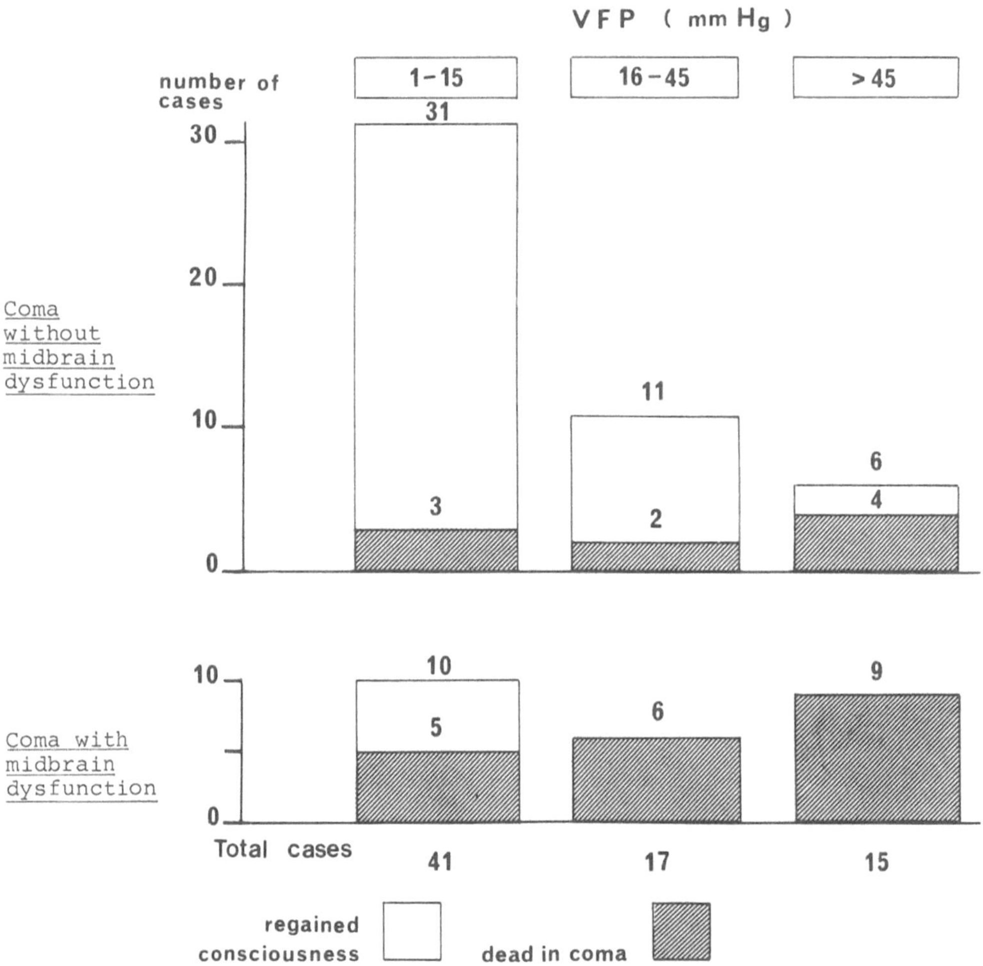

Fig. 1. Initial or preoperative syndromes, VFP (highest values of base line) and outcome in all 73 patients studied (for the 22 operated cases only postoperative recordings were considered). Moreover, six patients who fully regained consciousness died in a late stage from extracerebral complications; four patients died 45 to 130 days subsequent to the injury, after having regained wakefulness but no consciousness

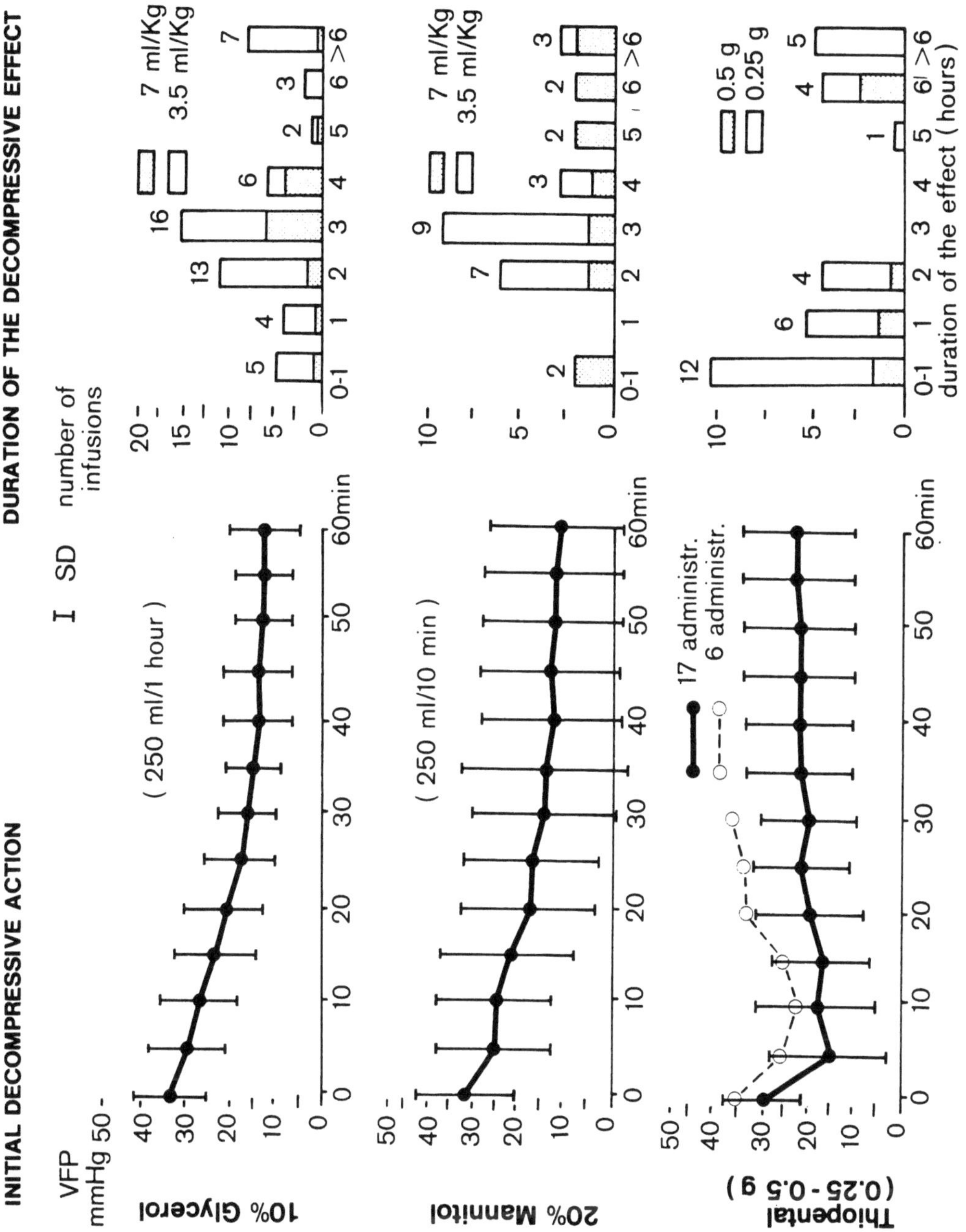

Fig. 2. Effect of 10% glycerol, 20% mannitol, and thiopental on VFP. Only tracings without interruptions or artefacts were considered: that is 56 glycerol infusions in 9 cases and 28 mannitol infusions in 8 cases for both initial decompressive action and duration of decompressive effect; 32 thiopental injections in 9 cases for duration of effect, and 23 injections in 9 cases for initial action (moreover, 6 out of 23 thiopental injections were analyzed separately because after their administration ICP returned at pretreatment level in 30 min and at this time a new dose was used)

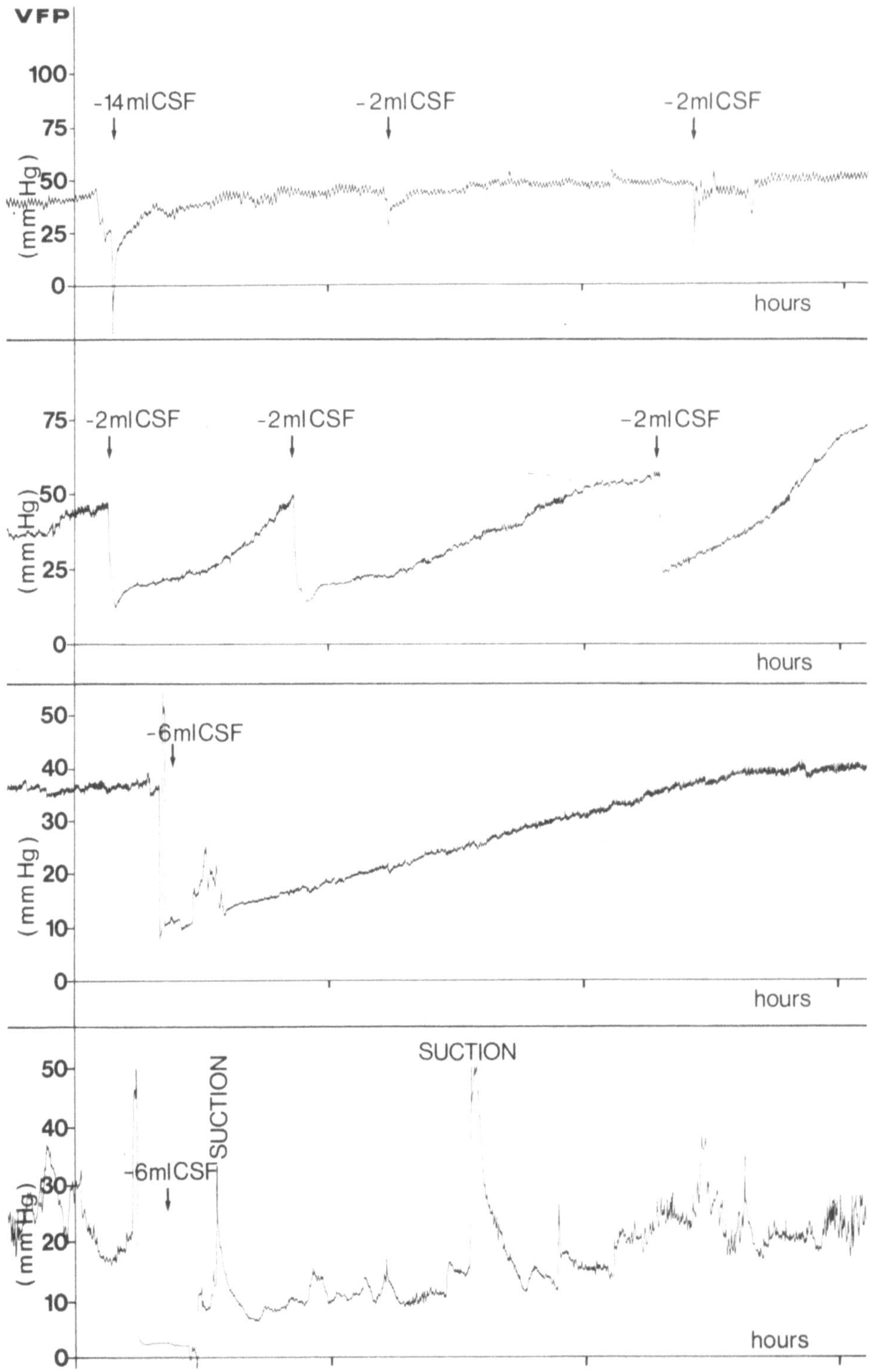
VFP
100
75
50
25
0
(mm Hg)
-14ml CSF
-2ml CSF
-2ml CSF
hours
75
50
25
0
(mm Hg)
-2ml CSF
-2ml CSF
-2ml CSF
hours
50
40
30
20
10
0
(mm Hg)
-6ml CSF
hours
50
40
30
20
10
0
(mm Hg)
-6ml CSF
SUCTION
SUCTION
hours

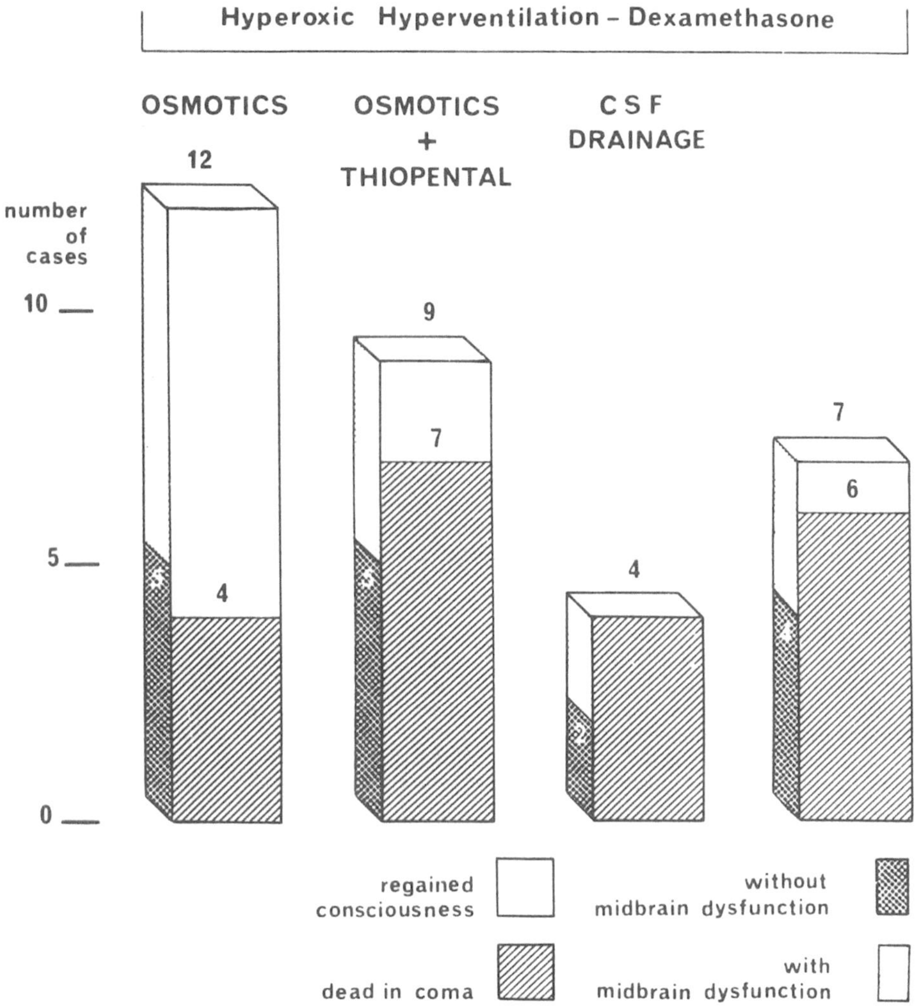

Fig. 4. Final outcome related to therapy in 32 cases with HICP

◁ Fig. 3. Effect of CSF withdrawals on VFP in four cases with HICP

Intracranial Pressure Monitoring in Intensive Care Patients Suffering from Acute Head Injuries

I. Papo and G. Caruselli

Introduction

We have reviewed a relatively homogenous group of patients with severe head injuries on intensive care, almost all of them undergoing early and long-term respirator treatment. Our aim was to try to make an overall assessment of the practical value of long-term intracranial pressure (ICP) monitoring as a guide to management. We have also tried to ascertain whether ICP recording alone or correlated to clinical examination could provide some reliable data for prognosis. In our study we have not considered ICP in untreated patients (admission pressure).

Material and Methods

ICP was monitored in 72 comatose patients suffering from severe head injuries. Of these 14 patients were operated upon but they remained in a coma state after the operation and 43 patients exhibited bilateral decorticate or decerebrate posturing. Oculo-vestibular reflexes were tested serially in 22 patients. When ICP recording was started 71 patients had already been intubated. In 40 patients ICP recording started on the 1st day after the injury, only in five patients ICP recording started after the 3rd day. The time of recording ranged from a few hours to 34 days (average 6.5 days). ICP was monitored until the patients improved definitely with stable base line, or died. In 63 patients ICP was measured with LUNDBERG's conventional intraventricular technique, in 9 patients ICP was measured only in the upper spinal space (C1-C2) approached anterolaterally. The patients were classified in three groups according to the values of mean ICP: I. patients with ICP below 20 mm Hg; II. patients with ICP ranging from 20 to 50 mm Hg; III. patients with ICP exceeding 50 mm Hg. Early and long-term respirator treatment was undertaken in 67 patients. The volumes of ventilation ranged from 10 to 15 l/m (40% O_2) in adults. $paCO_2$ was kept between 20 and 30 torr and arterial pH between 7.45 and 7.55. In 36 patients, 10% glycerol in saline was given. In 26 patients different amounts of cerebrospinal fluid (CSF) were withdrawn. In 6 patients a continuous CSF drainage was instituted, eventually 3 of them underwent permanent shunt procedures.

Results

As far as prognosis is concerned, no correlation whatsoever was found between ICP values and outcome (Table 1), when ICP did not exceed 50 mm Hg. All the patients with sustained pressure above 50 mm Hg died. In all of them autoregulation was lost, ICP following systemic arterial pressure (SAP) passively. When decerebrate posturing and age are also taken into account (Tables 2 and 3), we observed that posturing with pressure above normal values appears to have a definitely bad prognostic significance, but all the patients over 40 years with decerebrate

Table 1. ICP values and outcome: 72 patients

ICP values	Recovered	Severely disabled	Vegetative survival	Dead
0-20 mm Hg (24 patients)	4	3	-	17
20-50 mm Hg (49 patients)	9	5	2	33
50 mm Hg (9 patients)	-	-	-	9

Table 2. ICP, decerebrate posturing, and outcome: 63 patients

ICP values	Alive	Vegetative survival	Dead
0-20 mm Hg			
Posturing (12 patients)	3		9
No posturing (12 patients)	3		9
20-50 mm Hg			
Posturing (24 patients)	5	2	15
No posturing (17 patients)	10		7

Table 3. Age, ICP values, decerebrate posturing, and outcome: 72 patients

Age	ICP	Posturing	Alive	Vegetative survival	Dead
0-20 years	0-20 mm Hg	+	2		2
		-	2		1
	20-50 mm Hg	+	4	1	4
		-	4		1
	50 mm Hg	+			6
20-40 years	0-20 mm Hg	+			1
		-	1		5
	20-50 mm Hg	+	2	1	6
		-	3		1
	50 mm Hg	+			1
Over 40 years	0-20 mm Hg	+			4
		-	1		4
	20-50 mm Hg	+			7
		-	2		4
	50 mm Hg	+			2

posturing died regardless of their pressure. In our experience oculocephalic and oculovestibular reflexes could not provide useful information, as they never gave normal responses. In deeply comatose patients in whom we were unable to tap the ventricles, ICP was recorded only in the upper spinal space. As classical LANGFITT's (3) experiments showed, this way of recording proves reliable as long as the supratentorial pressure is freely transmitted to the infratentorial compartment and to the upper spinal space. Later on when ICP continues to rise and a progressive herniation of brain tissue into tentorial notch occurs, supratentorial pressure is no longer transmitted and Queckenstedt's maneuver becomes negative. In a further stage, pulsation disappears and the tracing becomes flat at a lower level. This might indicate a massive herniation into the foramen magnum, as SCHNEIDER et al. (5) described in brain death. All the patients in whom ICP was measured in the spinal space died. In 27 patients ICP was recorded before starting artificial ventilation: $paCO_2$ gradients between spontaneous and artificial ventilation were usually small (2-5 torr). In 10 out of 16 patients in whom ICP was raised, controlled ventilation was able to reduce it significantly, but in 8 patients ICP rose again to its initial value in a few hours. The effects of discontinuation of artificial ventilation were tested in 29 patients. In each patient the artificial ventilation pattern was kept constant. After switching off the ventilator, broad $paCO_2$ gradients (9-10 torr) were rare, being observed only in hypoventilating patients. In four patients no gradients were found on repeated examinations. Artificial ventilation was never discontinued when mean ICP exceeded 35 mm Hg. With base lines ranging from 20 to 35 mm Hg (15 patients) a steep rise in ICP took place in most patients: after the initial peak, ICP tends to decrease slowly, reaching its initial value in 1-2 h (Fig. 1). In some occasions, mainly in the first phase, the base line remains somewhat higher than its level prior to stopping the artificial ventilation (Fig. 2). In patients in whom there was no gradient of $paCO_2$, ICP remained unmodified. When base line shifted within normal limits the ICP variations were rather unpredictable: ICP sometimes rose abruptly as in hypertensive cases, but sometimes there was only slight, if any, modification in ICP values (Figs. 3-4). In 10 patients we studied serially the response to stopping the respirator treatment: we noticed that with the same base line and the same $paCO_2$ gradients, the ICP elevation was small after glycerol infusion or CSF withdrawal, while some time later a very steep increase in ICP occurred. In the first days after the head injury, ICP usually rose up to very high levels, whereas even with higher base lines, only slight variations were recorded some days later.

In two patients who had undergone decompressive procedures, only slight increases in ICP were recorded.
In 36 patients 10% glycerol was given in different ways: with single, repeated, and chronic administrations. Usually the effect of 250-500 ml lasted about 4-6 h, but in some patients it was much shorter. In the latter cases a repeated administration was usually ineffective. Glycerol was also given chronically (1000-1500 ml in four to six supplies): this procedure proved effective for 2-3 days at most. In 5 patients with early conjunctival edema, urine hyperosmolality, and a tendency to widespread edemas, glycerol failed to modify ICP. Intracranial hypertension could be controlled only by reducing fluid intake. Only one of these patients survived. Altogether glycerol proved to have some effectiveness in 25 patients: 14 of them survived. Only 2 patients survived when glycerol had failed, both remaining severely disabled.
In 26 patients different amounts of CSF were withdrawn. In patients in whom glycerol failed, CSF withdrawal had only slight effect.

In 9 cases we calculated the amount of CSF to be removed to keep ICP within normal limits: this quantity ranged from 100 to 500 ml/24 h. In 6 patients we left the drainage open, draining 250-500 ml in 24 h. After resetting the system at 15 mm Hg, in 3 patients the quantity of fluid drained decreased spontaneously in a few days. In 3 patients who continued to drain large amounts we put in a CSF shunt (ventriculoatrial in 2 and ventriculoperitoneal in the last one). All patients operated upon recovered quickly.

Summary

ICP alone cannot provide reliable data for a prognostic assessment. By contrast, as BECKER et al. (1) observed, ICP monitoring correlated to clinical data may provide very valuable information.
In our experience the respirator treatment does not appear to produce long-lasting ICP reduction. We feel, however, that the advantages of respirator treatment that ROSSANDA (4) and GORDON (2) have stressed, should not be considered only in terms of ICP reduction.

The discontinuation of artificial ventilation might provide some data of practical value. The effects of this maneuver depend on many factors: $paCO_2$ gradients, vascular reactivity to CO_2, brain elastance, etc. When $paCO_2$ gradients are constant in the same patient, the ICP variations should depend mainly on brain elastance.

This rough, but very simple, test could be of practical use to establish when artificial ventilation can be stopped safely. ICP monitoring appears to be very useful anyway when respirator treatment is undertaken. As a matter of fact, blind discontinuation of artificial ventilation may cause ICP to rise up to dangerous levels, at which cerebral perfusion pressure (CPP) would be seriously impaired.
Patients in whom glycerol is ineffective usually have a poor outcome.

In some of these cases ADH secretion disturbances are likely to play a role and CSF dynamics disturbances are far from rare even in the first phase of head injuries. Temporary drainage or permanent shunt procedures have a definite place in the management of these complications, although further studies are needed to outline their indications.

References

1. BECKER, D.P., VRIES, J.K., YOUNG, H.F., WARD, J.D.: Controlled cerebral perfusion pressure in human mechanic brain injury: Prevention of progressive brain swelling. In: Intracranial Pressure II (N. LUNDBERG, U. PONTEN, M. BROCK, eds.), pp. 480-484. Berlin-Heidelberg-New York: Springer 1975.

2. GORDON, E.: Controlled respiration in the management of patients with traumatic brain injuries. Acta anaesth. scand. 15, 193-208 (1971).

3. LANGFITT, T.W., WEINSTEIN, J.D., KASSEL, N.F., SIMONE, F.A.: Transmission of increased intracranial pressure. I. Within the craniospinal axis. J. Neurosurg. 21, 989-997 (1964).

4. ROSSANDA, M., COLLICE, M., PORTA, M., BOSELLI, L.: Intracranial hypertension in head injury. Clinical significance and relation to respiration. In: Intracranial Pressure II (N. LUNDBERG, U. PONTEN, M. BROCK, eds.), pp. 475-479. Berlin-Heidelberg- New York: Springer 1975.

5. SCHNEIDER, H., MATAKAS, F., SIMON, R.S., CERVOS NAVARRO, J.: Hypertension intracrânienne et infarctus ischémique total du cerveau. Neurochirurgie 18, 159-170 (1972).

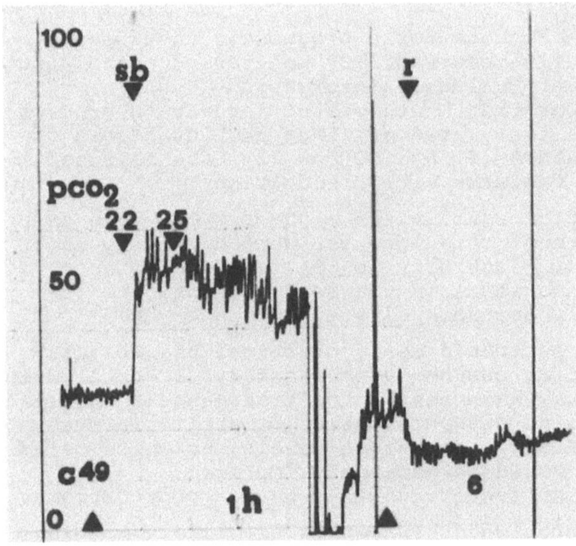

Fig. 1. Raised ICP base line during controlled ventilation. Initial peak and spontaneous reduction of ICP, after switching off ventilator. Recording interrupted for 10 min for technical reasons. $paCO_2$ gradient: 3 torr. sb spontaneous breathing, r respirator treatment

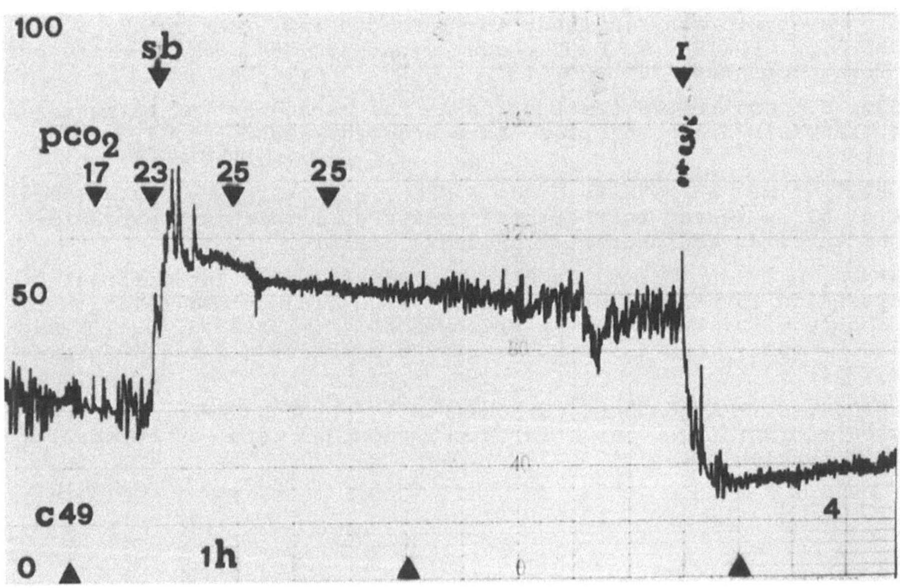

Fig. 2. Raised ICP base line during controlled ventilation (strong artificial hyperventilation). Initial peak followed by a long plateau after switching off ventilator. Incomplete spontaneous reduction of ICP. $paCO_2$ gradient: 6 torr

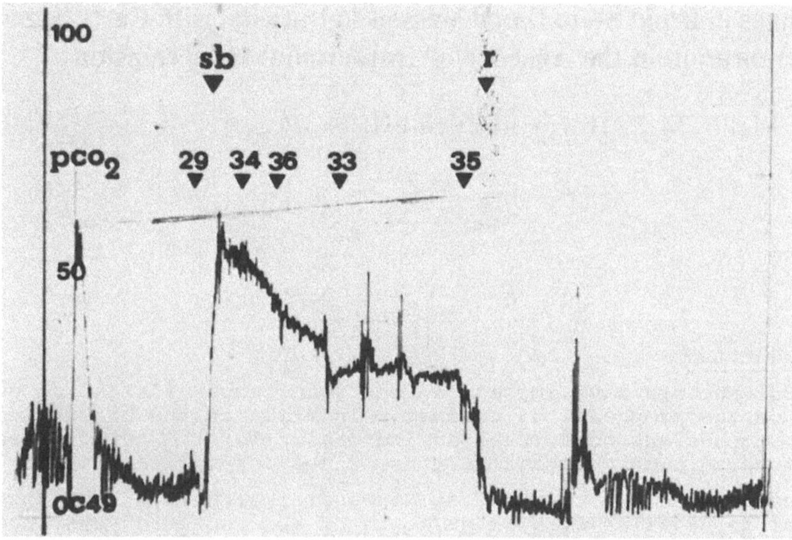

Fig. 3. Lower ICP base line during controlled ventilation: very steep peak and only partial reduction of ICP after switching off ventilator. $paCO_2$ gradient: 5 torr. sb spontaneous breathing, r respirator treatment

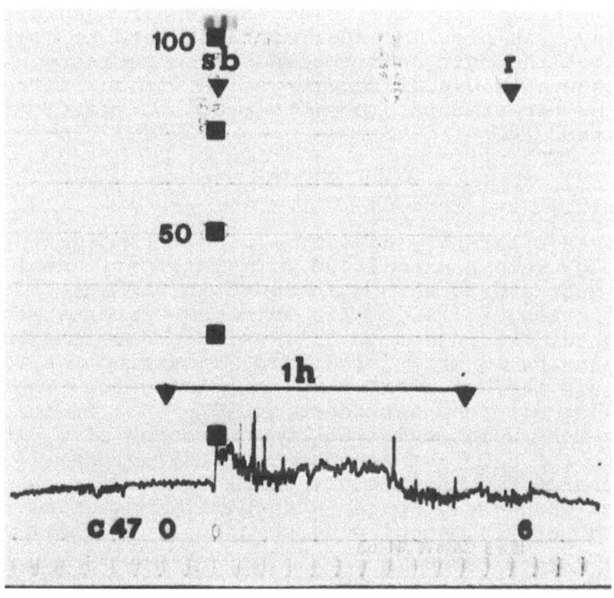

Fig. 4. Low ICP base line during controlled ventilation. Very small and short-lasting variation of ICP after switching off ventilator. $paCO_2$ gradient: 4 torr

Changes in Brain Stem Blood Vessels in Patients with Early Signs of Decerebration in the Absence of Intracranial Hypertension

P.A. Mello, M.P. Horta, and I. Leão

Introduction

Several authors have emphasized the importance of signs of decerebration on the prognosis of traumatic injuries to the brain. In some centers, such signs constitute an indication for the performance of extensive radiologic investigations or even exploratory surgery (2).

All casualties admitted to the Neurosurgical Unit of the Hospital Distrital de Brasilia with frank signs of decerebration are submitted to continuous monitoring of VFP subsequent to exploratory trepanation. If VFP is elevated, conservative measures to reduce it are started at once. If the pressure fails to decrease in response to high doses of dexamethasone and diuretics, a bilateral decompressive craniectomy is performed.

Our attention was drawn to the fact that in some of the patients treated in this way, decerebration is not necessarily accompanied by a marked increase in VFP (Fig. 1). The opinion has been expressed (2) that vascular changes rather than pure mass displacement, might be responsible for the clinical symptomatology under such circumstances. In order to study this problem experimentally, and to compare our findings with histopathologic data obtained from patients who died as casualties and presented signs of decerebration without increase in VFP, we developed a new experimental model to produce impaction on the central nervous system.

Material and Methods

Eleven apparently healthy albino rats of both sexes (average weight 130 g) were anesthetized with intraperitoneal Nembutal (30 mg/kg body weight) and an abrupt increase in ICP was induced by rapid (free hand) injection of 1 ml of air into the cisterna magna. Just before completion of the injection, all animals developed sudden tremors and stopped breathing. Shortly afterward, breathing was resumed but the rats died within the 1st h after the air injection. Their brains were fixed in 4% formalin and sectioned at 50 μ in a freezing microtome. The frozen sections were submitted to the action of 3,3-diaminobenzidine in presence of H_2O_2 and stained by cresyl violet (3). These animals were compared to controls not submitted to air injection. The histologic sections were compared with similar material obtained from patients with early signs of decerebration and submitted to exploratory burr holes followed by monitoring of VFP. These patients died in decerebration despite having normal or only moderately elevated pressure. Their brains were treated in the same way as that of the experimental animals.

Results

All animals that received cisternal air injection showed consistent increase in vascularization in the brain stem, mainly the superior colliculus and adjacent to the aqueduct. In no animal were microscopic hemorrhages observed. The stained blood vessels appeared to be highly congested. As opposed to this, the histologic sections of the brain stem of the patients who died in decerebration in the absence of increased ICP displayed no changes in vascularization and no signs of congestion. There had been no hypocampal or tonsillar herniation.

Discussion

The presence of early signs of decerebration in patients with low intracranial pressure justifies the search for primary cellular changes in the brain stem. These changes would indicate that the cause of decerebration in such cases is a direct traumatic damage to brain stem centers instead of secondary necrosis and hemorrhage consequent to herniation and brain stem compression or distortion. In fact, this group of patients already had serious (primary) respiratory dysfunction on admittance. This picture contrasts with the secondary (late) alterations in brain stem function observed in patients who decerebrate upon development of intracranial hypertension. The latter situation is mimicized by our experimental animals, all of which died with signs of secondary brain stem failure and all of which had marked vascular alterations in the brain stem, similar to those observed by GOODMAN (1) under similar conditions.

Summary

The authors have continuously monitored ventricular fluid pressure in patients with severe head injuries and early signs of decerebration. Special attention is deserved by those who have normal intracranial pressure levels despite a very severe clinical picture. Such patients do not present the histologic picture of vascular congestion of the brain stem. Their primary and severe brain stem dysfunction is believed to be due to direct traumatic damage to brain stem centers.

References

1. GOODMAN, S.J., BECKER, D.F.: Vascular pathology of the brain stem due to experimentally increased intracranial pressure, noted changes in the micro- and macrocirculation. J. Neurosurg. 38, 601-609 (1973).
2. GUTTERMAN, P., SHENKIN, H.: Prognostic features in recovery from traumatic decerebration. J. Neurosurg. 32, 330-335 (1970).
3. LA VAIL, J.H., LA VAIL, M.M.: Retrograde axonal transport in the central nervous system. Science 176, 1416-1417 (1972).

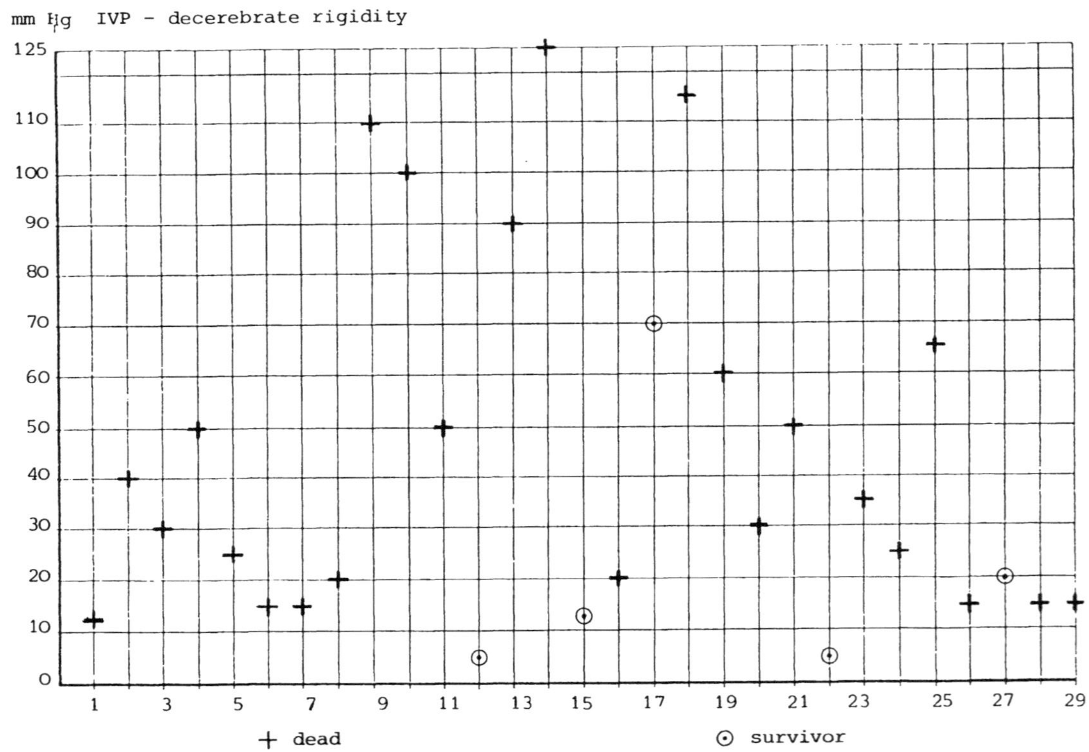

Fig. 1. ICP values in overall material of 29 patients with decerebrate rigidity. Those with ICP below 20 mm Hg were studied in this report

The Brain Vasomotor Tone Index as Prognosis Leader in Severe Head Injuries

J. de Rougemont, A. L. Benabid, J. P. Chirossel, and M. Barge

Introduction and Principle

Prognostical significance of intracranial pressure (ICP) is today a question which is still discussed. The problem lies mainly in the quest of ICP data that could have a statistical use. The rough value of ICP is certainly not sufficient, nor is the cerebral perfusion pressure (CPP): the data are not normalized and cannot be used in a statistical way. Referring to the well-known BURTON's diagram (2) it can be said, that the radial component Tr of the vasomotor tone exactly equilibrates the gradient between the mean ICP (MICP) and the mean arterial blood pressure (MABP). Then: Tr = MABP - MICP = CPP.

It can be written: Tr/MABP = 1 - MCIP/MABP.
We have named Brain Vasomotor Tone Index (BVMI) the ratio MICP/MABP.
Then: BVMI = MICP/MABP = 1 - Tr/MABP.

BVMI actually is an index because it is normalized, varying between 0 (when Tr = MABP, corresponding to a complete vasospasm) and 1 (when Tr = 0, corresponding to a complete vasoplegia). It is also an index of the brain vasomotor tone because it expresses the ratio between the radial component of arterial vasomotor tone and the MABP, which characterizes the vasomotor state of the brain. So far, the BVMI could show a statistical prognosis and check at any time the efficiency of the treatment. On a nonselected series of neurosurgical patients 4 years ago, the authors (5) showed that the remarkable value 0.5 of BVMI represented a true prognostical line: above this line, all patients went to brain death and reached, at the time of circulatory arrest, a BVMI equal to 1. Under this line, two areas were recognized: the upper, between BVMI 0.5 and 0.3, presented a 43% rate of mortality; the lower, under BVMI 0.3, was free of death. *The present work deals with the use of the BVMI in the intensive neurosurgical care of severe head injuries.*

Materials and Methods

Among 430 patients whose ICP was recorded, 64 patients, suffering from severe head injuries, without hematomas and not operated upon, were selected. In the intensive care unit, they had ICP (epidural device (4) or intraventricular catheter) and ABP (femoral catheter) monitoring. Blood gases were measured in blood samples two or three times a day, artificial ventilation was done when necessary. The net differences between liquid perfusions and fluid losses were daily calculated, and the clinical status of the patients was continuously checked by the medical team.

Results

BVMI and Outcome of Patients (Fig. 1A). (1) No cerebral death due to a cerebral origin occurred under the BVMI 0.25. (2) No surviving patient had a BVMI higher than 0.5. Patients who died from extracerebral causes were widespread between BVMI 0.5 and 0.1. (3) All patients who had a circulatory arrest, controlled by angiography and flat EEG, had their BVMI between 0.8 and 1.

A statistical prognosis can be outlined from this plot: The mortality rate is 100% above BVMI 0.5; between BVMI 0.5 and 0.25, this rate is 22% if cerebral causes are only concerned, and 41% when considering the whole mortality. Under 0.25, it is 25%, only due to extracerebral causes.

BVMI and Arterial Blood Pressure (Fig. 1B). The mean value of MABP is about 100 mm Hg: so far, *the BVMI 0.5* corresponds to a MICP equal to 50 mm Hg, or to a CPP equal to 50 mm Hg. This value is the same as that which has been reported to be the boundary after which cerebral blood flow (CBF) starts to be impaired (3, 7) and the EEG begins to flatten or alter (1). So far, *this 0.5 line bears a particular significance* on a physiopathologic ground also.

BVMI and ICP Patterns (Fig. 2). Stable records are always encountered for the lower values of BVMI, under 0.3, and no difference is induced by the type of ventilation; on the other hand, records showing waves (A, B, C) were situated in a higher range of BVMI, between 0.2 and 0.6, mainly in the remarkable area of BVMI 0.25 - 0.5. In this range A-Waves and B-Waves were often observed in patients freely breathing, but never under artificial ventilation, except for one A-Wave. Patients with higher BVMI needed artificial ventilation, and had the worst prognosis. So far, *the BVMI area 0.25 - 0.5 appears to be a range of poorly regulated vasomotor tone,* showing signs of damaged autoregulation.

BVMI and Brain Damage (Fig. 3). When the BVMI is correlated with the anatomical lesions, determinated on clinical or autopsic findings, an ascending relationship is found. (1) *Isolated brain stem lesions* give no reason to elevation of ICP, except for one case which had a tegmen hemorrhage with compression of the aqueduct, and who died with a BVMI of 0.42. (2) *Unilateral hemispheric lesions,* even when associated with brain stem lesions were observed to have a BVMI that could remain low, but also could reach the 0.5 value; the global mortality in this category was 28%. (3) *Bilateral hemispheric lesions* had a higher BVMI, ranging between 0.25 and 1, and all these patients died.

BVMI, Duration of Coma, Time of Death. (1) *Deaths from cerebral causes* had a BVMI higher than 0.25; all of them occurred before the 10th day, except for one case who was brought up to 17 days, by a particularly intensive care; the higher the BVMI, the earlier the death. (2) *Deaths from extracerebral causes* occurred after 8 days, and all of them had a BVMI ranging between 0.1 and 0.5. (3) *Surviving patients* had a duration of coma ranging from 1 to 134 days, without any correlation with the BVMI, which was always lower than 0.5. Somewhere around the tenth days there seems to be a critical period as far as the final outcome of the patients is concerned.

BVMI and Water Movement (Fig. 4). It has been observed in this study that when patients got worse, except for space-occupying lesions developing, always a positive difference between perfusion and fluid losses could be found during the previous days. *This difference was called the water movement. During the impairing phase,* the BVMI increased in direct correlation with the net amount of fluid which was stored; in many cases, this newly impaired BVMI, following a positive water movement, settled the prognosis and the patient died. *Improvement of the clinical status* of the patients corresponded both to decrease in BVMI and negative water movement, i.e., fluid losses that were higher than the amount of perfusions.

Discussion

Significance of the Critical Values of BVMI. At first glance, the BVMI seems to bear a strong prognostic significance: the mortality rate, only due to extracerebral causes under a BVMI of 0.25, varies between 22% for cerebral causes and 41% for all causes in the BVMI range of 0.25 - 0.5. Above 0.5, the mortality rate is 100%. So far, *a BVMI of 0.5 represents a very critical step.* Indeed, it has been shown that CBF is altered when ICP reaches the diastolic blood pressure, (1) or when ICP is equal to 50 mm Hg (3). These values correspond roughly to a BVMI of 0.5 which is found here. Moreover, it has been shown in the present work that ICP waves occurred preferentially in a BVMI range of 0.25 - 0.5. So far, it can be supposed that *this special area of 0.25 - 0.5 corresponds to the field where autoregulation begins to be damaged*, showing signs of disregulation like C waves or bursts of paroxysmal failure as are the A waves. Under a BVMI of 0.25, the mechanism of autoregulation should work well; above a BVMI of 0.5, it should be abolished, leading to a complete vasoplegia; CBF decreases quickly and then the circulatory arrest occurs when BVMI equals 1.

Significance of the Time Course of BVMI during Water Movements. The influence of the water movement on the BVMI supposedly may reflect the effect of the water content of the brain on cerebral blood dynamics. Then, as it is changing, it must be looked at as an index of the present state of the vasomotor tone, or as an index of the extent of the brain damage at the time when the BVMI is checked. Its prognostic value must not be looked at as a fixed prognosis that could not vary after it had been evaluated; in fact, at any time, the prognosis is settled by the actual anatomical state of the brain, but this can be either impairing or improving, especially by the way of therapeutic measures. When a high BVMI is not corrected, it bears a poor prognosis; if it is corrected, hope is permissible. When the BVMI is low, it indicates that the treatment is well done or efficient; when it is high, it reflects the severity of the lesion, either primarily brought about by the head injury, or later by therapeutic iatrogenic injury.

Use of the BVMI for a Therapeutic Schedule of Severe Brain Injuries. So far, the BVMI assessment provides a guide to the type of treatment to be done as well as an index reflecting the efficiency of the therapeutic procedures. (1) *Above a BVMI of 0.5*, the therapy is today unefficient if this value is overpassed for a long enough time. (2) *Under a BVMI of 0.5* the treatment must consist of three procedures: water restriction, checking of blood gases (essentially $paCO_2$), and long-lasting anesthesia. They must be balanced according to the range of BVMI in which the patient is situated:

1. *Between 0.25 and 0.5*, the treatment is difficult and must be handled with precision. *Water restriction* must be drastic even if it leads temporarily to functional kidney deficiency. *Blood gases* must be carefully checked to normocapnia, it was shown (6) that at this level hypocapnia is poorly efficent on increased ICP but decreases the CBF. *Long-lasting anesthesia*, eventually associated with controlled hypothermia, must be used in order to lower nociceptive stimulations and brain metabolism as well as vegetative disorders.
2. *Under a BVMI of 0.25*, the intensive care of the head injuries is easy and must try to prevent BVMI rising up: (1) *Water restriction* must be slight or even nil, with an hydric equilibrium well checked.

(2) *Blood gases* must be in slight hypocapnia as it is efficient on ICP and decreases it. (3) *Long-lasting anesthesia* as well as hypothermia are not required here.

Summary

The ratio MICP/MABP is theoretically shown to be an index of the brain vasomotor tone (BVMI). Its prognostical usefulness was studied on 64 severe head injuries. Three main ranges were recognized: *under 0.25*, no death from cerebral cause occurred, ICP records were stable and the management of the patient was easy. *Above 0.5*, all patients died, regardless of the treatment. *Between 0.25 and 0.5*, the mortality rate was between 22 and 41%; ICP records often showed waves, autoregulation appeared to be damaged, and the therapy was very difficult to handle. The 0.5 level of BVMI is tightly connected with water movements inside the brain tissue, and this leads to a therapeutic schedule.

References

1. BALDY-MOULINIER, M., FREREBEAU, Ph.: Blood flow of the cerebral cortex in intracranial hypertension. International Symposium on "CSF and CBF", Lund and Copenhagen, May 9-11, 1968. Scand. J. Clin. Lab. Invest., 22, Suppl. 102, XV:G (1968).
2. BURTON, A.C.: Physical principles of circulatory phenomena: The physical equilibria of the heart and blood vessels. In: Handbook of Physiology. Section 2: Circulation, Volume 1 (J. FIELD, ed.). Washington D.C., American Physiological Society, 85-106 (1962).
3. HAGGENDAL, E., JOHANSSON, B.: Effects of arterial carbon dioxide tension and oxygen saturation on cerebral blood flow autoregulation in dogs. Acta Physiol. Scand., Suppl. 258, 27-53 (1965).
4. ROUGEMONT, J. de, BARGE, M., BENABID, A.L.: Un nouveau capteur pour la mesure de la pression intracrânienne. Valeur de la dure-mère en tant que membrane susceptible de transmettre les pressions. Neurochir., 17, 579-590 (1971).
5. ROUGEMONT, J. de, BARGE, M., BENABID, A.L.: Correlative study of intracranial and systemic arterial pressures in neurosurgical patients. In: Intracranial Pressure, First International Symposium on Intracranial Pressure, Hannover, 1972 (M. BROCK and H. DIETZ, eds.). Berlin-Heidelberg-New York: Springer 1972.
6. RUNDENBERG, F.H., McGRAW, C.P., TINDALL, G.T.: Effects of hyperventilation, CO_2, and CSF pressure on internal carotid blood flow in the baboon. J. Neurosurg., 44, 347-352 (1976).
7. ZWETNOW, N.N.: CBF autoregulation to blood pressure and intracranial pression variations, International Symposium on "CSF and CBF", Lund and Copenhagen, May 9-11, 1968. Scand. J. Clin. Lab. Invest., Suppl. 102 V:A (1968).

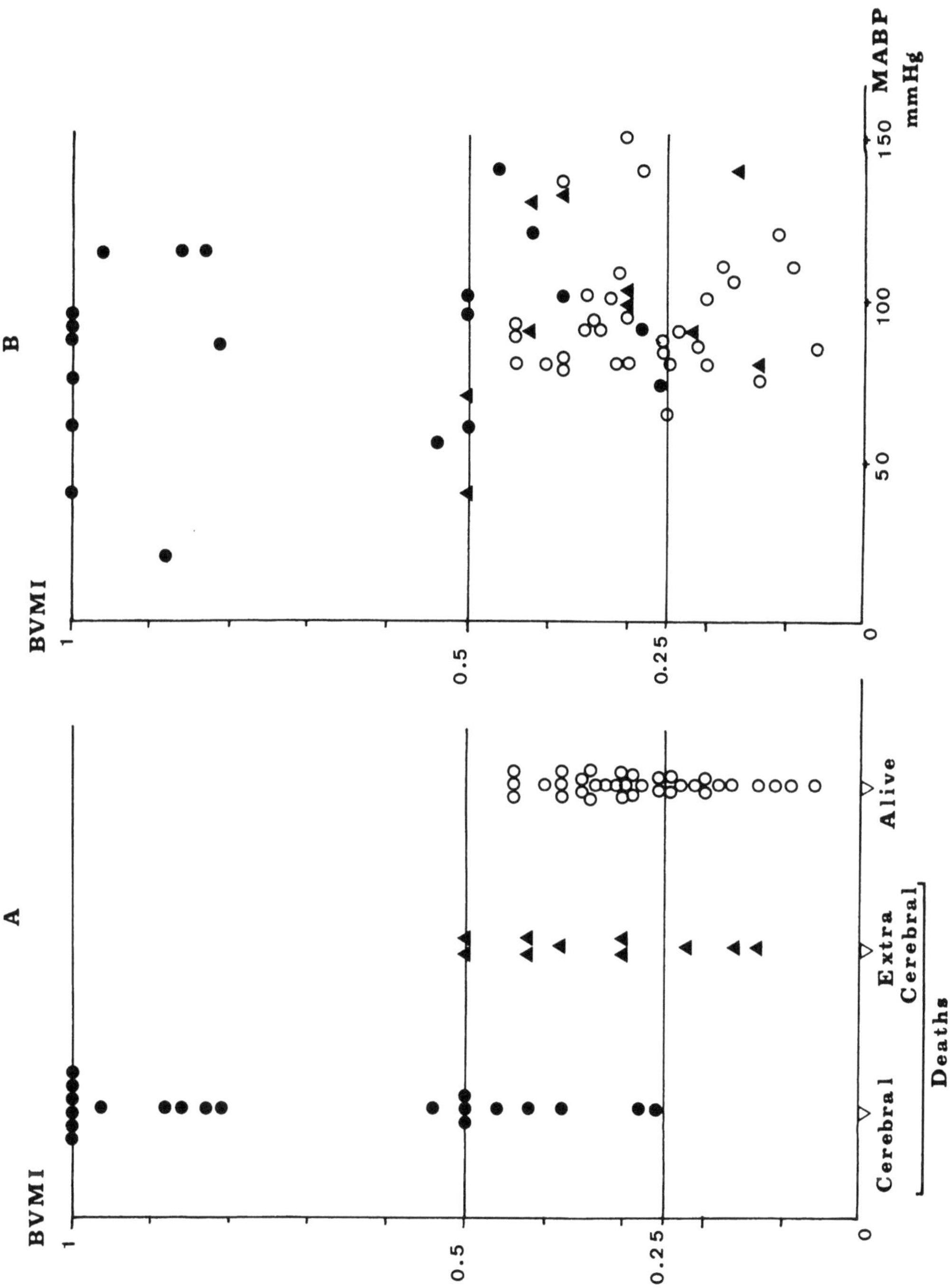

Fig. 1. BVMI and mortality. (A) Statistical distribution of BVMI according to outcome of patients (● death from cerebral causes (C). ▲ death from extracerebral causes (E.C.). ○ surviving patients). (This convention is same for all figures)
(B) Statistical distribution of BVMI according to MABP

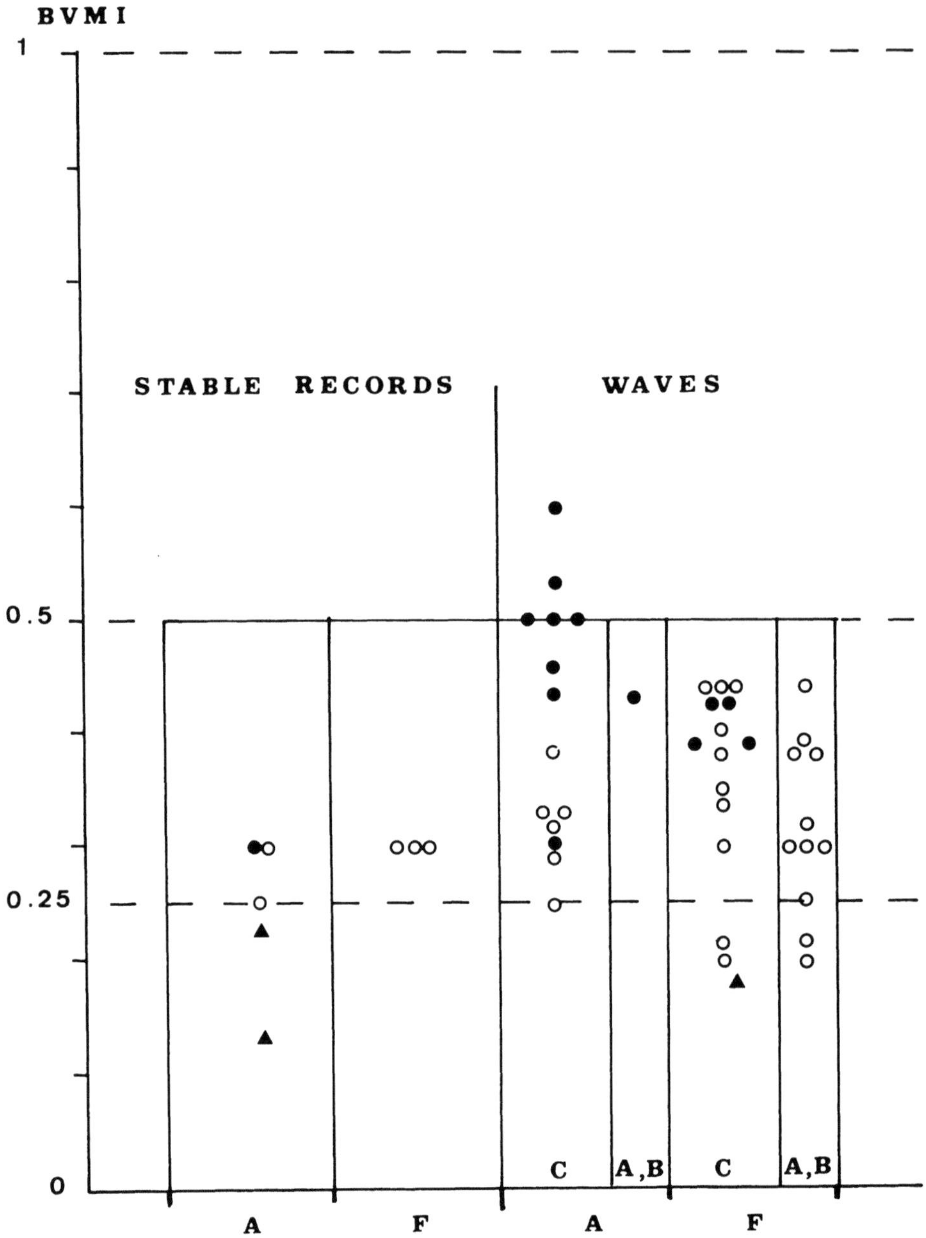

Fig. 2. BVMI and ICP patterns. Records showing waves (A, B, C) are more influenced by type of ventilation (A assisted, F free) as far as A and B waves are concerned. BVMI of these records is higher than in stable ICP records

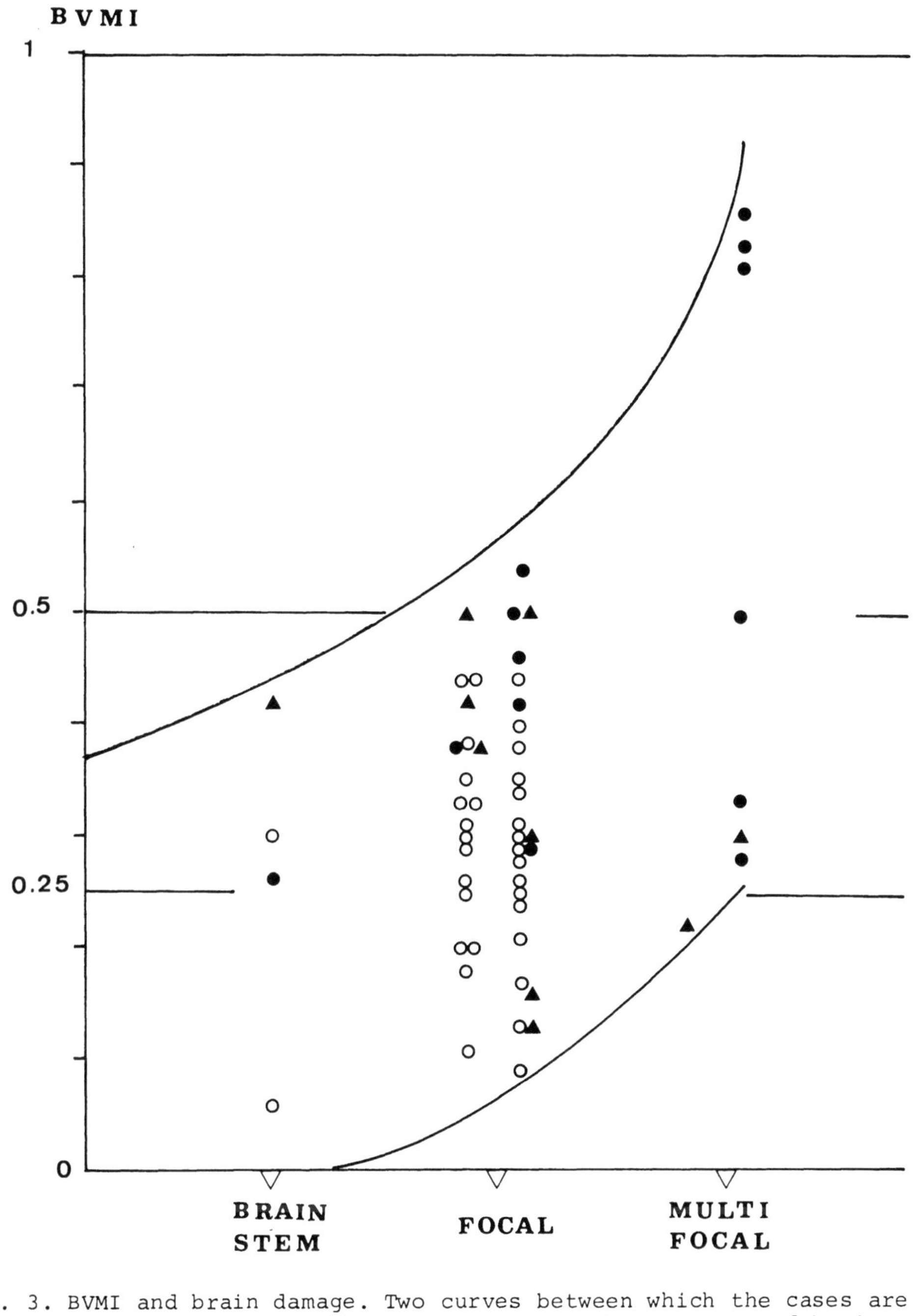

Fig. 3. BVMI and brain damage. Two curves between which the cases are situated show ascending relationship between BVMI and type of brain lesion, together with an increase in mortality rate

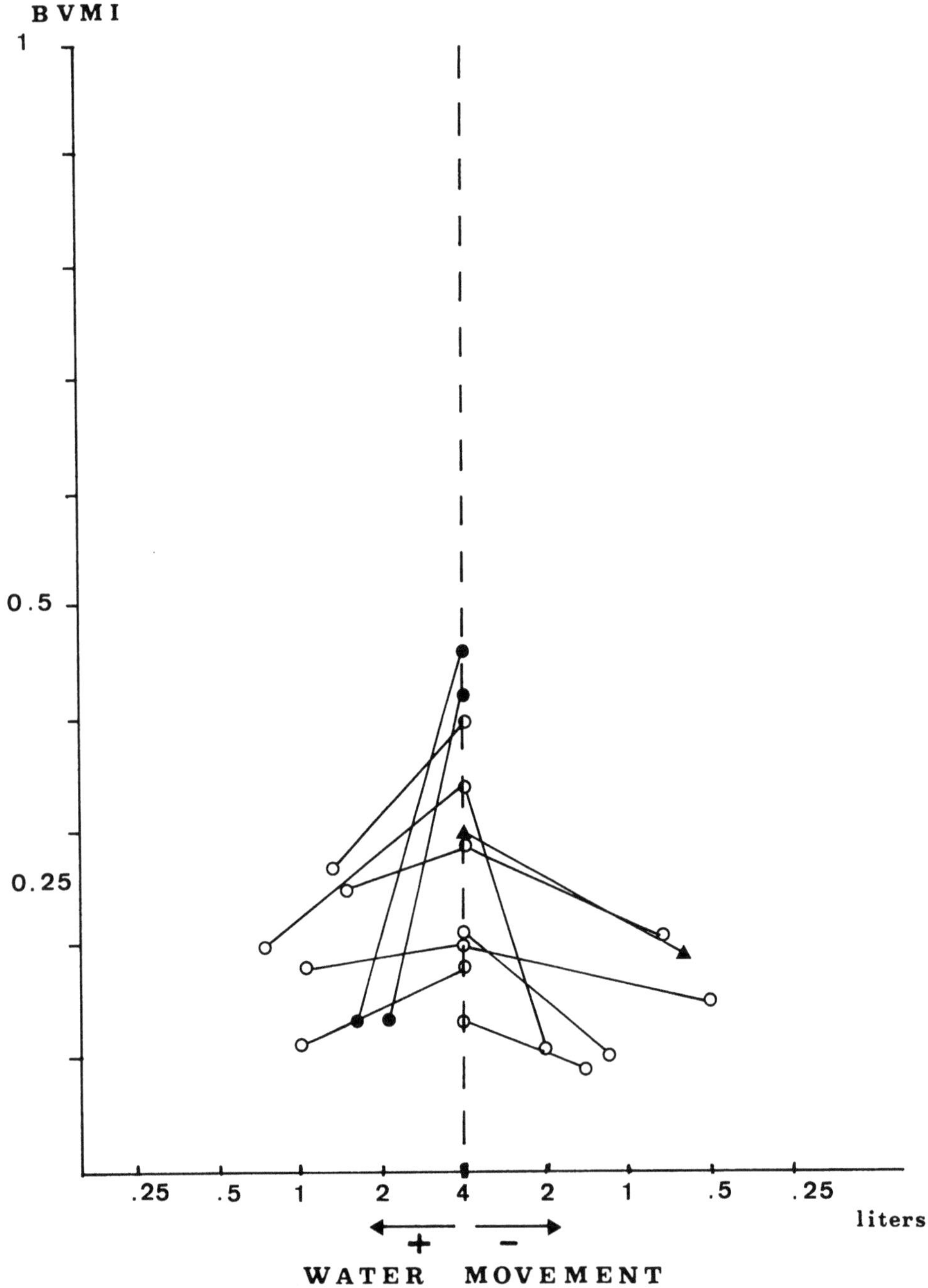

Fig. 4. BVMI and water movement. Scale of water movement (difference between liquid perfusion amounts and fluid losses) is logarithmic and inversed: a positive water movement is plotted on the left part of scale, and reversely. Line in middle corresponds to BVMI in the most imparing clinical period. On the left, values of BVMI before impairment, plotted with respect to positive water movement. On the right, values BVMI after improvement, according to negative water movement

The Relation Between Intracranial Pressure and Regional Cerebral Blood Flow in the Acute Phase of Severe Head Injury

E. M. Enevoldsen and F. T. Jensen

Introduction

The aim of this study was to investigate the relation between intracranial pressure (ICP), regional cerebral blood flow (rCBF), and brain metabolism in patients with acute severe brain injuries in order to evaluate how much the intracranial pressure could be increased if brain ischemia was to be avoided.

Materials and Methods

There were 23 patients studied during the acute phase after severe head injury, the period of study lasting from 3-21 days (2). All patients were deeply comatose on admission, and only those who, after the initial neursurgical treatment, were still so comatose that they needed artificial ventilation were included in the series. The study was concluded when respirator treatment could be stopped. The ventilation was maintained with positive pressure and controlled respiration. Arterial carbon dioxide tension ($paCO_2$) was maintained at a constant level in the individual patient, but interindividually the levels varied between 25 and 45 mm Hg, depending on the patient's need for hyperventilation (see below). The oxygen tension was kept above 100 mm Hg. Sedatives used were meperidine, chlorpromazine and diazepam. A total of 18 patients were treated with dexamethasone, 24 mg daily, and 4 patients had an additional dose of 48 mg because of high ICP. Also 4 patients underwent surgical decompression. The ICP was measured continuously in all patients during the entire study by the method of LUNDBERG (6). The intraventricular pressure (IVP) was measured through a catheter inserted into one of the lateral ventricles of the brain and kept below 45 mm Hg by means of the following methods of treatment:

1. Tracheal toilet followed by manual hyperventilation for 5 min.
2. Meperidine plus chlorpromazine intravenously.
3. Increased continued hyperventilation.
4. Mannitol by continuous infusion with a number of drops depending on the effect on the IVP.
5. Nembutal or pentothal in dosis of 50-100 mg.
6. Dexamethasone in a single dose of 48 mg.
7. Continuous ventricular drainage.
8. Surgical decompression with removal of lacerated and severe edematous brain tissue and bone over the injured area.

In each patient the rCBF was measured one to four times during the study, and always before carotid angiography. The time intervals depended on the indications for angiography. A total of 203 blood flow runs were done in 66 separate cerebral blood flow studies. The intra-arterial isotope injection technique devised by LASSEN and INGVAR (5) was used for the measurements. The clearance of ^{133}Xe was recorded, using a 16 detector unit placed extracranially over the brain area to be studied. The flow values were calculated by computer from the 1st min of the clearance curves as the initial slope flow index. The computer automatically compensated for residual radioactivity. All CBF measurements were done under local anesthesia, and prior to each CBF study the patient was given meperidine, chlorpromazine, and pancuronium bromide. If required, administration of these drugs was repeated during the study. Before each CBF measurement, arterial pCO_2, pH, pO_2, and hemoglobin were determined.

Brain metabolism was evaluated from the ventricular fluid (CSF) lactate, pyruvate, pH, pCO_2, and pO_2. CSF was collected anaerobically from the ventricular system, and lactate and pyruvate were immediately precipitated in 3% metamorphoric acid, and later determined enzymatically. The other parameters were determined by radiometric method. A total of 92 samples of ventricular fluid were studied.

Results

No correlation was found between IVP and rCBF in the series as a whole, but if a group of patients with brain stem symptoms, but without signs of cortical lesions, was selected, this group showed a positive correlation between IVP and rCBF, the coefficient of correlation being 0.50, significant at $P < 0.05$. This group consisted of only five patients in whom 19 separate CBF studies were performed.

Neither in the group as a whole, nor in the selected group of patients with brain stem symptoms, was there any correlation between CSF, pH, and IVP, or between CSF lactate and IVP, but high CSF lactate and low pH were found to precede pronounced increases in IVP.

In four patients in whom continuous IVP measurements and repeated rCBF measurements were performed during a period of increasing IVP referable to the development of edema, high CSF lactate and low pH as well as increased rCBF *preceded* the increase in IVP. One of these cases is described below.

Case 1. Cortical Lesion, Hemorrhagic Shock, and Secondary Brain Stem Symptoms

A 14-year-old boy sustained closed head injury without fractures. On admission craniotomy revealed a subdural hematoma and diffuse edema in the right frontal and temporal regions. Burr holes on the left side showed a normal cortex. At the initial craniotomy, severe venous bleeding occurred, during which the blood pressure dropped and was unobtainable for 3-5 min. During the first few days after the injury, the IVP was about 20 mm Hg. From the 4th day it gradually increased to about 45 mm Hg. Between the 6th and the 9th day, numerous plateau waves of a duration of 30 min occurred, accompanied by attacks of decerebrate rigidity and dilatation of the right pupil. On the eighth day, carotid angiography revealed a mass lesion in the right temporal region. Craniotomy disclosed massive edema of the temporal lobe, but neither hematomas nor malacia was found. Decompression was performed in the right temporal region, and the anterior part of the lobe was removed. Postoperatively, the IVP again increased to above 40 mm Hg, and the patient was given a single dose of dexamethasone, 48 mg. The IVP was 20 mm Hg 5 h later, and during the next 6 days it stabilized at 15 mm Hg. The relation between IVP, CBF, and metabolism in this patient is shown in Figure 1.

Discussion

In agreement with other authors (1, 3) we found that intracranial hypertension did not limit rCBF, at least not if IVP was kept below 45 mm Hg, as it was in all our patients. On the contrary, high IVP was often accompanied by increased rCBF, and in a group of patients with brain stem symptoms, but without signs of cortical lesions a positive correlation between rCBF and IVP was found. Correlation did not exist between IVP and CSF pH or between IVP and CSF lactate. On the other hand, CSF acidosis with high CSF lactate and high CBF preceded high IVP, but the CSF acidosis might subside at a time when the IVP was still increasing. This might indicate that the acidosis in the brain provokes vasoparalysis with an increase in rCBF (4), causing a secondary increase in IVP owing to the development of edema. The high rCBF removes the acidosis, and simultaneously with the IVP increase and the decrease of acidosis the rCBF again decreases (case 1).

Summary

Correlation did not exist between IVP and rCBF or between IVP and CSF acidosis with high lactate, but CSF acidosis (low pH and high lactate) as well as high rCBF preceded the increase in IVP caused by the edema of the brain tissue.

Key words

Intraventricular pressure, Regional cerebral blood flow, Brain metabolism.

References

1. BRUCE, D.A., LANGFITT, T.W., MILLER, J.D., SCHUTZ, H., VAPALAHTI, M.P., STANEK, A., GOLDBERG, H.I.: Regional cerebral blood flow, intracranial pressure, and brain metabolism in comatose patients. J. Neurosurg. 38, 131-144 (1973).

2. ENEVOLDSEN, E.M., COLD, G., JENSEN, F.T., MALMROS, R.: Dynamic changes in regional CBF, intraventricular pressure, CSF pH and lactate levels during the acute phase of head injury. J. Neurosurg. 44, 191-214 (1976).

3. FIESCHI, C., BATTISTINI, A., BEDUSCHI, L., BOSELLI, L., ROSSANDA, M.: Regional cerebral blood flow and intraventricular pressure in acute head injuries. J. Neurol. Neurosurg. and Psychiat. 37, 1378-1388 (1974).

4. HJELM, M., OVERGÅRD, J., LASSEN, N.A., TWEED, W.A.: Brain tissue lactacidosis of hyperemic regions around brain tumors. In: Blood Flow and Metabolism (A.M. HARPER, W.B. JENNETT, J.D. MILLER, J.O. ROWAN, eds.), pp. 13, 41-42. Edinburgh-London-New York: Churchill Livingstone 1975.

5. LASSEN, N.A., INGVAR, D.H.: The blood flow of the cerebral cortex determined by radioactive krypton-85. Experientia (Basal) 17, 42 (1961).

6. LUNDBERG, N.: Continuous recording and control of ventricular fluid pressure in neurosurgical practice. Acta Psychiatr. Scand. (Suppl.) 149, 1-193 (1960).

Subdural Hematoma and Edema in the Right Frontal and Temporal Regions

A

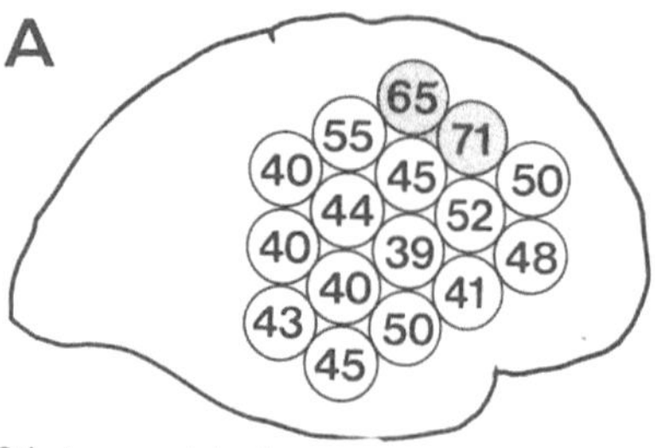

24 h postinjury

Consciousness: Deep coma

Average $F_{initial}$ 48

Mean SAP 109
" IVP 19
" CPP 90
$PaCO_2$ 36

CSF lactate 4.04
" pH 7.27

B

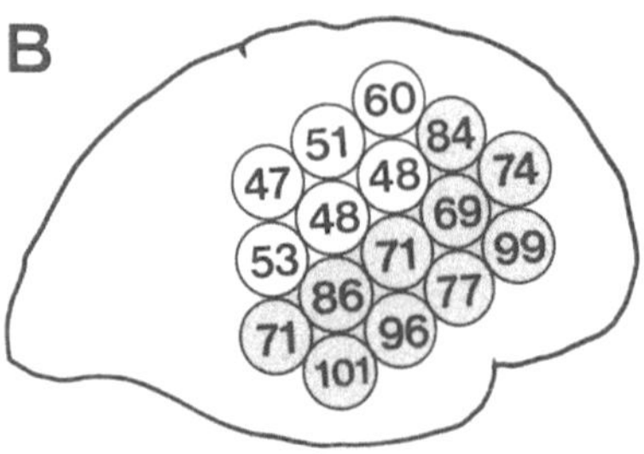

3 days postinjury

Consciousness: Deep coma

Average $F_{initial}$ 71

Mean SAP 90
" IVP 26
" CPP 64
$PaCO_2$ 34

CSF lactate 4.56
" pH 7.28

C

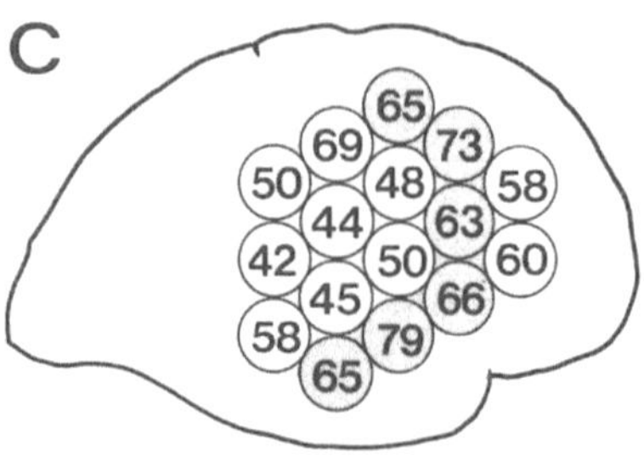

5 days postinjury

Consciousness: Deep coma, pronation–extension movements

Average $F_{initial}$ 59

Mean SAP 86
" IVP 35
" CPP 51
$PaCO_2$ 28

CSF lactate 1.96
" pH 7.32

D

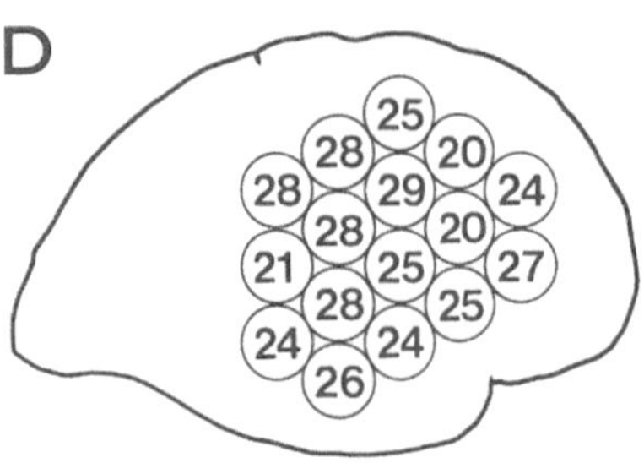

12 days postinjury

Consciousness: Deep coma

Average $F_{initial}$ 25

Mean SAP 84
" IVP 25
" CPP 59
$PaCO_2$ 32

CSF lactate 2.45
" pH 7.31

◁ Fig. 1 (case 1). Regional CBF (left), average CBF, cerebral perfusion pressure (CPP), $paCO_2$, amd CSF lactate and pH (right), in a patient who initially had a subdural hematoma and edema of the right frontal and temporal regions. Blood flows are expressed in ml/100 g/min, pressure in mm Hg.

A. Flow values were relatively low, on average 48 ml/100 g/min, 24 h postinjury and 15 h postoperation when IVP was 19 mm Hg. Only in two areas in the upper frontal region was flow above normal value of 60 ml/100 g/min. CSF lactate was high (4.04 mmol/L) and CSF pH low (7.27). CSF lactate increased to 4.7 mmol/L and the pH decreased to a level as low as 7.06 2 days postinjury.

B. At 3 days postinjury IVP had increased to 26 mm Hg, and flow values had increased in areas from which hematoma was removed initially to above normal values on average 71 ml/100 g/min. Ventricular fluid lactate was still high (4.56), but pH had increased again, to 7.27. At 5 days postinjury, IVP had further increased of 59 ml/100 g/min and CSF lactate had decreased to 1.96 mmol/L. CSF pH had increased to normal values, 7.32. Thus, CSF acidosis had been returned at a time when IVP was still increasing.

At 12 days postinjury (4 days after a period with high IVP and plateau waves simultaneous with attacks of decerebrate rigidity and followed by decompression in temporal region) IVP had decreased to 25 mm Hg and flows had decreased to very low values, averaging 25 ml/100 g/min. CSF lactate had again slightly increased. Case shows that edema with high IVP is preceded by high CSF lactate, low CSF pH, and high CBF

Summary

M. Brock and D.P. Becker

The papers presented in this session elicited a vivid discussion for two main reasons:

1. They deal with a subject of immediate interest to the neurosurgeon, and
2. they present "challenging" data.

The general consensus was reached that (1) continuous monitoring of intracranial pressure is indicated in patients with severe brain trauma, and (2) ICP monitoring can steer therapy in this type of patients. This is so in part because deleterious changes in ICP are unpredictable from the clinical symptomatology and from the type and/or intensity of the trauma, and because of the individual variations in the way each patient reacts to trauma. Increasing experience in this field has shown that there is something like a "critical level" of ICP at which brain function is still upheld but in a very unstable equilibrium. This critical level appears to lie at 30-40 mm Hg. An increase in ICP to this level in a patient who underwent a brain trauma should lead to energetic therapeutic activity.

On the other hand, clinical deterioration in the absence of intracranial hypertension following a brain trauma is a bad prognostic sign - a fact to which JENNETT already called attention at the first ICP Symposium in Hannover. In this group of patients, primary traumatic lesion of vital brain stem centers rather than secondary damage of these structures by intracranial hypertension and mass displacement is responsible for the symptoms (and for the outcome).

Cerebral circulation is, perhaps, the main factor determining outcome in patients with brain trauma. Not only the amount of regional edema formation and resolution, but also metabolism and recovery of function strongly depend on the maintenance of CBF. Here, also, a "critical level" exists. Nevertheless, it has been shown during this session that - at least for brain trauma patients - the "classical" concept that CBF decreases when ICP increases does not always hold. Cases have been presented in which tissue acidosis and CBF displayed changes in apparent contradiction to the ICP values. The presence of blood in the subarachnoid space, giving rise to spasm and to alterations in vascular reactivity further complicates the analysis of this topic.

No specific comments on complications due to the methodology of ICP monitoring itself were made during this session. This is probably due, on the one hand, to the fact that pressure is usually recorded from the epidural space in such cases and, on the other hand, to the dramatic clinical condition in which most of these patients are. At any rate, the advantages of monitoring ICP in patients with brain trauma by far outweight the possible risks of the procedure in itself.

Session E

Subarachnoid Hemorrhage

Chairman: L. Symon
Co-chairman: E. Pasztor

Incidence of Hydrocephalus and Increased Ventricular Fluid Pressure in Patients with Ruptured Supratentorial Aneurysms[1]

M. Vapalahti, V. Nieminen, and K. Kari

Introduction

The amnestic syndrome may often complicate the results of aneurysm surgery and even after a technically perfect operation the slow deterioration of the patient may turn early success into a disaster. There are many causes of the organic psychosyndrome, including accidental ligation of important vessels: pericallosal arteries, Heubner's artery, or small perforating arteries. There may be spasm, postoperative hematoma or edema, or bleeding from possible multiple aneurysms. The most common cause is hydrocephalus which may develop either preoperatively or postoperatively. The differential diagnosis is possible only after control angiography, and the planning of the treatment is facilitated by information on intracranial pressure relationships. To study the incidence of hydrocephalus and increased intracranial pressure, we measured in a prospective study the VFP in all patients operated on for aneurysms and who had symptomatic angiographically diagnosed hydrocephalus.

Material and Methods

During 1973-1975 111 consecutive patients were operated on for supratentorial intracranial aneurysms in the University Central Hospital, Turku. The patients usually came into the Neurosurgical Service at about 1 week after their initial bleeding episode, and the operation was performed after angiography, usually during the 2nd or 3rd week (mean 15-16 days) after the SAH. There were 10 patients operated on during the 1st week and 16 after the 3rd week. If there was angiographically verified spasm, the operation was postponed until the symptoms were over. Patients over 60 were not included. The mean age at the series was 42 years, 48 out of 111 were women. The location of the ruptured aneurysm is presented at Table 1. A total of 16 patients had multiple aneurysms and 12 out of 22 intact aneurysms were ligated, usually at the same sitting. All verified ruptured aneurysms were operated on by two neurosurgeons using microtechnique and controlled hypotension. The aneurysm was clipped intracranially in 102 cases, wrapped in 5 cases, and in 3 cases with aneurysm of the ophthalmic artery the common carotid was ligated. One patient died during the induction of the anesthesia from repeat hemorrhage. Total mortality was 17. There were 4 deeply unconscious patients operated acutely, and the removal of their hematomas did not improve the poor outcome. Others had later complications, pulmonary embolism in 2 and infection in 3. There were 9 patients who died from acute complications of surgery, 5 with rupture before or during the clipping and 4 with occlusion or spasm of one major vessel.

[1]This work was supported by a grant from the Emil Aaltonen Foundation.

Table 1. Incidence of hydrocephalus and location of aneurysm in 111 patients

Location of aneurysm	Total Material	Hydrocephalus Patients	incidence
Anterior area	44	13	30%
Anterior cerebral	4	1	
Anterior comm.	35	11	
Pericallosal	5	1	
Middle cerebral	43	5	12%
Internal carotid	24	3	13%
Ophthalmic	3	0	
Posterior comm.	16	3	
Bifurcation	5	0	
Total	111	21	19%

Hydrocephalus was diagnosed from the venous phase of the preoperative or control angiography, the latter being always performed on the second postoperative day.

If the ventricles were enlarged and there were symptoms of hydrocephalus a ventricular (HOLTER) catheter was inserted during the aneurysm operation, VFP-recording was started, and continued 3-4 days. In patients with postoperative symptoms and enlarged ventricles the VFP-recording was started immediately after angiography. If a shunt operation was needed, ventriculoauriculostomy was performed using the same ventricular catheter already in place.

Results

There was marked ventricular enlargement in 21 patients, with preoperative hydrocephalus in 15 and postoperative only in 6 patients. The incidence was significantly higher in aneurysms of the anterior area (30%) as compared with middle cerebral or internal carotid aneurysms having an incidence of 12-13% (Table 1). The VFP-recording was normal in 9 patients (Table 2), in 4 of them the size of the ventricles decreased and these patients made a good recovery. In 5 others the ventricles remained enlarged, the patients got slowly better, but had some residual defect, and all of them clearly had had some vascular complications during SAH or operation. In 12 patients with VFP-record-

Table 2. Ventricular fluid pressure in 21 patients with hydrocephalus after SAH and operation

VFP normal Constantly below 15 mm Hg at end of recording	9
VFP increased	12
Basic VFP normal, small nightly waves over 15 mm Hg	2
Basic VFP increased, pressure waves up to 25 mm Hg	6
Basic VFP constantly over 25 mm Hg, or high plateau waves	4

ing the pressure was increased, 3 of them died before any treatment could be started for their hydrocephalus. In 9 others the pressure was treated by a shunt-operation; 7 made a good recovery and 2 died from later infectious complications one of which was caused by the shunt. Of the 18 patients with both pre- and postoperative angiograms there was verified spasm in 8. The VFP was increased in 7 out of 8 spasm patients but in only 2 out of 10 patients without spasm.

Discussion

The incidence of hydrocephalus after SAH depends on the time after the bleeding at which the ventricular size is evaluated and upon the definition of hydrocephalus. We did not measure the ventricular index (2) prospectively, but it was over 0.30 in all our patients diagnosed with hydrocephalus.

Early hydrocephalus - during the first few days after the SAH - can be seen very frequently, even as often as in 43% of patients (5), and when there is lowered consciousness the VFP certainly will be very high as shown by others (3, 4, 6). Early hydrocephalus may disappear spontaneously, or during treatment such as drainage, but our figures show that the incidence after the 2nd week is still 14%. The operation significantly increases the danger of hydrocephalus, in our series to 19%, which is the same as has been found by others in the subacute phase (2, 9). One possible explanation for postoperative hydrocephalus may be the spasm, even new blood in the CSF. On the other hand, there certainly are patients in whom the opening of basal cisterns will facilitate the recirculation of CSF. Hydrocephalus per se, even with symptoms, is no indication for shunt surgery. In almost half of our patients the VFP was normal and because even the simple shunt operation carries a certain risk, only patients with increased pressure should be operated upon.
Two patients in the material were treated late, 4-5 weeks after the SAH. They both had a NPH-type of pressure recording (7), with normal basic pressure but spontaneous nightly plateaus over 15 mm Hg. It may be possible that those waves totally disappear if measured later (8).

Awaiting the certainly important information of serial computerized tomography studies, the combination of angiography and VFP-recording will be enough to draw the lines of the treatment of these hydrocephalic patients. Symptomatic hydrocephalus with increased VFP is an indication for a shunt 2 weeks after the SAH, and a quick recovery should be the rule. In our material the significantly high correlation of spasm and increased VFP needs further analysis and more material. However, in vitro studies have shown that the combination of high ICP and active vasoconstriction could produce a marked spasm with low blood flow (1).

We do measure VFP in all our aneurysm patients to get more information on the possible role of spasm in developing hydrocephalus and to follow the postoperative course of the patients. We see VFP-recording as especially important in patients with ACA-aneurysms where the incidence of hydrocephalus is high, and differential diagnosis from other complications may be difficult

Summary

The incidence of hydrocephalus in 111 consecutive patients operated on for supratentorial aneurysms, mainly during the 2nd or 3rd week after SAH, was 19%. The incidence was highest, 30%, with anterior communicating aneurysms and 12-13% elsewhere. VFP measured a few days after the operation was normal in 9 and raised in 12 out of 21 hydrocephalic patients. Of the patients with increased VFP, 3 died from primary operation, 9 others were subjected to shunt surgery; 7 patients made a good recovery and 2 others died later. There was a correlation between increased VFP and the incidence of spasm.[2]

References

1. FARRAR, Jr., J.K.: Chronic cerebral arterial spasm. J. Neurosurg. 43, 408-417 (1975).
2. GALERA, R.G., GREITZ, T.: Hydrocephalus in the Adult Secondary to the Rupture of Intracranial Arterial Aneurysms. J. Neurosurg. 32, 634-641 (1970).
3. HAYASHI, M., MARUKAWA, S., FUJII, H., KOBAYASHI, H., YAMAMOTO, S.: Intracranial hypertension in acute stage of ruptured intracranial aneurysms. In: Intracranial Pressure III (J.W.F. BEKS, D.A. BOSCH, M. BROCK, eds.), pp. 162-167. Berlin-Heidelberg-New York: Springer 1976.
4. KUSSKE, J.E., TURNER, P.T., OJEMANN, G.A., HARRIS, A.B.: Ventriculostomy for the treatment of acute hydrocephalus following subarachnoid hemorrhage. J. Neurosurg. 38, 591-595 (1973).
5. PERTUISET, B., HOUTTEVILLE, P., GEORGE, B., MARGENT, B.: Dilatation ventriculaire précoce et hydrocéphalie consécutives à la rupture d'anévrysmes artériels sus-tentoriels. Neurochirurgie 15, 113-126 (1972).
6. SUNDBÄRG, G., PONTEN, U.: ICP and CSF absorption impairment after subarachnoid hemorrhage. In: Intracranial Pressure III (J.W.F. BEKS, D.A. BOSCH, M. BROCK, eds.), pp. 139-146. Berlin-Heidelberg-New York: Springer 1976.
7. SYMON, L., DORSCH, N.W.C.: Use of long-term intracranial pressure measurement to assess hydrocephalic patients prior to shunt surgery. J. Neurosurg. 42, 258-273 (1975).
8. TROUPP, H.: Intracranial Pressure in Hydrocephalus after Subarachnoid Haemorrhage. Zbl. Neurochir. 36, 10-17 (1975).
9. YASARGIL, M.G., YONEKAWA, Y., ZUMSTEIN, B., STAHL, H.-J.: Hydrocephalus following spontaneous subarachnoid hemorrhage. J. Neurosurg. 39, 474-479 (1973).

[2] We thank Dr T. Törmä for allowing patients under his care to be included in this study.

ICP and CSF Absorption Impairment After Subarachnoid Hemorrhage

G. Sundbärg and U. Pontén

Introduction

Subarachnoid hemorrhage (SAH) implies an immediate potential catastrophy but also a high risk of later complications with fatal outcome or lasting morbidity. Raised intracranial pressure (ICP) after SAH has been frequently observed (2, 6, 7, 8). The cause is usually obvious in cases with intracerebral hematomas (5) and/or massive invasion of blood into the ventricular system. In some cases the high ICP is explained by ischemic lesions due to arterial spasm, causing focal cerebral edema. In the long run the development of so-called normal pressure hydrocephalus (NPH) is well known. However, except for this late manifestation of cerebrospinal fluid (CSF) absorptive difficulties, problems appertaining to the CSF dynamics in SAH have been given comparatively little consideration until recent years. It has been shown (1) that posthemorrhagic ventricular dilatation roentgenologically is a frequent finding. Apparently clinically manifest NPH is much more unusual. Several investigators (3, 8, 10) have recently published their experiences with ventricular drainage (VD) *early* after SAH.

Material and Procedures

Most patients with SAH in the region served by the neurosurgical department at the University Hospital in Lund, are admitted early. Since the later part of 1972 patients with clinical signs that might reflect raised ICP, mainly drowsiness, stupor, and coma but also restlessness and/or severe and intolerable headache, underwent continuous ventricular fluid pressure (VFP) recording performed according to LUNDBERG (4). Until October 1975, 127 patients had been investigated according to these indications. The series included 8 patients in very good condition, who were subjected to early aneurysm surgery (day 3-5), as well as 13 patients, who were operated for their aneurysms on the 9th day or later and were subjected to peroperative VFP recording. Table 1 gives the angiographic findings in all 148 patients. Intracranial hematomas were operated according to customary rules in 10 out of the 88 aneurysm patients.

In all patients with a VFP above 15 mm Hg, ventricular fluid was continuously drained into a closed system to a level of 15 mm Hg. The daily amounts of CSF drained were measured. The drain was kept open until the volumes of CSF drained per day were less than 10 ml. If the ventricular catheter was blocked by blood clots and if flushing with small amounts of saline did not restore communication, a new catheter was inserted. Patients who did not spontaneously cease draining within 4 weeks after the last SAH, were treated with a shunt, except two cases, in whom the VFP normalized during digoxin treatment.

Table 1. Angiographic findings in VFP-recorded patients. Hematomas in the "no source of bleeding" group were only minimally expansive

	Indications for VFP recording		
	Symptoms of high ICP	Peroperative	
		Early operation	Late operation
Aneurysm	88	8	12
(Hematoma)	(8)		
Arteriovenous malformation	10		1
(Hematoma)	(2)		
No source of bleeding	29		
(Hematoma)	(14)		
Total	127	8	13
(Hematoma)	(24)		
Total	148		

Results

The initial VFP levels are presented in Figure 1. In 7 of the 127 symptomatic cases and 2 of the 21 peroperative ones the initial VFP was not properly recorded for different reasons and accordingly not presented in the figure. The upper normal limit is considered as 10 mm Hg. Only 8 patients of the remaining 120 in the symptomatic group had an entirely normal initial VFP; 4 of those later had an increased VFP and were drained. The other 4 as well as 6 patients with an initial VFP between 10 and 15 never exceeded 15 mm Hg. In all other patients of the "symptomatic" group an attempt was made to drain CSF. Continuous VD was possible in 99 of 117 cases. Intermittent VD was achieved in 8. In 10 patients VD proved completely unsuccessful; 9 of those died within a few days of massive intraventricular hemorrhage, as found at autopsy. Among the 19 peroperative VFP's there were 7 between 10 and 20 and 1 above 20 mm Hg.

Only 2 of the 127 patients died from purely ischemic complications. Their initial VFP's were not dramatically elevated but the course was that of a progressive intracranial hypertension and finally VD proved impossible. In general the highest VFP's predominated during the first week. In 71 cases continuous VD was uninterrupted by rebleeding (RB), operation, or death of the patient. Of the 8 patients operated within 5 days after the SAH, 7 needed postoperative VD and were included into this group.

1. Of the 71 patients (the early operated cases included), 56 spontaneously ceased draining and showed no signs of hydrocephalus later in the course. The duration of the VD is presented in Table 2. The day of spontaneous cessation of drainage (median 14.5, range 7-22 days) was not influenced by the time that had elapsed between the bleeding and the start of VD. The daily amounts of CSF drained varied widely (Fig. 2). The volume during the 1st day of VD (often less than 24 h) was taken into account only if it exceeded the following volume. Mean daily volumes in this group of patients were around 170 ml during the 1st week. In the course of the 2nd week

Table 2. Duration of ventricular drainage in 56 patients who spontaneously ceased draining and did not develop permanent signs of hydrocephalus. Day 1 refers to last bleeding

```
1 2 3 4 5 6 7 8 9 10 11 12 13 14 15 16 17 18 19 20 21 22 Day

1-----------------10
1-----------------------------14
1-----------------------------14
1--------------------------------------17
  2---------7
  2-----------------11
  2-----------------11
  2-----------------------13
  2-----------------------13
  2--------------------------14
  2--------------------------14
  2--------------------------14
  2-----------------------------15
  2-------------------------------------18
    3----------9
    3------------------------------16
    3------------------------------16
      4------8
      4----------10
      4------------------13
      4--------------------------16
      4--------------------------16
        5-----8
        5-------9
        5-------9
        5---------10
        5------------------13
        5--------------------14
        5--------------------------16
        5-------------------------------------19
          6-------10
          6----------11
          6----------11
          6-------------12
          6-------------12
          6----------------------15
          6-------------------------16
            7--------11
            7--------11
            7--------------13
            7--------------------15
            7--------------------15
            7--------------------15
              8------11
              8------------13
              8------------13
              8---------------14
                9-----------13
                  10----------14
                  10-------------15
                  10----------------16
                     11----------15
                     11---------------------------------22
                        12----14
                        12--------------17
                        12---------------------20
```

mean volumes gradually decreased and toward the end of the 3rd week only a few patients were still draining. In this group of patients 7 had rebled but only 1 was drained before the last bleeding.

2. The remaining 15 patients continued to drain after the 3rd week or developed NPH later on, although they had finished VD within 3 weeks. Of those, 13 required a shunt but 2 of the 15 cases ceased draining within 10 days after digoxin treatment was started. Of the 15 cases, 6 were rebleeders, 4 of the rebleeders had been drained before the last bleeding. The mean volume drained per day during the 1st week did not differ significantly from the "uncomplicated" 56 patients (Fig. 3).

In the total series of 127 patients there were altogether 54 recent RB's in 34 patients (30 aneurysm cases and 4 with arteriovenous malformations). Of these RB's, 20 occurred during continuous VD in 12 patients. Of these 12 patients, 8 died from the RB, 5 of whom had suffered repeated bleedings. Of the remaining 22 rebleeding patients, 5 died of the RB, 3 of whom had repeated bleedings. The overall incidence of RB was highest during the first 5 days after the initial bleeding. Later on the number was low until after the 20th day, when a moderate increase was noted. Table 3 shows the mortality rate in relation to the number of RB's.

Table 3. Mortality rate in relation to number of rebleedings

Rebleedings	No. of patients	Mortality
1	22	5 (23%)
2	5	2 (40%)
3	5	4 (80%)
4	2	2 (100%)
Total	34	13 (38%)

Discussion

The symptoms used in this study as indications for VFP recording are known to occur in connection with actually increased ICP but they may also be explained by previous brain stem lesions or meningeal irritation. The fact that 9 of 10 patients in the symptomatic group had significantly, sometimes considerably increased VFP while only 4 of the 9 almost asymptomatic patients in the early operated group had a slightly increased VFP corroborates our and others notion that raised ICP is of importance for the symptomatology during the first weeks after SAH. A marked improvement often occurred during VD, especially in patients with very severe headache, restlessness, and high fluctuating BP. Dramatic improvement was also noted in some severely ill patients with acute brain stem stress. A protracted course occurred in many cases, however, and the therapeutical value of VD was difficult to evaluate in these cases.

In this material it was possible to control the VFP at almost normal levels by long-term. continuous VD in all patients with SAH uncomplicated by massive blood invasion in the ventricles or by ischemic brain lesions. The explanation for the increased VFP in the uncomplicated cases must be an increased resistance to the resorption of CSF caused by the blood in the subarachnoid space since large expansive processes were excluded angiographically or operatively removed.

When VD takes place against a constant outflow resistance the amounts of CSF drained per day will indicate the degree of resorption block prevailing. The normal production of CSF in man is around 0.5 l/day (11). The volumes drained were less indicating that the CSF block was only partial. The CSF pathways cleared spontaneously over a 2-3 weeks period in the majority of the patients. The clearance of the CSF pathways most likely was due to the fibrinolytic activity of the CSF and it seemed unrelated to the duration of the VD.

The time course for the resolution of the CSF block and the normalization of the VFP agrees with a vast clinical experience that most patients are not in an optimal condition for operation until 2-3 weeks after a severe SAH and with the recommendation of KLAFTA and HAMBY (2) to wait with operation until ICP is normal.

Almost all patients who did not cease draining within 3 weeks subsequently needed a shunt. The risks of shunt failures are great as long as the CSF is bloody. From a practical point of view it thus seems appropriate to rely upon an external drainage when needed during the first 3-4 weeks after the last SAH, but to insert a permanent shunt as soon as possible later on, if the ICP still is increased.

Repeated RB's worsened the prognosis which is in agreement with previous findings (9).

It has been argued (7) that reduction of ICP might cause an aneurysm to rerupture due to an increased transmural pressure difference. The number of RB's in the present series did not have the magnitude to suggest that RBs were provoked by the VD but no firm conclusions can be drawn on this point. It was often found, however, that previously high and fluctuating arterial pressures tended to normalize and usually decreased more than did the VFP, thus diminishing the transmural pressure and probably lessening the risk for a RB. The systolic hypertension provoked in some patients by the raised ICP and the restlessness is probably more dangerous than a controlled and continuous VD.

It is impossible to statistically assess if VD had any influence upon the incidence or the extent of brain ischemia due to arterial spasm. It should be pointed out, however, that many of these patients are on the brink of focal or global permanent tissue damage. They probably use their autoregulatory capacity to its maximum. In this situation it seems reasonable to assume that even small changes in the perfusion pressure are critical and that continuous VD is a rational treatment. It should be started, however, before ischemic lesions have occurred, which might cause ventricular narrowing and prevent an adequate drainage.

Summary

Increased ICP due to a block in the CSF resorption pathways was found in most patients with recent nontraumatic subarachnoid hemorrhage (SAH) and impairment of consciousness. Usually the pathways cleared spontaneously in about 2 weeks. If CSF resorption still was impaired 4 weeks after the last SAH a permanent shunt was needed. Ventricular drainage is easily accomplished in cases uncomplicated by large hematomas, intraventricular clots or severe ischemic brain lesions. It is the rational treatment when control of the increased ICP is needed in these patients.

References

1. BERGVALL, U., GALERA, R.: Time relationship between subarachnoid haemorrhage, arterial spasm, changes in cerebral circulation and posthaemorrhagic hydrocephalus. Acta Radiol. 9, 229-237 (1969).
2. KLAFTA, L.A., HAMBY, W.B.: Significance of cerebrospinal fluid pressure in determining time of repair of intracranial aneurysms. J. Neurosurg. 31, 217-219 (1969).
3. KUSSKE, J.A., TURNER, P.T., OJEMANN, G.A., HARRIS, A.B.: Ventriculostomy for the treatment of acute hydrocephalus following subarachnoid hemorrhage. J. Neurosurg. 38, 591-595 (1973).
4. LUNDBERG, N.: Continuous recording and control of ventricular fluid pressure in neurosurgical practice. Acta Psych. Scand. Suppl. 149, 1-193 (1960).
5. MILHORAT, T.H.: Intracerebral hemorrhage, acute hydrocephalus and systemic hypertension. J.A.M.A. 218, 221-225 (1971).
6. NORNES, H., MAGNAES, B.: Intracranial pressure in patients with ruptured saccular aneurysms. J. Neurosurg. 36, 537-547 (1972).
7. NORNES, H.: The role of intracranial pressure in the arrest of hemorrhage in patients with ruptured intracranial aneurysms. J. Neurosurg. 39, 226-234 (1973).
8. PONTEN, U., KÅGSTRÖM, E., SUNDBÄRG, G.: Ventricular fluid drainage after subarachnoid hemorrhage. Excerpta Med. 293, 49 (1973).
9. STEINER, L.: Recurrent subarachnoid hemorrhage. An experimental study. Stockholm: Thesis 1975.
10. SUZUKI, J., YOSHIMOTO, T., HARI, S.: Continuous ventricular drainage to lessen surgical risk in ruptured intracranial aneurysm. Surg. Neurol. 2, 87-90 (1974).
11. WELCH, K.: The principles of physiology of the cerebrospinal fluid in relation to hydrocephalus including normal pressure hydrocephalus. In: Advances in Neurology, Vol. 13: Current Reviews (W.J. FRIEDLANDER, ed.), pp. 247-332. New York: Raven Press 1975.

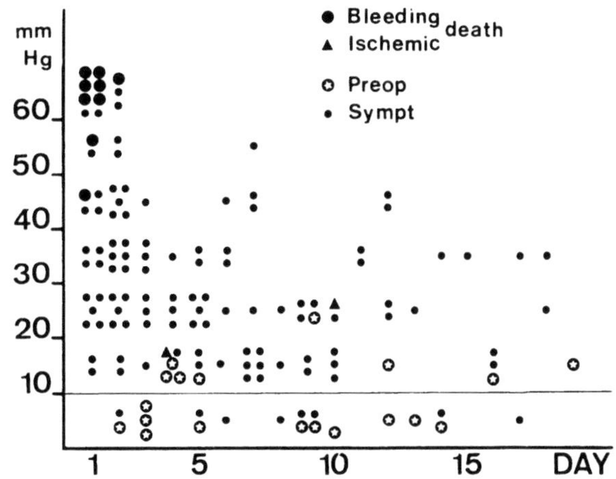

Fig. 1. Initial VFP levels after subarachnoid hemorrhage. Day 1 refers to last bleeding. Individual pressures are grouped according to pressure intervals of 10 mm Hg and day after SAH. All values above 60 are grouped together

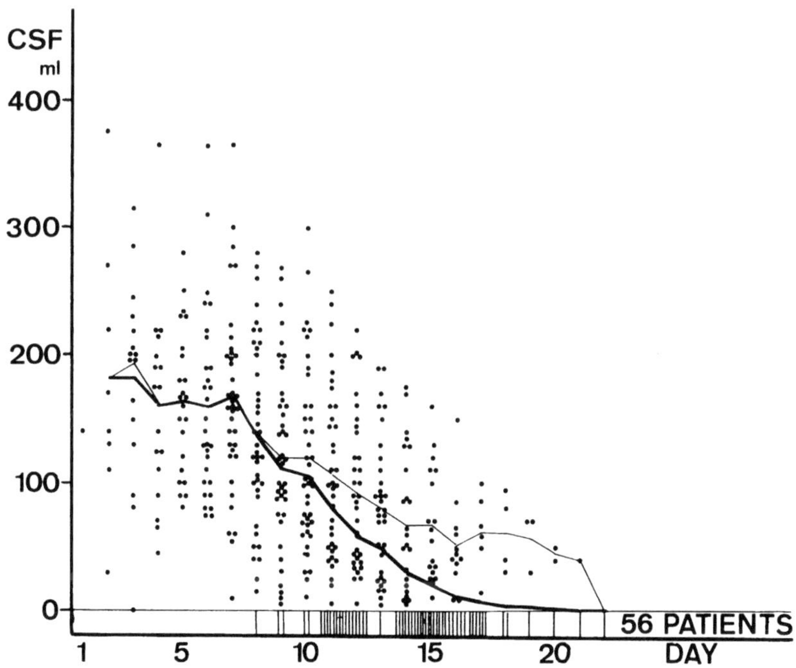

Fig. 2. CSF volumes drained per day in 56 patients, who spontaneously ceased draining and showed no signs of hydrocephalus in the long run. Thick line denotes mean values for all patients, thin line mean drained volumes, zero-drainage excluded. Vertical lines below zero-line denote when individual patients ceased to drain. Day 1 refers to day of last bleeding. Causes of SAH: Aneurysm 35 (7 early operated patients), AVM 3, unknown source 18

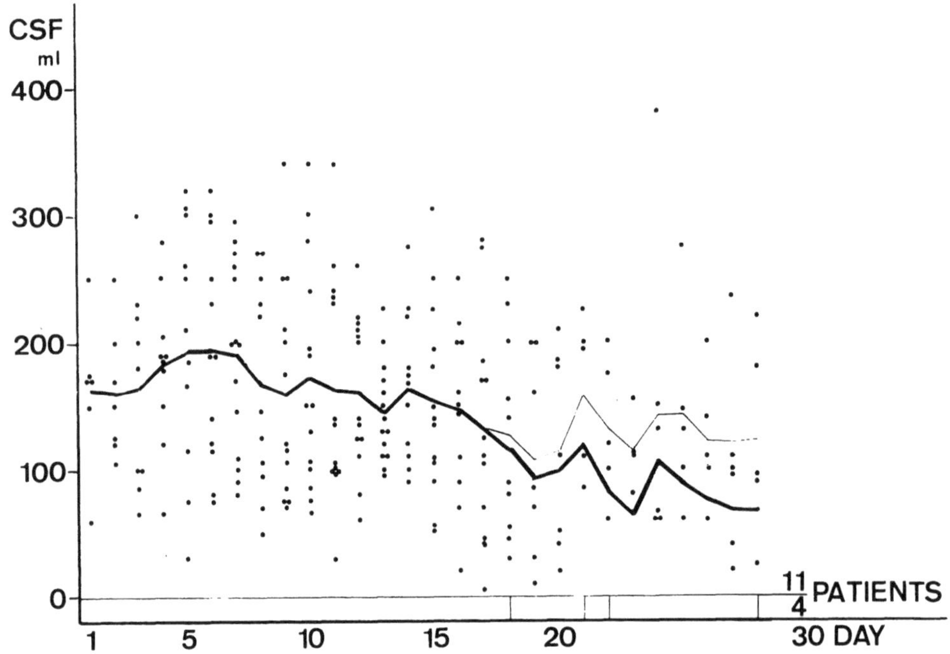

Fig. 3. CSF volumes drained per day in 15 patients, who did not cease drainage within 3 weeks or who later on developed normal pressure hydrocephalus. There were 13 patients shunted and 2 ceased draining during digoxin treatment. Thick line denotes mean values for all patients, thin line mean drained volumes, zero-drainage excluded. Vertical lines below zero-line denote when 4 patients ceased to drain. Day 1 refers to day of last bleeding. Causes of SAH: aneurysm 10, unknown source 5

ICP, Aneurysms, and Subarachnoid Hemorrhage

N.F. Kassell, S.J. Peerless, and P.L. Reilly

Introduction

The overall morbidity and mortality in subarachnoid hemorrhage (SAH) and intracranial aneurysm surgery remains unacceptably high. Pathophysiologically, SAH is complicated out of proportion to the benign anatomical appearance of the underlying vascular lesion. The final common factors producing an unfavorable outcome are decreased cerebral blood flow, ischemia, and infarction. Perfusion pressure is the major variable related to cerebral blood flow and accessible to therapeutic manipulation, thus, ICP should be as important as systemic blood pressure in the management of these patients. Furthermore, a slack brain is essential for satisfactory surgical results. ICP should be an important parameter in anticipating the state of the brain.

Material and Methods

The patients in this series were randomly selected from those cases of cerebral arterial aneurysm and/or SAH admitted to the Neurosurgical Unit in London, Ontario between July 1, 1975 and April 15, 1976. ICP was measured from the lateral ventricle, cerebral subdural space, or spinal subarachnoid space alone or in combination for comparison. ICP catheters were connected to Bentley Trantec transducers zeroed at the level of the external auditory meatus. Pressures were monitored with an HP digital pressure module. Wave forms were displayed on an oscilloscope and permanent records made on a Gould Model 280 strip chart recorder. ICP was transcribed to the patients chart at intervals along with other vital parameters.

Results

A total of 30 patients with SAH and/or aneurysm had ICP monitored from between 1 and 10 days (mean = 3.2). In 5 patients ICP was measured from the lateral ventricle, in 7 from the spinal subarachnoid space, in 1 from the cerebral subdural space, in 2 simultaneously from the lateral ventricle and spinal subarachnoid space and in 15 from the cerebral subdural space and spinal subarachnoid space. There were no infections, hematomas, or other complications attributable to the ICP measuring techniques. Pressure measured from the spinal subarachnoid space accurately reflected intracranial pressure, although there was moderate damping of the wave form (2). Another 6 patients had ICP monitored preoperatively between 1 and 10 days (mean = 6.83), 23 postoperatively between 1 and 5 days (mean = 2.18), and 1 both pre- and postoperatively for 5 days total (Table 1). In the 7 patients monitored preoperatively the mean ICP was 51.3 ± 19.3 and in the 24 patients monitored postoperatively 29.7 ± 9.4. A variety of pressure waves were observed. B waves were most common; plateau waves occurred in 1 patient.

Table 1. Distribution of ICP

	ICP					
	15	16-30	31-45	45-60	60	Total
Preoperative	0	1	3	1	2	7
Postoperative	0	13	10	1	0	24
Total	0	14	13	2	2	31

Table 2. Postoperative ICP and timing of surgery

	Recent	Old and Intact
No.	13	11
Mean	30.1	23
SD	6.8	8.9

Table 3. ICP and aneurysm location

	Anterior	Posterior
No.	11	18
Mean	37	32.6
SD	21	11.3

Table 4. ICP and clinical grade

	III	IV
No.	3	4
Mean	33.3	58.2
SD	3.1	24.7

Table 5. Postoperative ICP and early outcome

	Excellent	Good	Poor
No.	10	7	7
Mean	24	30.3	37.1
SD	6.3	5.6	11.5

Patients with recent SAH (totalling 6) were monitored preoperatively, 13 postoperatively, and 1 in both periods; 11 patients with intact aneurysms (7) or old SAH (4) were monitored postoperatively. Patients with recent SAH had higher ICP's (mean 36.1 ± 6.8) postoperatively than patients operated with intact aneurysms or old SAH (mean 23.0 ± 8.9) (Table 2).

There were 11 patients who had anterior circulation aneurysms, 18 posterior circulation, and 1 none. There were no differences in ICP based on site of aneurysm (Table 3).

In the 7 preoperative patients 3 were Grade III with a mean ICP of 33.3 ± 3.06 and 4 were Grade IV with a mean ICP 58.3 ± 24.72 (Table 4). The postoperative ICP in patients with excellent results were significantly lower than those with good results which in turn were lower than those with poor results (Table 5). An ICP greater than 40 torr, pre- or postoperatively was ominous and all patients exhibiting ICP greater than 50 torr had a poor outcome.

In 3 patients rebleeding occurred during the preoperative period. In 2 this occurred during spinal fluid drainage to less than 15 torr, and 1 patient exhibited multiple "warning episodes" (3) prior to rebleeding fatally.

The most frequent causes of elevated ICP were spasm, hydrocephalus, and brain swelling alone or in combination (Table 6). During the preoperative period intracranial pressure required treatment in 5 patients and in the postoperative period in 3 (Table 7). All patients with elevated ICP received dexamethasone. CSF drainage to less than 25 torr was used in 6 patients, 5 preoperatively and 1 postoperatively. Mannitol at 1 gm/kg was used in 5 patients and Furosemide in 2.

Table 6. ICP and pathology

	Preoperative	Postoperative	Total
Brain swelling	0	0	0
Hydrocephalus	2	2	4
Spasm	0	2	2
Spasm and brain swelling	2	4	6
Spasm and hydrocephalus	2	0	2
Intracerebral hematoma	0	1	1
Subdural hematoma	0	0	0
Epidural hematoma	0	1	1

Table 7. Treatment of increased ICP

	Preoperative	Postoperative	Total
Decadron	5	3	8
Mannitol	2	3	5
Furosemide	2	0	2
CSF drainage	4	1	5
Hyperventilation	0	1	1

Discussion

Is ICP a valuable parameter in the management of patients with SAH and/or aneurysm? Does the information gained justify the effort and risks involved? In which patients should it be measured? How? When? What does it mean?

The value of ICP measurements in these patients can be determined definitively only by a randomized controlled series studying the morbidity and mortality in cases with and without ICP monitoring. It is unlikely that such a study will ever be performed, since the importance of monitoring ICP has firm theoretical basis, there is abundant anecdotal evidence supporting its value, and the measurements can be accomplished with minimal effort and risk (1, 4).

Many of the poor results in these patients are clearly the result of ischemic events. Therefore, any parameter directly related to perfusion pressure and blood flow is obviously important. The basic pathophysiologic processes operant in SAH and aneurysm surgery are similar to those in other conditions of neurosurgical interest where measurement of ICP is a well-established and accepted practice.

In this series only patients Grade III or IV were monitored preoperatively. While they were helped by having ICP measurements, irreversible deficit had occurred by the time monitoring and therapy were instituted. It is perhaps the Grade I and II patients who can benefit most. Postoperatively, ICP was measured until the patients were clinically stable and angiography had been performed.

ICP may be measured from the lateral ventricle, cerebral subdural space, or spinal subarachnoid space. In patients with SAH it is important to be able to sample and drain CSF. Intraventricular pressure is most useful in preoperative patients with extremely high ICP and/or mass effect. Spinal subarachnoid pressure is appropriate for Grade I and II patients preoperatively and all patients postoperatively. A continuous recording of ICP is desirable; however, intermittent measurement along with other vital parameters is probably satisfactory although more sophisticated display and analysis techniques may prove beneficial.

In conclusion, ICP is a useful parameter in timing of surgery (along with clinical Grade and degree of spasm), prediction and detection of rebleeding, determining etiology of neurological deterioration, and rational use of CSF drainage, diuretics, hyperventilation, etc., in the control of intracranial hypertension.

Measurement of ICP does not entail undue risks. Spinal subarachnoid space pressure is safe and reliable in selected patients. ICP monitoring techniques provide direct additional diagnostic and therapeutic benefits with access to the CSF for sampling and drainage.

Preoperatively, increased ICP is common. Postoperatively, it is also common, but when it exceeds 40 torr, it often forewarns of a complicated course. CSF removal is an effective means of controlling intracranial hypertension, but drainage to less than 15 torr may precipitate rebleeding (5). Small reductions in increased ICP may be accompanied by significant clinical improvement. Pressure waves are common; except for plateau waves, their clinical significance was uncertain.

Summary

ICP was monitored in 30 patients with SAH and/or aneurysms. Intracranial hypertension was common both pre- and postoperatively. Pressure waves were frequent, but plateau waves rare. Postoperative ICP was highest with recent SAH. There was no relationship between ICP and aneurysm location. A positive correlation existed between ICP and outcome. ICP greater than 50 was uniformly associated with a poor outcome. The most common findings in increased ICP were spasm, hydrocephalus, and brain swelling. ICP monitoring was safe and provided ready access to CSF sampling and drainage.

References

1. JOHNSTON, I.H., JENNETT, W.B.: The place of continuous intracranial pressure monitoring in neurosurgical practice. Acta Neurochirurgica 29, 53-63 (1973).
2. KASSELL, N.F., PEERLESS, S.J.: ICP monitoring from spinal subarachnoid space in intracranial aneurysms and subarachnoid hemorrhage. In preparation.
3. NORNES, H.: Intracranial pressure in patients with ruptured saccular aneurysm. J. Neurosurg. 36, 537-547 (1972).
4. NORNES, H.: Monitoring of patients with intracranial aneurysms. In: Clinical Neurosurgery, Vol. 22 (R.H. WILKINS, E.B. KEENER, J.C. MAROON, H. FRIEDMAN, G. MAGID, P.W. CARMEL, eds.), pp. 321-331. Baltimore: Williams and Wilkins 1975.

5. PONTEN, U., KAGSTROM, E., SUNDBARG, G.: Ventricular fluid drainage after subarachnoid hemorrhage, In: 5th International Congress of Neurological Surgery, Congress Series, No. 253 (R. CARNEA, S. ISHII, D. LeVRY, eds.), p. 49. Amsterdam: Excerpta Medica 1973.

An Analysis of Postoperative Time Course of ICP in 35 Cases with Intracranial Aneurysms

H. Takagi, K. Yada, T. Ohwada, and T. Saito

Introduction

The purpose of this study is to analyze the correlation between preoperative factors and the postoperative time course of ICP following intracranial surgery of aneurysms.

Material and Methods

This study consists of 35 patients admitted with subarachnoid hemorrhage (SAH) due to rupture of aneurysms. Cases that had aneurysms of the vertebrobasilar artery were excluded from this study because there were many complicating factors. The necks of all aneurysms were clipped successfully with microsurgical technique. There were no cases that developed a postoperative hematoma. There was one postoperative death.

To measure ICP, a small rubber balloon was placed under the dura at the time of dural closure (2). The balloon was inflated with 0.2-0.3 ml of normal saline and was connected to the strain gauge pressure transducer via a polyethylene catheter. The ICP then was recorded by using a pen writing oscillograph with a laboratory recorder. The paper speed has been set at 2 cm/h. By using low speed, it became possible to observe at a glance the pattern of the postoperative time course of ICP over a long period. Duration of recordings in this series ranged from 16 h to 22 days.

The postoperative time course thus recorded was analyzed according to the elevation curves and the level of maximum ICP following the surgery of aneurysms.

Relationships between preoperative factors and the types of postoperative time course of ICP were analyzed. Preoperative factors that have been subjected to this analysis are the following: (1) number of SAH, (2) site of aneurysm, (3) arterial spasm as demonstrated by angiography, (4) clinical grade as described by HUNT and HESS (1), and (5) interval from last SAH to operation.

Results

1. Postoperative Time Course of ICP

According to the types of postoperative time course of ICP the authors found that these types fell into the following four groups (Fig. 1).

Group 1: ICP gradually elevates to reach a first plateau approx. 10-12 h after the operation and does not exceed 18 mm Hg throughout the time course. There were 11 such cases.

Group 2: Pattern of elevation of ICP is similar to that of group 1, but the range of the first plateau is higher than that of group 1 (18-30 mm Hg). There were 8 such cases.

Group 3: ICP elevates more rapidly than in groups 1 and 2 and ICP at the moment of the first plateau exceeds 37 mm Hg. There were 3 such cases. Two cases required administration of a hypertonic solution to control ICP.

Group 4: All those cases required ventricular drainage to control ICP as judged at the time of surgery. There were 13 such cases. Among the 13 cases, 6 cases required a hypertonic solution to control ICP as the ventricular drainage was obstructed due to severe cerebral swelling. All the cases required a ventricular drainage to control ICP for at least 3 days following surgery.

2. *Relationships Between the Preoperative Factors and the Types of ICP as Grouped Above*

By analyzing the relationships between the above-mentioned five factors and the types of postoperative ICP, we couldn't find statistically significant relationships between either number of SAH or site of aneurysms and postoperative ICP patterns. The authors found that the following three factors have a statistically significant influence upon the postoperative ICP (Tables 1, 2, 3).

Table 1. Correlation between preoperative arterial spasm and postoperative time course of ICP

	Arterial spasm	Recognized	Not recognized
ICP Group	Group 1	1	10
	Group 2	4	4
	Group 3	3	
	Group 4	3	10
		P < 0.02	Total 35

Table 2. Correlation between clinical grade (HUNT and HESS) and postoperative time course of ICP

	Clinical grade	I	II	III	IV	V
ICP Group	Group 1	6	4	1		
	Group 2	2	6			
	Group 3	1	2			
	Group 4	3	2	2	2	4
		P < 0.05		Total 35		

Table 3. Correlation between interval from last SAH to operation and postoperative time course of ICP

	Interval	-1	1-3	4-7	8-14	15-28	29- days
ICP Group	Group 1					1	10(1)
	Group 2			1	2(2)	2(2)	3
	Group 3			1(1)	2(2)		
	Group 4	5	4	4(3)			
		P < 0.001			Total 35		

( ): Arterial spasm.

(1) arterial spasm ($P < 0.02$), (2) clinical grade ($P < 0.05$), and (3) interval from last SAH to operation ($P < 0.001$).
Although of these three factors each in itself seems to have a statistically significant influence upon the postoperative ICP, one must consider that these factors have close relationships among themselves also. As shown in Table 3, 8 out of 11 cases with arterial spasm were operated upon within 14 days. Furthermore, as demonstrated in Figure 2, all the cases in clinical grade IV and V were operated upon within 7 days following the last SAH. Therefore, it can be concluded that the most significant one among these three factors is the interval from last SAH to operation.

Discussion

By measuring ICP following SAH, NORNES and MAGNES (3) have pointed out that the optimal time for radical surgery should be 8 to 14 days after the last SAH, when the ICP falls down to 15-30 mm Hg. The results of the present study also suggest that the patients who are operated upon in early stages must be watched carefully for marked elevation of ICP following surgery.

Presence of arterial spasm and low clinical grade must also be considered seriously as adding factors to facilitate the elevation of postoperative ICP. However, the authors have become convinced that the elevation of ICP following surgery in these cases can be well controlled by monitoring ICP with the use of the subdural balloon method. When using this method, combination of ventricular drainage and administration of a hypertonic solution can be applied adequately for controlling ICP. As a result, although many of our cases were operated upon in early stages and in low clinical grades, only one operative death occurred in this entire series.

Summary

By observing the postoperative time course of ICP in cases with aneurysms, four groups could be recognized.

Preoperative factors such as interval from last SAH to operation, arterial spasm and clinical grade, as described by HUNT and HESS (1), showed a significant correlation to these four groups of ICP types. The authors would like to stress that continuous monitoring of ICP is effective to lessen the operative mortality of those patients whose clinical grade is lower than III, or whose operation is performed within 7 days following the last SAH.

Key Words

Intracranial pressure, Subarachnoid hemorrhage, Intracranial aneurysm.

References

1. HUNT, W.E., HESS, R.M.: Surgical risk as related to time of intervention in the repair of intracranial aneurysm. J. Neurosurg. 28, 14-20 (1968).
2. NAKAGAWA, T., YADA, K., MITSUO, T.: Clinical significance of ICP measurements following intracranial surgery. In: Intracranial Pressure II (N. LUNDBERG, U. PONTEN, M. BROCK, eds.), pp. 350-354. Berlin-Heidelberg-New York: Springer 1975.
3. NORNES, H., MAGNES, B.: Intracranial pressure in patients with saccular aneurysm. J. Neurosurg. 36, 537-547 (1972).

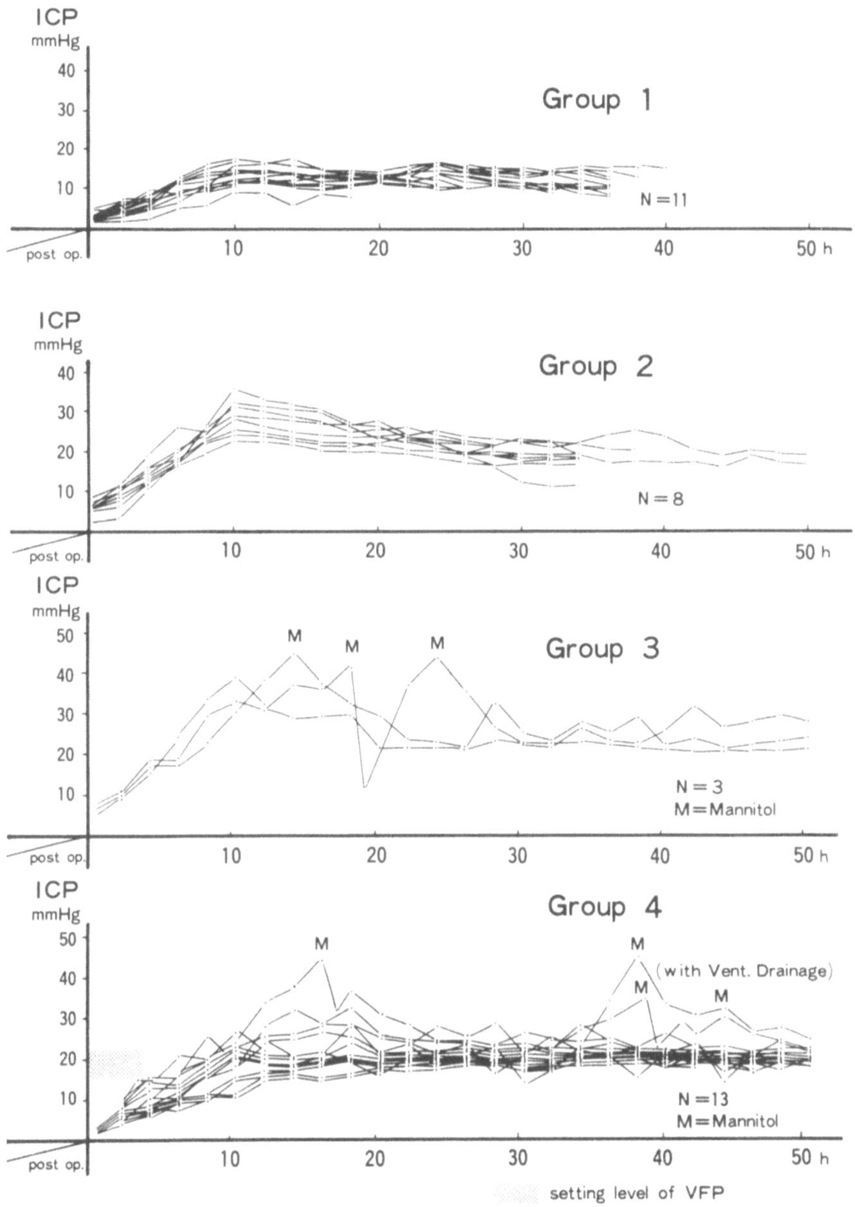

Fig. 1. Four groups of postoperative time course of ICP in 35 patients with aneurysm

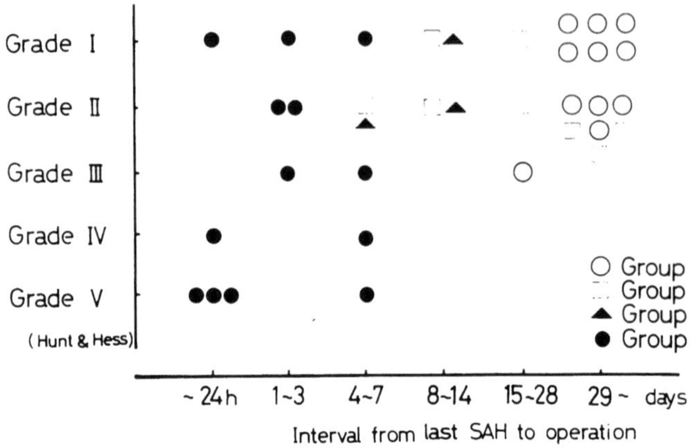

Fig. 2. Distribution of each postoperative ICP group in relationship with clinical grade (HUNT and HESS) and interval from last SAH to operation

Mean Intracranial Resting Pressure, Episodic Pressure Fluctuations, and Intracranial Volume/Pressure Response in Patients with Subarachnoid Hemorrhage

J. Hamer and A. Kühner

Introduction

It is well known that craniotomy for direct repair of ruptured cerebral aneurysms in patients with grade IV and V according to the grading system of HUNT and HESS (1) has a high operative mortality. For this reason, grade IV and V patients are usually excluded from surgery. A special problem, however, is the neurosurgical management of grade III patients. In these cases, too, operative risk is much higher than in grade I or II where early operation is indicated. On the other hand, there exists always the danger for grade III patients to deteriorate and to fall into the next most unfavorable groups IV and V and to suffer a lethal rebleeding. In this group it is particularly difficult to assess the right time for neurosurgical intervention. Thus, better knowledge about the causes for the operative risks is most desirable. KLAFTA and HAMBY (2) have shown in grade III patients that operative mortality was considerably reduced when the CSF pressure had fallen below 200 mm H_2O (i.e., 15 torr). Furthermore, KUSSKE and coworkers (3) have recently observed that external drainage of ventricular CSF may improve the patient's condition from grade V or IV to the next lower grade. These findings would suggest that raised intracranial pressure plays a significant role in patients with grade III to V.

The present clinical investigations were limited to patients with grade III in the acute stage of SAH (i.e., 1 to 10 days after the first aneurysmal rupture). This study contributes to the questions: (a) whether and to what extent raised intracranial pressure is involved, (b) whether episodic pressure waves do occur, and (c) how is the intracranial pressure-volume relationship.

Materials and Methods

From this series of grade III patients, all cases with arterial hypertension, disturbances of arterial blood gases, and with angiographically verified intracerebral hematoma were excluded. Thus, seven patients form the basis of the present clinical study. Intraventricular fluid pressure (VFP) was measured according to the LUNDBERG technique and continuously monitored from 1 to 5 days with the mean being 3 days. VFP was recorded both as electronically determined mean pressure (mVFP) and as pressure pulsations. During the total period of continuous pressure recording the mean pressures were stored in time-intervals of 15 min. Later, the basal resting pressure for each patient was calculated as the arithmetical mean of the total sum of the stored mean pressure values. Ventricular size was examined by ventriculography or by echoencephalography. In none of the cases, marked hydrocephalus (i.e. a dilatation of the third ventricle over 10 mm) was observed. 24 h after continuous intracranial pressure monitoring has been started, the intraventricular pressure-volume relationship was tested as described by MILLER et al. (5,6). The upper limit of artificially increased mVFP was kept to about 40 mm Hg. Altogether, 19 volume-pressure tests could be performed in this series. In no instance was the clinical condition worsened by this pressure-volume test. During the time of continuous pressure recording no aneurysmal bleeding occurred. The patients did not receive steroids or dehydrating agents. Ventricular CSF drainage was not instituted.

Results

The mean resting intraventricular fluid pressure (mVFP) varied in the range of 10-25 mm Hg, the mean value (n=7) being 14.1 mm Hg (SD ± 4.6 mm Hg). Plateau waves with markedly increased intracranial pressures were never observed. Episodic pressure fluctuations with a mean pressure increase of about 10 mm Hg and a mean duration of 100 s were frequently seen, in particular during sleeping (Fig. 1). There was a close linear correlation between the resting mVFP and the pressure increase after artificial intraventricular volume addition (Fig. 2). Another very close correlation was found between the pressure increase and the corresponding rise in CSF pulse amplitude (Figs. 3 and 4).

Discussion

The present findings indicate that in the acute stage of SAH in grade III patients intracranial base line pressure is moderately increased or at the upper limit of normal. These pressure values are consistent with recent findings in grade III patients by KUSSKE et al. (3) who found pressures bwtween 14 and 30 torr. In accordance with the observations of NORNES et al. (7), plateau waves of type A did not occur in this series. As there was no rebleeding in our patients, we neither observed the marked pressure increases of the so-called "warning episodes" that, as NORNES (7) has shown, may occur some hours before a rupture of the aneurysm. The episodic short lasting pressure variations in our case material resemble the B waves. The occurrence of similar waves has also been demonstrated during long-term intracranial pressure measurement in adult patients with nontumorous hydrocephalus (8), but the relatively small pressure increase of such B waves is probably of minor pathophysiologic significance. The present findings show that the clinical condition of grade III patients, in the acute phase of SAH, is not explained by high intracranial pressures or by episodic marked pressure waves. KLAFTA and HAMBY (2) have already emphasized that in these cases "the elevated pressure is not considered to be primarily significant, but rather, that it indicates a brain remaining in a state of injury." The pressure-volume relationship in our cases allows us to describe this "state of injury" as a disturbed intracranial volumetric compensatory capacity due to a marked change in cerebral compliance. LÖFGREN (4) has shown that the pressure-volume curve of the intracranial CSF spaces has a critical breakpoint at about 15 mm Hg. Beyond this pressure, intracranial elastance rapidly changes from a state of low to a state of high elastance. These experimental findings would fit in with the present clinical observations in grade III patients whose mean resting pressure varied just in this critical pressure range. The causes for disturbed cerebral compliance may be related to three main factors: (a) to brain edema as the sequel of high intracranial pressure at the time of bleeding and of ischemic hypoxia, (b) to disturbed CSF passage in the basal cisterns due to blood in the CSF, and finally (c) the third important factor may be altered cerebrovascular reactivity with a diminished damping of the systemic arterial pressure head in the arteriolar and capillary bed of the brain. This is indicated by the close relationship between the increase of intracranial pressure and the marked rise in cerebral pulse amplitude. The disturbance of the volumetric compensatory capacity easily explains why, in grade III patients, even a moderate increase of arterial blood pressure or moderate hypercapnic or hypoxemic cerebral hyperemia must have a considerable and deleterious pressure raising effect in the brain.

As to practical therapy, some questions are still open to discussion. The results of KUSSKE and coworkers (3) would favor the temporary external shunting of ventricular CSF. On the other hand, one should take into account the risk of a rebleeding, in particular when the pressure is rapidly dropped in the first days after aneurysmal rupture. Recently MILLER and LEECH (6) have shown in patients that betamethasone favorably alters the volume-pressure curve. If this can be confirmed in grade III patients, we would have a rational and probably causal therapy for treating altered cerebral compliance.

Summary

The present findings show that in grade III patients suffering from SAH, intracranial pressure is moderately increased or at the upper limit of normal. The volume-pressure response in these cases demonstrated an altered volumetric compensatory capacity of the brain. The close relationship between pressure increase and rise in cerebral pressure pulse amplitude indicated a disturbed cerebrovascular reactivity with diminished damping of the systemic arterial pulse in the cerebral vasculature.

Key Words

Subarachnoid hemorrhage, Volume-pressure relationship, Cerebral pulse amplitude.

References

1. HUNT, W.E., HESS, R.M.: Surgical risk as related to time of intervention in the repair of intracranial aneurysms. J. Neurosurg. 28, 14-20 (1968).
2. KLAFTA, L.A., HAMBY, W.B.: Significance of cerebrospinal fluid pressure in determining time for repair of intracranial aneurysms. J. Neurosurg. 31, 217-219 (1969).
3. KUSSKE, J.A., TURNER, P.T., OJEMANN, G.A., HARRIS, B.: Ventriculostomy for the treatment of acute hydrocephalus following subarachnoid hemorrhage. J. Neurosurg. 38, 591-595 (1973).
4. LÖFGREN, J., VON ESSEN, C., ZWETNOW, N.N.: The pressure volume curve of the cerebrospinal fluid spaces in dogs. Acta Neurol. Scand. 49, 557-574 (1973).
5. MILLER, J.D., GARIBI, J., PICKARD, J.D.: Induced changes of cerebrospinal fluid volume. Effects during continuous monitoring of ventricular fluid pressure. Arch. Neurol. 28, 265-269 (1973).
6. MILLER, J.D., LEECH, P.: Effects of mannitol and steroid therapy on intracranial volume-pressure relationships in patients. J. Neurosurg. 42, 274-281 (1975).
7. NORNES, H., MAGNES, B.: Intracranial pressure in patients with ruptured saccular aneurysm. J. Neurosurg. 36, 537-547 (1972).
8. SYMON, L., DORSCH, N.W.: Use of long-term intracranial pressure measurement to assess hydrocephalic patients prior to shunt surgery. J. Neurosurg. 42, 258-273 (1975).

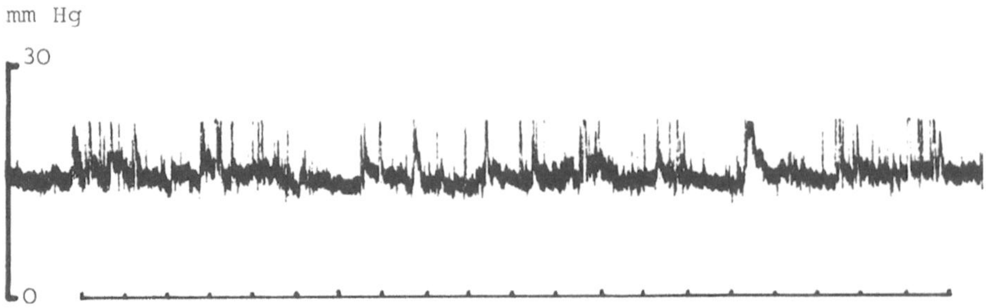

Fig. 1. Episodic intracranial pressure fluctuations with B-wave activity during sleep. Time scale: 2 min

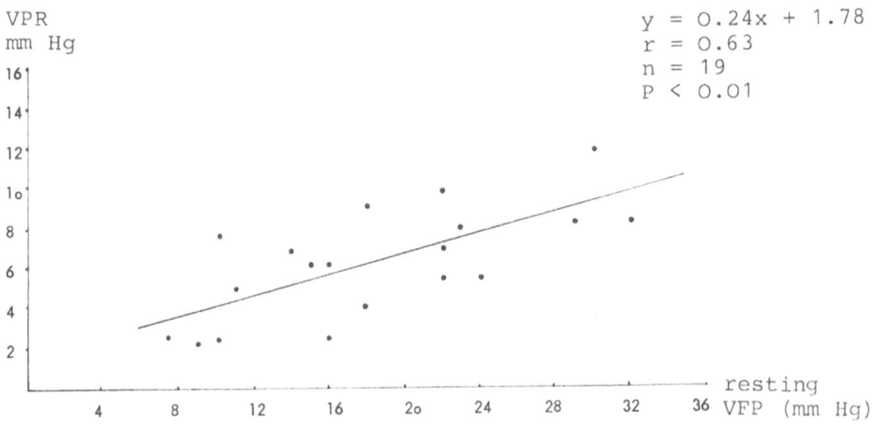

Fig. 2. Relationship between mean resting ventricular fluid pressure (VFP, abscissa) and increase in VFP/2 ml of saline solution injected into lateral ventricle (volume-pressure response, VPR, ordinate). Regression line is drawn and equation is given

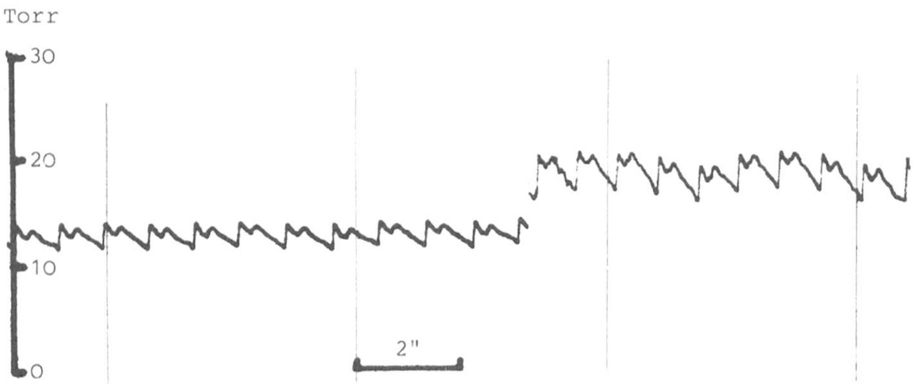

Fig. 3. This figure shows the increase in cerebral pulse amplitude after artificial elevation of ventricular fluid pressure (Time scale: 2 s)

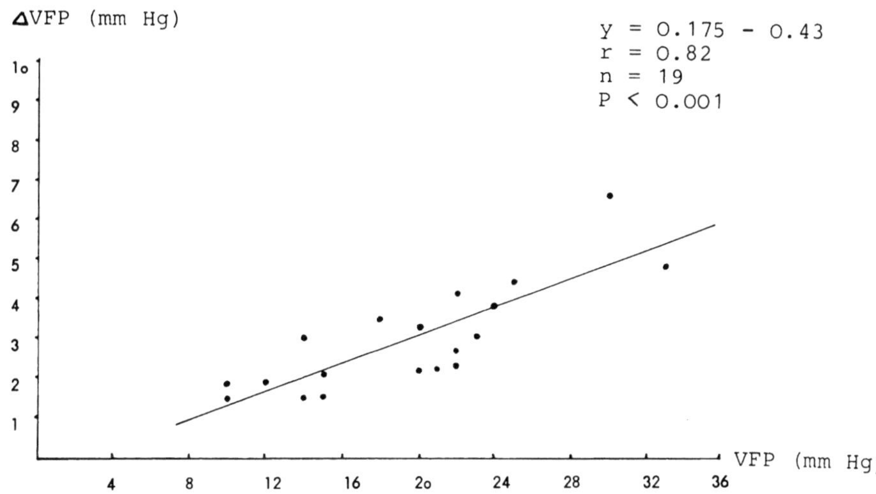

Fig. 4. Relationship between mean ventricular fluid pressure (VFP) and increase in pulse amplitude (ΔVFP). Regression line and equation are shown

Intracranial Hypertension in Acute Stage of Ruptured Intracranial Aneurysm

M. Hayashi, S. Marukawa, H. Fujii, T. Kitano, H. Kobayashi, and S. Yamamoto

Introduction

The purpose of this investigation is to study the correlations between the level of consciousness, the rate of intracranial pressure (ICP), and the prognosis in patients with recently ruptured intracranial aneurysm.

Material and Methods

The series consists of 26 patients admitted within 1 week after subarachnoid hemorrhage due to a ruptured intracranial aneurysm; each of these patients was unfit for immediate surgery. Patients were graded according to the method of HUNT and HESS (1). Patients with the complication of an intracerebral hematoma were omitted in this report.

ICP was recorded with the aid of an indwelling ventricular and/or lumbar subarachnoid catheter connected with a pressure transducer. Ventricular fluid pressure recording was made in the 3 Grade III patients and all 13 of the Grade IV and V patients. Lumbar subarachnoid pressure recording was made in the 10 Grade III patients. The lumbar subarachnoid pressure recording method was used only for the Grade III patients who showed no signs of obstruction of cerebrospinal fluid pathways.

Systemic blood pressure (SBP) was recorded simultaneously in all patients through an intra-arterial catheter placed in the femoral artery. ICP and SBP were continuously recorded on a two channel paper-chart recorder for 1 to 5 days.

In this series, intracranial direct operation was carried out in 22 patients using the microsurgical technique, and in the remaining 4 patients, who were in a Grade V state, only continuous ventricular drainage was done.

Results

Satisfactory recordings were obtained in all patients. There have been no complications attributed to the indwelling catheters, such as intracerebral hemorrhage or infection.

Clinical Grade and Mean ICP

Figure 1 shows a correlation between the clinical grade and mean ICP. The mean ICP level ranged from 15 to 40 mm Hg in Grade III patients, from 30 to 75 mm Hg in Grade IV patients and exceeded 75 mm Hg in Grade V patients. Only 1 of the 15 Grade III patients died of diffuse vasospasm that developed after surgery. The remaining 14 patients of this group survived and the quality of survival was good in all of them.

All 4 of the Grade IV patients survived, but 3 of them showed severe residual neurologic deficits. All the Grade V patients died of severe intracranial hypertension within 5 days after the last rupture.

Cerebral Vasospasm

At arteriography cerebral vasospasm was observed in 12 of the 26 patients (46%); one out of the 5 Grade V patients; 5 out of the 8 Grade IV patients; and 6 out of the 13 Grade III patients. In all the cases the vasospasm was of the localized type. There was no definite correlation between the severity of vasospasm and the clinical grade.

Pressure Patterns in Grade III and IV Patients

The continuous ICP recording in the 21 Grade III and IV patients showed a marked tendency to rapid variations superimposed upon the increased ICP base line. These pressure variations were in fact recurring increases in ICP to values of 15-20 mm Hg in Grade III and 30-45 mm Hg in Grade IV patients. Analysis of the waves revealed only two types of variations, one related to periodic breathing of the Cheyne-Stokes' type (B-wave) and the other to Traube-Hering-Mayer waves of SBP (C-waves), as described by LUNDBERG (4). In our series of ICP recordings, we never observed a typical plateau wave. Figure 2 shows an example of marked ICP fluctuations in Grade IV patients.

Pressure Patterns in Grade V Patients

Figure 3 shows the trace of ICP in a patient going worse from Grade IV to V. Frequent ICP fluctuations were seen in the period of Grade IV. But, once in a state of Grade V, the ICP fluctuations seen previously were replaced by high amplitude monotonous waves derived from the arterial pulses. They were registered upon the extremely increased ICP base line exceeding 80 mm Hg. Tachycardia and tachypnea have usually been seen in this stage. This high level of ICP dropped concomitantly with falling SBP in the terminal stage. Such a pattern of ICP holds true for all Grade V patients, and is supposed to indicate a state of cerebral vasomotor paralysis.

ICP during Subarachnoid Hemorrhage

Figure 4 shows an incidence of rupture of an aneurysm during ICP recording. The patient deteriorated to a state of Grade IV after the first attack. Continuous ventricular drainage was applied to keep ICP constant at about 20-30 mm Hg (Fig. 4A). On the ventricular drainage, ICP showed a steep rise to about 80 mm Hg (Fig. 4B) 20 h later, and effusion of fresh blood was seen from the ventricular catheter. The patient suddenly entered into a deep coma and ICP started to show the typical vasomotor paralytic pattern. The patient died and subsequently ICP decreased concomitantly with falling SBP.

Discussion

The increase in ICP following rupture of intracranial aneurysms contributes to the arrest of the hemorrhage (6, 7). Increased ICP, when exceeding a critical level in rate as well as duration, produces fatal brain swelling due to cerebral vasomotor paralysis (3). When patients tolerate the high ICP at the time of the hemorrhagic attack, subsequently ICP falls to a considerable lower level with little or no formation of intracerebral hematoma, but thereafter a slow increase in ICP occurs in the course of the next hours (6). Our study shows that this secondary increase in ICP will continue for several days.

NAGAI et al. (5) reported that, when ICP was raised to about 40 mm Hg in dogs, cerebral blood flow decreased slightly, and that, at about 75 mm Hg, the blood flow in the brain stem began to decrease and brain function became irreversibly damaged. LANGFITT et al. (3) stated that acute elevation of ICP causes cerebral vasodilatation and the vasopressor mechanism fails in the ultimate state. Our data show that impaired consciousness in patients with recently ruptured aneurysm is much more dependent on the increased ICP rather than on the cerebral vasospasm. Our mean ICP levels have been in the range of 15-40 mm Hg in Grade III patients, 30-75 mm Hg in Grade IV patients, and exceeded 75 mm Hg in Grade V patients. It is likely that the autoregulatory mechanism of the cerebrovascular system may still be preserved in a state of Grade III, while the cerebral blood flow may be much more reduced in a state of Grade IV and the autoregulatory mechanism is lost in the last stage.

In acute intracranial hypertension in Grade III and IV patients, the more impaired the consciousness, the more frequent and the higher the amplitude of B- and C-waves. The B- and C-waves are supposed to be related to an intrinsic rhythmic activity of medullary centers that are disconnected from the influence of higher centers in the upper brain stem (2), and are therefore regarded to be a sign of brain stem dysfunction (4). The fact that the frequent and continuing B- and C-waves have been found in Grade III and IV patients suggests that the cerebral vasomotor instability may play an important role in these stages. Such a condition of vasomotor instability may still be reversible. On the other hand, the high amplitude ICP changes derived from arterial pulses seen in Grade V patients indicate a state of loss of cerebral vasomotor mechanism, i.e., the vasoparalytic state that is no longer reversible.

Summary

(1) The more impaired the consciousness, the higher the rate of ICP increase in acute stages of ruptured intracranial aneurysm. (2) A definite correlation between vasospasm, as found at cerebral arteriography, and the clinical grade was not observed. (3) In our series of ICP recordings, we never observed a typical plateau wave. The variations of ICP seen in Grade III and IV patients were in fact B- and C-waves as described by LUNDBERG (4), and those in Grade V patients were high amplitude monotonous waves derived from the arterial pulses. These phenomena may indicate that the patients graded III and IV in subarachnoid hemorrhage are in a state of cerebral vasomotor instability, and the patients graded V in a state of cerebral vasomotor paralysis.

References

1. HUNT, W.E., HESS, R.M.: Surgical risk related to the time of intervention in the repair of intracranial aneurysm. J. Neurosurg. 28, 14-19 (1968).

2. KJÄLLQUIST, A., LUNDBERG, N., PONTEN, U.: Respiratory and cardiovascular changes during rapid spontaneous variations of ventricular fluid pressure in patients with intracranial hypertension. Acta Neurol. Scand. 40, 291-317 (1964).

3. LANGFITT, T.W., WEINSTEIN, J.D., KASSELL, N.F.: Cerebral vasomotor paralysis produced by intracranial hypertension. Neurology (Minneap) 15, 622-641 (1965).

4. LUNDBERG, N.: Continuous recording and control of ventricular fluid pressure in neurosurgical practice. Acta Psychiat. Scand. 36 (Suppl. 149), 1-193 (1960).

5. NAGAI, H., IKEYAMA, A., FURUSE, M., MAEDA, S., BANNO, K., HASUNO, M., KUCHIWAKI, H.: Effect of increased intracranial pressure on cerebral hemodynamics. Europ. Neurol. 8, 52-56 (1972).

6. NORNES, H., MAGNAES, B.: Intracranial pressure in patients with ruptured saccular aneurysm. J. Neurosurg. 36, 537-547 (1972).

7. NORNES, H. : The role of intracranial pressure in the arrest of hemorrhage in patients with ruptured intracranial aneurysm. J. Neurosurg. 39, 226-234 (1973).

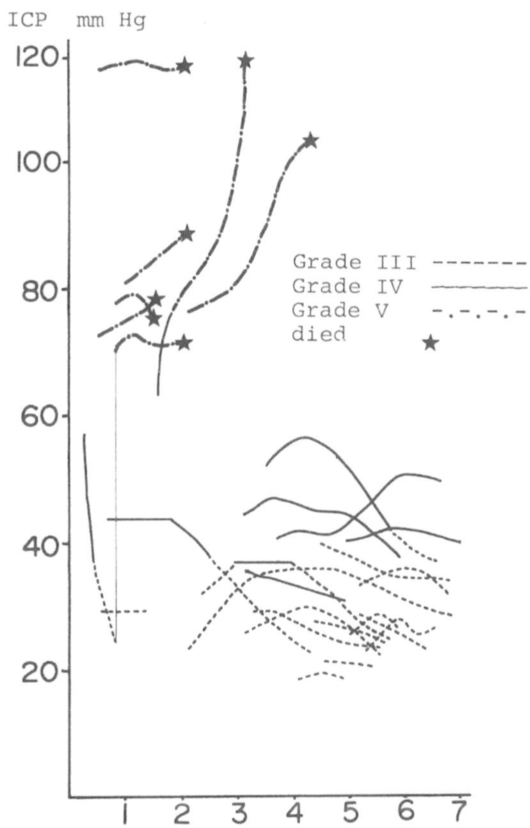

Fig. 1. Correlation between clinical grade and mean intracranial pressure (ICP) in 26 subarachnoid hemorrhage patients. SAH: subarachnoid hemorrhage

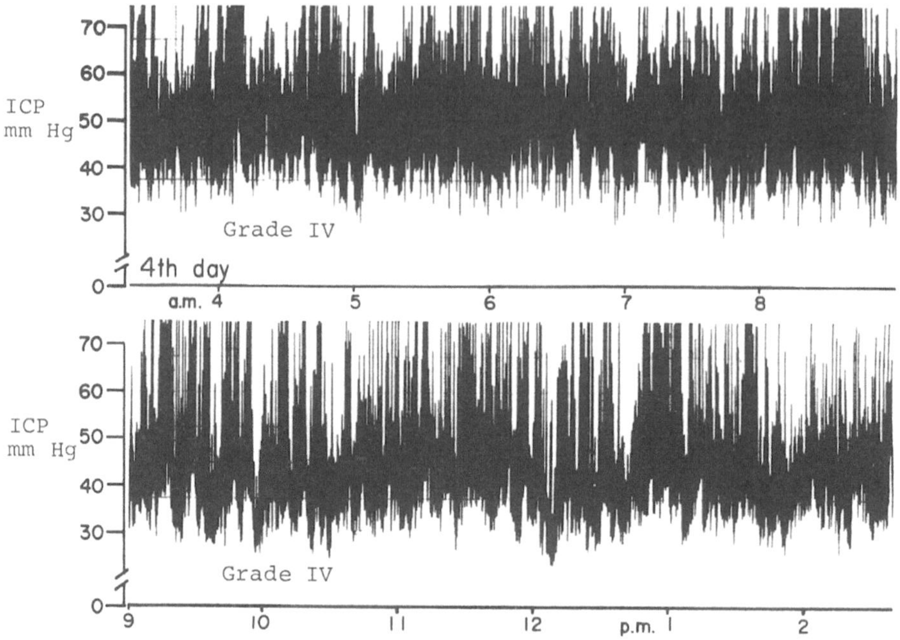

Fig. 2. 43-year old man with left internal carotid-posterior communicating aneurysm. Recording of ICP on the 4th day after subarachnoid hemorrhage. State of Grade IV. Frequent ICP variations with extremely high amplitude are seen

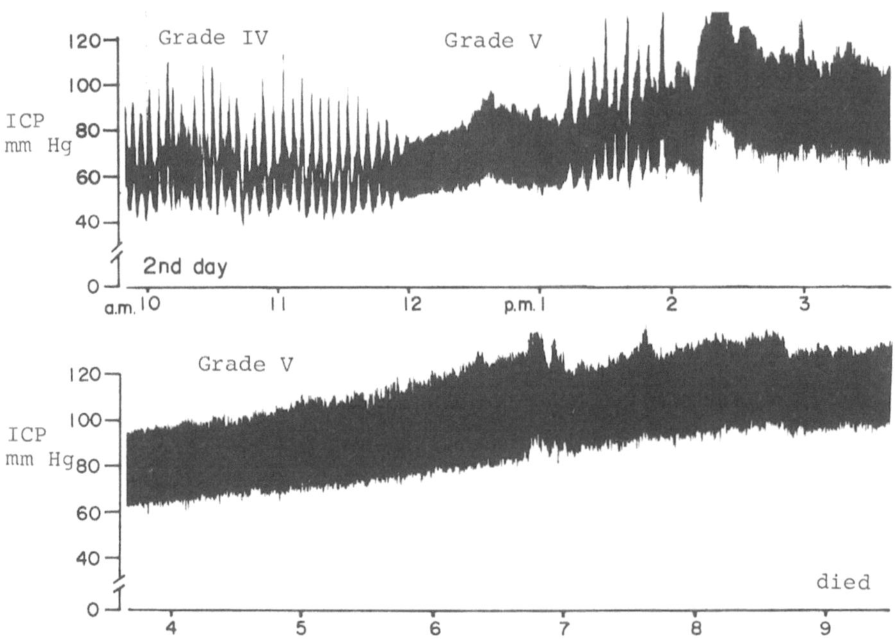

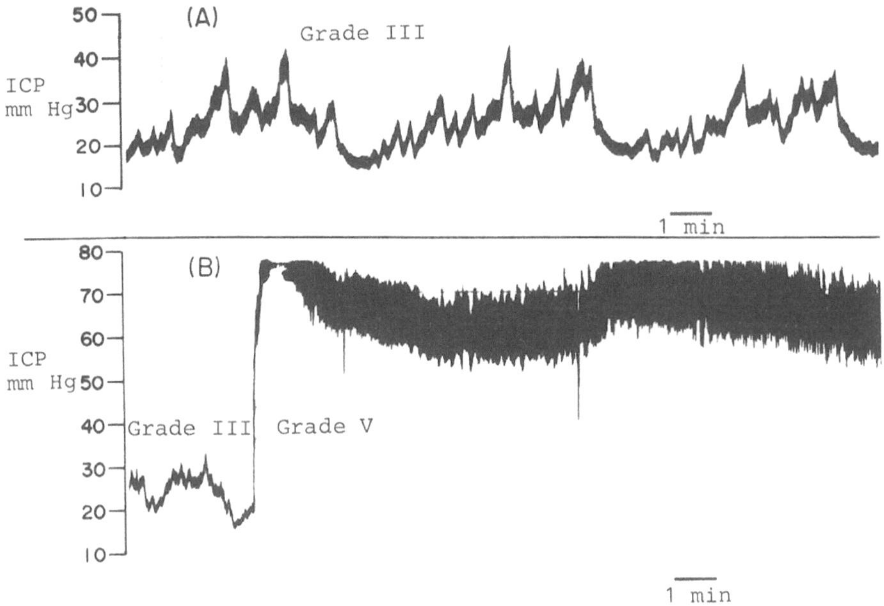

Fig. 4. 43-year old man with left internal carotid-posterior communicating aneurysm. Recording of ICP before (A) and during rupture (B) of aneurysm. Monotonous high amplitude waves of ICP after rupture. Paper-chart speed is 2 cm/min

◁ Fig. 3. 52-year old man with right internal carotid-posterior communicating aneurysm. Recording of ICP from the 1st day to the second day after subarachnoid hemorrhage. State developing from Grade IV to V. ICP fluctuations with moderate durations are remarkable in Grade IV, and they are replaced by high amplitude monotonous waves derived from arterial pulses in Grade V

Summary

L. Symon and E. Pasztor

This session contained six papers concerned primarily with two problems: the development of intracranial hypertension associated with communicating hydrocephalus after subarachnoid hemorrhage, and pressure phenomena which might be indicative, even predictive, of the probable state of the brain following hemorrhage.

The first of the problems is well recognized and has been assessed so frequently that the figure of around 10% of cases of subarachnoid hemorrhage which will develop long-lasting, absorptive deficits is now well accepted. VAPALAHTI emphasized again, however, the early and transient nature of communicating hydrocephalus in a high proportion of cases, especially those with anterior communicating artery aneurysms.

The advantages of continuous venting of CSF were discussed following SUNDBÄRG's paper but unfortunately, partly no doubt because his data included a variety of pathologic conditions whose pathophysiology was very clearly different from that of intracranial aneurysm, his advocacy of a 15 mm Hg threshold for drainage appeared difficult to sustain. In our opinion, drainage raises several further major problems. The possible contribution of continuous drainage to rebleeding from aneurysms was discussed. The data do not admit authoritative denial of this possibility but, as SHULMAN pointed out, it seems unlikely from the figures presented that any significant effect was produced. PONTEN stated in discussion that, as soon as rebleeding appeared, drainage usually became blocked. If this did not happen, he indicated that drainage should at once be stopped. A further problem which should be considered is the effect of drainage upon clearance of the subarachnoid pathways. The general agreement of the conference was that the magnitude of the hemorrhage was a major factor in the occurrence of "vasospastic" complications, but no evidence could be adduced at this time to suggest that ventricular drainage in any way impaired clearance of the CSF pathways. The detailed analysis of CSF constituents under the two circumstances, raised and normalized pressure, must be studied further.

The work of the London, Ontario, group presented by KASSELL, the Heidelberg experiences of HAMER, and a thoughtful and carefully executed study by YADA's group in Kanagawa, emphasized that there already appears to be a link established between raised pressure, the appearances of impaired perfusion (though none had actual regional CBF analysis), and a generally unsatisfactory clinical state. The link appears to hold true either in assessment of preoperative grade or in the development of the clinical deterioration so familiar to aneurysm surgeons in the postoperative period and generally called "vasospasm."

A third and final problem which is familiar in the concept of compartmentalized elastance in the intracranial space, emerged with the demonstration that where raised intracranial pressure was associated with brain swelling, and (by inference) "vasospasm" or perfusion deficit, CSF drainage was often insufficient to restore intracranial pressure to normal, and other measures to increase perfusion were necessary. Hyperosmolar agents had been effective in this regard, but it was emphasized by the CHAIR, KASSELL, and others, that induced hypertension under these circumstances need not be associated with increased intracranial pressure and that, under these special conditions, with careful intracranial pressure monitoring, induced hypertension could be attended by the resolution of focal deficits. The work of COLLINS in the United States was mentioned in this regard.

Our view for the future, which emerged both from the papers and from the discussions of this session, points to these main problem areas: the problems of accumulation of CSF, of diminished perfusion and of brain swelling. It seems clear that over the next few years continuous intracranial pressure monitoring must be used to analyze these problems more fully. We feel it necessary to emphasize, however, that the data which will be collected must have clear associated clinical description. It seems strange, in 1976, that data concerned with subarachnoid hemorrhage should still be presented without clear clinical grading and, however imperfect the HUNT and HESS system of grading may be, its widespread acceptance leads us to believe that such description of cases, with specification of clinical grade and of time from hemorrhage when the patient was studied, constitutes an essential measurement in the analysis of the phenomena of subarachnoid hemorrhage. It certainly must be stated in relation to our more sophisticated modern techniques.

Session F

Hydrocephalus

Chairman: U. Pontén
Co-chairman: G. M. Hochwald

An Explanation of the Reversible Memory Defect in Hydrocephalus

L. Granholm

Introduction

Subarachnoid hemorrhage (SAH) may cause mental changes similar to those found in a Korsakow's syndrome (KS), e.g., a severe dysmnesia, particularly affecting the capacity to retain recent memories (9). A curable form of KS following SAH is connected with hydrocephalus. Bilateral damage to structures of the limbic system may result in a KS. Some structures of this system, e.g., the hippocampal formations, are located in the periventricular areas. GREITZ and HINDMARSCH (7), found a narrow zone of relatively low attenuation (indicating increased water content) adjacent to the dilated ventricles, when they studied intracranial cerebrospinal fluid (CSF) circulation in hydrocephalus by means of computer tomography. This observation probably localizes the lesion for the short-term memory defect in hydrocephalus.

Materials and Methods

Patients with hydrocephalus were chosen from a large number of cases studied with computer tomography (EMI-scanner). All examinations were performed employing 120 kV, a 160 by 160 matrix, and a scanning time of 4.5 min. Cases of cerebral atrophy were excluded but the series contains patients with both normal pressure hydrocephalus (NPH) and those with increased pressure. Scans were done before and after a shunt procedure aiming at a reduction of intraventricular pressure. Efforts were made to maintain the same orientation of the patient during different studies.

The attenuation of brain tissue is higher than that of CSF, whereas the attenuation number of edematous brain tissue falls somewhere between tissue and CSF. Attenuation numbers from the data print-out were plotted against position along a transversal axis across the ventricular wall. The thought line of interest was drawn perpendicularly to the ventricular wall of the frontal horns. The obtained curve can be described as an attenuation profile. In the present study no attempts have been made to examine the attenuation profile over the ventricular wall in the hippocampal region. Technique and results will be described more thoroughly elsewhere (4).

Results

Prerequisites for the demonstration of the suggested mechanism are 1. hydrocephalus due to increased intraventricular pressure, 2. amelioration of symptoms following a shunt procedure, and 3. high quality computer tomograms pre- and postoperatively. Only few cases have so far fulfilled all these criteria. The semischematic Figure 1 demonstrates, however, findings preoperatively (30/10) and postoperatively (17/11) in a case of hydrocephalus. The drop in attenuation number shown in the profile, occurs much more rapidly over the ventricular wall postoperatively than preoperatively. Preoperatively there is a gradual fall in attenuation periventricularly toward the ependyma and corresponding to the periventricular zone of increased water content.

Discussion

An occasional feature of the clinical picture of SAH is a short-term memory defect, frequently mimicking that of a KS (9). This memory defect might in some cases be connected with posthemorrhagic hydrocephalus (see, e.g., 13). Shunting of CSF then frequently produces rapid and substantial improvement in short-term memory. Spontaneous recovery is also known to occur, however, and sometimes "over night" (14). This tendency to rapid improvement indicates that the symptoms are caused by a nondestructive lesion, which could inter alia presumably consist in localized edema.

In hydrocephalus, ventricular dilatation occurs chiefly at the expense of the periventricular white matter. A study of the vascular pattern in experimental hydrocephalus indicates a relative loss of the smaller vessels - capillary and precapillary - in all the structures around the dilated ventricle (1, 15). The extent of ischemia varies directly with the degree of dilatation of the ventricles. This circumscribed ischemia is accompanied by hypoxic changes, detectable in CSF samples (6). Hypoxia leads to edema in or CSF penetration into the white matter in experimental hydrocephalus (2). This edema is strictly confined to the periventricular area (3, 11), and has sometimes been described as indicative of transventricular CSF absorption. Periventricular edema has also been found in clinical hydrocephalus, both by light microscopy (10) and by computer tomography (7). Ventricular dilatation and periventricular ischemia in hydrocephalus are related to raised intraventricular pressure. As the intraventricular pressure is increased also in NPH in spite of the designation of this entity (5), identical pathophysiologic mechanisms must be operative in various forms of hydrocephalus.

Evidence shows that the temporal lobes and especially the hippocampal areas contribute to the mechanisms of memory recording, memory recall, and the capacity of comparing the present experience with that of the past (see, e.g., 12). Bilateral lesions to the hippocampus thus result in a remarkably clearcut symptom complex including a pronounced short-term memory defect. Recent literature in this field is extensive. Hippocampus actually forms part of the wall of the temporal horn of the ventricular system and is thus exposed to local ischemia in hydrocephalus. It seems likely that ischemia and the demonstrated edematous lining of the ventricular system in hydrocephalus could interfere with the axonal function of hippocampus.

The present investigation reveals that the previously demonstrated periventricular zone of low attenuation is a common finding in hydrocephalus. It also shows that periventricular edema disappears following shunting concomitantly with clinical improvement. A reduced cerebral blood flow in NPH frequently also normalizes following a shunt procedure (8) and concomitantly with clinical improvement.

Summary

It is suggested that the dysmnesic state found in hydrocephalus is due to periventricular edema affecting hippocampal function. A reduction in intraventricular pressure, e.g., by a shunt procedure, ameliorates perfusion in ischemic regions. This results in the absorption of periventricular edema or penetrated CSF. Whenever dysmnesia is cured by a shunt, the ischemic edematous damage to the limbic system must be at least partially reversible.

References

1. DE, S.N.: A study of the changes in the brain in experimental internal hydrocephalus. J. Path. Bact. 62, 197-207 (1950).
2. FISHMAN, R.A., GREER, M.: Experimental obstructive hydrocephalus. Arch. Neurol. 8, 156-161 (1963).
3. GRANHOLM, L.: On water shifts in the hydrocephalic brain. Develop. Med. Child Neurol. Suppl. 16, 1-2 (1968).
4. GRANHOLM, L., HINDMARSH, T., LEVANDER, B.: Periventricular changes in hydrocephalus studied by computer tomography. To be printed in 1976.
5. GRANHOLM, L., LÖFGREN, J.: A discussion on the intracranial pressure-volume relationship in normal pressure hydrocephalus. In: Intracranial Pressure II (N. LUNDBERG, U. PONTEN, M. BROCK, eds.), pp. 137-140. Berlin-Heidelberg-New York: Springer 1975.
6. GRANHOLM, L., SIESJÖ, B.K.: Signs of tissue hypoxia in infantile hydrocephalus. Develop. Med. Child Neurol., Suppl. 22, 73-77 (1970).
7. GREITZ, T., HINDMARSH, T.: Computer assisted tomography of intracranial CSF circulation using a water-soluble contrast medium. Acta Radiol. Diagnosis 15, 497-507 (1974).
8. GREITZ, T., GREPE, A.O.L., KALMER, M.S.F., LOPEZ, J.: Pre- and postoperative evaluation of cerebral blood flow in low-pressure hydrocephalus. J. Neurosurg. 31, 644-651 (1969).
9. HALL, A.J.: Three cases of spontaneous subarachnoid hemorrhage: with special reference to the occurrence of massive albuminuria and Korsakoff's syndrome. Brit. Med. J. 3570, 1025-1028 (1929).
10. KWITNITSKY-RYJOV, Y.N.: The problem of edema and swelling of the cortical substance in occlusive hydrocephalus. Z. Nevropath. Psich. S.S. Korsakova 61, 848 (1961).
11. LUX, W.E., Jr., HOCHWALD, G.M., SAHAR, A., RANSOHOFF, J.: Periventricular water content. Arch. Neurol. 23, 475-479 (1970).
12. PENFIELD, W., MILNER, B.: Memory deficit produced by bilateral lesions in the hippocampal zone. Arch. Neurol. Psychiat. 79, 475-497 (1958).
13. THEANDER, S., GRANHOLM, L.: Sequelae after spontaneous subarachnoid hemorrhage, with special reference to hydrocephalus and Korsakoff's syndrome. Acta Neurol. Scand. 43, 479-488 (1967).
14. WALTON, J.N.: The Korsakow syndrome in spontaneous subarachnoid hemorrhage. J. Ment. Sci. 99, 521-530 (1953).
15. WOZNIAK, M., McLONE, D.G., RAIMONDI, A.J.: Micro- and macrovascular changes as the direct cause of parenchymal destruction in congenital murine hydrocephalus. J. Neurosurg. 43, 535-545 (1975).

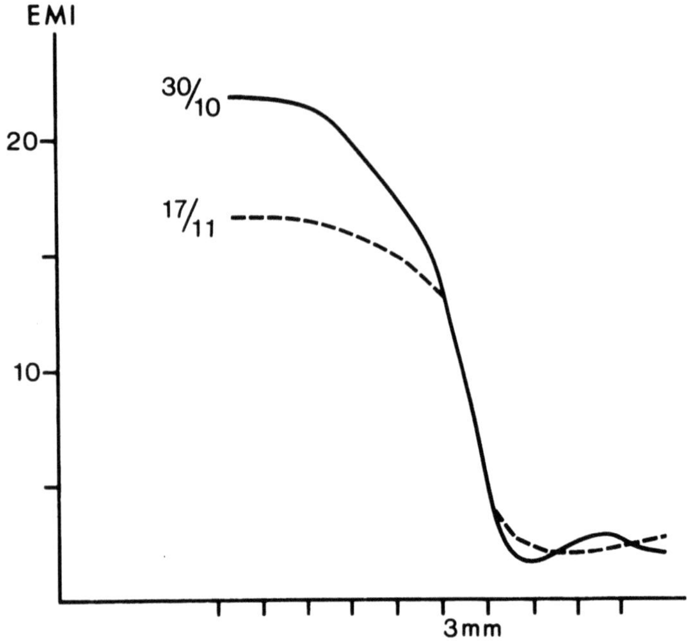

Fig. 1. Attenuation profile showing changes in attenuation (vertical axis) across ventricular wall (horizontal axis, distance markings every 3 mm) pre- and postoperatively. Brain tissue attenuation is found to the left and CSF attenuation to the right. Postoperatively (November 17, 17/11) there is a much more abrupt change in attenuation than preoperatively (October 30, 30/10), probably because of absorption of periventricular fluid

CSF Hydrodynamics Especially in the Adult Hydrocephalus Syndrome[1]

J. Ekstedt and H. Fridén

Introduction

The adult communicating hydrocephalus syndrome has been subjected to intense scientific study all over the world since HAKIM and ADAMS drew attention to its existence (6, 7, 1). The initial enthusiasm of excellent surgical treatment results has, however, been replaced with a more subdued optimism (2, 12). No doubt, there are patients who dramatically respond to a shunt operation, but it is also obvious that many patients, fulfilling the original diagnostic criteria, do not benefit from the operation. The terms "normal-pressure hydrocephalus" and "low-pressure hydrocephalus" have been extensively used to characterize this syndrome. Systematic studies of CSF pressure have been rare. Many clinical reports have entirely lacked information of the CSF pressure values. There are reports (13) on episodic CSF pressure increase in the patients with otherwise normal pressure, and this condition has been considered to be pathogenetic. The original concept of HAKIM and ADAMS was that here has been, at one stage of the development of the syndrome, a period of increased CSF pressure causing a dilatation of the ventricles. When the pressure decreases again, the ventricles should remain dilated also at a lower pressure due to the law of surface tension.

Infusion tests with artificial CSF (9, 8, 11, 10, 14) and isotope cisternography (3) have been considered as aids to the pneumoencephalograms and computerized axial tomograms in selecting patients suitable to shunt surgery. This paper is intended to emphasize that the study of the CSF hydrodynamics might contribute to increased understanding of the adult hydrocephalus syndrome and be a valuable adjunct in the selection of patients for surgery.

Methods

The methods were described at the second ICP meeting in Lund (5) and will be published in detail elsewhere. In short: A double lumbar puncture is performed and recording made in the supine position with the sagittal center of the skull as the zero reference level (Fig. 1). *CSF resting pressure* (P_{clr}) is recorded for 60 min. Artificial CSF is then infused at 8-15 different constant pressure levels and the resulting flow is recorded. The relation between pressure and flow is, in most cases, linear (Fig. 2). The inclination of the regression line is a measure of the facility of outflow of CSF from the subarachnoidal space and is called the *conductance of the CSF outflow pathways* (C_{op}). By lowering the CSF pressure to a value (0.25 kPa) below the pressure in the sagittal sinus the pressure difference across the arachnoidal villi is reversed. This prevents CSF outflow to the sagittal sinus.

[1]Supported by the Medical Research Council (Grant No. 04X-4125).

Thus, all CSF formed is collected in the bottle and the *CSF formation rate* (q_f) determined. From these data the *pressure difference across the arachnoidal villi* may be calculated ($P_{dop} = q_f/G_{op}$) as well as the *sagittal sinus pressure* ($P_{ss} = P_{clr} - P_{dop}$). The normal values for these CSF hydrodynamic parameters will be given in detail elsewhere and are summarized in Table 1.

Table 1. Of 685 patients 58 adults were selected as probably not having any intracranial or circulatory disease. This group of patients has been considered as normal material. For the resting pressure the normal material is 100 patients. 1kPa = 7.5 mm Hg. 1 mm^3 = 0.06 ml min^{-1}. 1 $mm^3 kPa^{-1} s^{-1}$ = 0.008 ml mm $Hg^{-1} min^{-1}$

Normal values for CSF hydrodynamic parameters
58 patients (for P_{clr} 100) 15-83 years
Supine horizontal position. Reference level: Cranial sagittal center
Constant pressure infusion method with artificial CSF

	$\bar{M}$	SD	90% within
Lumbar resting pressure (P_{clr})	1.38 kPa	0.19	1.15-1.75
Conductance of CSF outflow pathways (G_{op})	17.98 $mm^3.kPa^{-1}.s^{-1}$	4.06	12.0-26.0
CSF formation rate (q_f)	6.67 $mm^3.s^{-1}$	1.39	4.5- 9.5
Pressure difference across outflow pathways (P_{dop})	0.37 kPa	0.10	0.25-0.55
Sagittal sinus pressure (P_{ss})	1.00 kPa	0.20	0.70-1.35

No sex differences in parameters nor any age dependence.

Material

The experience has been gained over a 6-year period, between 1970 and 1976 in Uppsala and thereafter in Umea. Moving to Umea has made follow-up of the Uppsala patients difficult and therefore only part of the total material is presented. To date no statistical analysis has been made. In total 765 hydrodynamic investigations have been performed on 685 patients with different diagnosis at ages 3 days to 93 years. In all cases the investigation has been made on suspicion of disturbed intracranial hydrodynamics.

Results

1. Seven of the patients who have been treated with ventriculoatrial shunt have shown a lasting and significant improvement. In these successful cases there has been preoperatively an increase of the CSF resting pressure. The cause of the CSF pressure increase was an increase of the pressure difference across the arachnoidal villi (P_{dop}) (Fig. 3). This, in turn, is due to a decreased conductance of the CSF outflow pathways (G_{op}). Different CSF production rates (q_f), of course, influence the value (Fig. 4). In these cases G_{op} has been below 8 mm^3 $kPa^{-1}s^{-1}$ (2.3-8.0) and P_{dop} within the range of 0.8-2.5 kPa. The resting CSF pressure has had a value between 2.15-3.25 kPa.

2. Seven patients have had CSF hydrodynamic parameters very similar to those described under 1, but the effect of the shunt operation has been zero or scarcely of importance.

3. There were 12 patients who had a considerable ventricular enlargement but their CSF hydrodynamic parameters were in all respects normal. The result of shunting in these cases has been of zero or unsignificant improvement. A patient with a primary cerebral atrophy and a resulting "hydrocephalus ex vacuo" does not benefit from a shunt operation.

4. There were 14 patients observed who, during a period of up to 6 years, have had a considerable increase of the CSF pressure, which proved to be due to an increase of the sagittal sinus pressure (P_{ss}) while the conductance of the CSF outflow pathways (G_{dop}) was normal. In none of these cases had hydrocephalus developed. An increase of sagittal sinus pressure with normal pressure difference across the arachnoidal villi is thus not a cause of hydrocephalus.

5. Six patients have proved to have CSF hydrodynamic parameters of the type described under 1., with increased resting pressure due to an increased pressure difference across the arachnoidal villi as well as having increased ventricle size but being devoid of serious symptoms from the central nervous system. These patients are followed with CSF hydrodynamic studies each 6 months. If and when the clinical symptoms develop the patients will be considered for shunt operation.

6. Six patients have had a hydrocephalus with a pressure within or close to the upper limit of normal pressure. The conductance of the CSF outflow pathways has been abnormally low. However, the CSF formation rate has also been very low and a normal pressure is thus maintained (Fig. 4). Of these patients, 3 were subjected to a shunt operation without obvious positive results. These patients have in fact compensated the lowered conductance with a decrease in the CSF formation rate. A shunt operation had no further effect on normalizing the intracranial pressure or on the symptoms.

7. In a considerable portion of the patients with shunts investigated years after the operation, the shunt has been nonfunctioning in spite of normal function judged by palpation. The hydrodynamic investigation offers a sensitive test for shunt function because of the nonlinearity of the pressure/flow properties of most shunt systems. Unsuspected shunt dysfunction may be one reason why a patient does not improve after the operation.

8. In most cases of adult hydrocephalus with symptoms that have been to different degrees reversed by shunt surgery, there is a very strong impression that the patients concomitantly have had a circulatory cerebral disturbance. It is possible that the combined effect of disturbed CSF hydrodynamics and, e.g., arterial disease may be, in some cases, responsible for the development of the hydrocephalus syndrome. This view has been advanced by EARNEST et al. (4). The results are summarized in Table 2.

Discussion

The question of selecting the patients who will benefit from shunt surgery has proved to be very difficult. It is our belief that the computerized axial tomogram, the pneumoencephalogram, and isotope cisternogram may be very important for selecting patients for further studies but do not give conclusive indications for surgery. It seems to us that an increased pressure difference across the arachnoidal villi (and thus also an increased pressure difference between the CSF and the postcapillary vascular bed in the brain) may be a common denominator for those who have benefited from shunt operation. A decreased conductance of the CSF outflow pathways seems to be the reason for the pressure increase. This frequent finding of grossly abnormal CSF hydro-

Table 2. A schematic summary of results. In column "Clinical symptoms", + means presence and - absence of symptoms that may be attributable to adult hydrocephalus syndrome. In column "Shunt results", + means significant and lasting improvement and - unsignificant or no improvement

CSF Hydrodynamic findings p_{clr}	p_{ss}	p_{dop}	G_{op}	q_f	Number of Patients	Ventricle volume	Clinical symptoms	Shunt results
					7	↑	+	+
↑	→	↑	↓	→	7	↑	+	—
					6	↑	—	No shunt
↗	→	↗	↓	↓	3	↑	+	No shunt
					3	↑	+	—
↑	↑	→	→	→	14	→	—	No shunt
→	→	→	→	→	12	↑	+	—

↑ means increase, ↗ means slight increase, → means normal, ↓ means decrease

dynamics of this kind in patients without symptoms attributable to altered CSF hydrodynamics makes it obvious that the clinical judgment regarding the patient shall be an important part of the total preoperative diagnosis.

The development of hydrocephalus symptoms is probably a very slow process, and it is possible that some additional factor is also needed for symptom development, such as, e.g., an arterial disease causing multiple embolic infarctions or multiple small hemorrhages.

Those patients who benefited from shunt operation had, at the time of operation, pathologic CSF hydrodynamics detectable with the constant pressure infusion method. It should, however, be stressed that the same information can be obtained with the method of constant rate infusion, e.g., according to KATZMAN and HUSSEY (9), but the experimental data should then be handled in terms of the hydrodynamic parameters, as done here. If so, the values of the parameters should be the same irrespective of the method.

It seems likely that the ultimate cause of the type of hydrocephalus which is amenable to therapy is a decreased conductance of CSF outflow, probably at the site of the arachnoidal villi. When the conductance of the CSF outflow pathways is low, even small changes in CSF formation rate result in considerable changes in the CSF pressure (Fig. 4). This might well be responsible for the fluctuations in CSF pressure that have been reported in adult hydrocephalus (13).

Summary

A patient with a primary cerebral atrophy and a resulting "hydrocephalus ex vacuo" does not benefit from a shunt operation. Such patients can be identified by normal CSF hydrodynamic parameters and unnecessary operations can thus be prevented.

The patients who benefited from operation had a CSF pressure above the normal caused by an increased pressure difference across the arachnoidal villi that was, in turn, caused by a decreased conductance of the CSF outflow pathways. Even if this finding was also made in patients who had not benefited from operations and in patients devoid of clinical symptoms, it seems possible that the CSF hydrodynamic parameters may be an aid in selecting patients who will benefit from a shunt operation.

References

1. ADAMS, R.D., FISHER, C.M., HAKIM, S., OJEMANN, R.G., SWEET, W.H.: Symptomatic occult hydrocephalus with "normal" cerebrospinal-fluid pressure: A treatable syndrome. New Eng. J. Med. 273, 117-126 (1965).

2. BANNISTER, C.M.: A report of eight patients with low pressure hydrocephalus treated by C.S.F. diversion with disappointing results. Acta Neurochirurgica 27, 11-15 (1972).

3. BANNISTER, R., GILFORD, E., KOCEN, R.: Isotope encephalography in the diagnosis of dementia due to communicating hydrocephalus. Lancet 1967 II, 1014-1017.

4. EARNEST, M.P., KARP, J.H.: Normal pressure hydrocephalus and hypertensive cerebrovascular disease. Arch. Neurol. 31, 262-266 (1974).

5. EKSTEDT, J.: CSF hydrodynamics studied by means of constant pressure infusion technique. In: Intracranial Pressure II (N. LUNDBERG, U. PONTEN, M. BROCK, eds.), pp. 35-41. Berlin: Springer-Verlag 1975.

6. HAKIM, S.: Algunas observaciónes sobre la presión del L.C.R. sindrome hidrocefalico en el adulto con "presión normal" del L.C.R. In: Tesis de grado. Universidad Javeriana, Bogotá, Colombia, 1964.

7. HAKIM, S., ADAMS, R.D.: The special clinical problem of symptomatic hydrocephalus with normal cerebrospinal fluid pressure. Observations on cerebrospinal fluid hydrodynamics. J. Neurol. Sci. 2, 307-327 (1965).

8. HUSSEY, F., SCHANZER, B., KATZMAN, R.: A simple constant infusion manometric test for measurement of CSF absorption. II. Clinical studies. Neurology 20, 665-680 (1970).

9. KATZMAN, R., HUSSEY, F.: A simple constant-infusion manometric test for measurement of CSF absorption. I. Rationale and method. Neurology 20, 534-544 (1970).

10. MARTINS, A.N.: Resistance to drainage of cerebrospinal fluid: Clinical measurement and significance. J. Neurol. Neurosurg. Psychiat. 36, 313-318 (1973).

11. NELSON, J.R., GOODMAN, S.J.: An evaluation of the cerebrospinal fluid infusion test for hydrocephalus. Neurology 21, 1038-1053 (1971).

12. STEIN, S.C., LANGFITT, T.W.: Normal-pressure hydrocephalus. Predicting the results of cerebrospinal fluid shunting. J. Neurosurg. 41, 463-470 (1974).

13. SYMON, L., DORSCH, N.W.C., STEPHENS, R.J.: Pressure waves in so called low-pressure hydrocephalus. Lancet 1974 II, 1291-1292.

14. TROTTER, J.L., LUZECKY, M., SIEGEL, B.A., GADO, M.: Cerebrospinal fluid infusion test. Identification of artifacts and correlation with cisternography and pneumoencephalography. Neurology 24, 181-186 (1974).

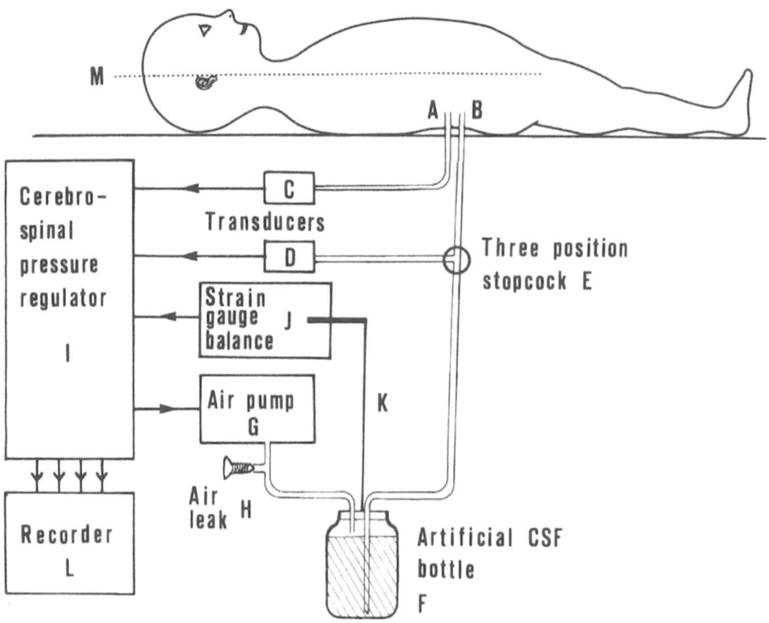

Fig. 1. Investigation set-up. Two lumbar needles A and B, filled with artificial CSF, are connected to pressure transducers C and D by tubes. Zero pressure reference level M is adjusted to sagittal center of cranium. Needle B can also be connected to bottle with artificial CSF (F) by means of stopcock E. Bottle is pressurized from air pump G, governed by one of the transducers (C, D) via regulator I. Flow through needle B is calculated from change of weight of bottle F, measured with strain gauge balance J. Airleak H sets maximally attainable pressure and permits a fast pressure regulation

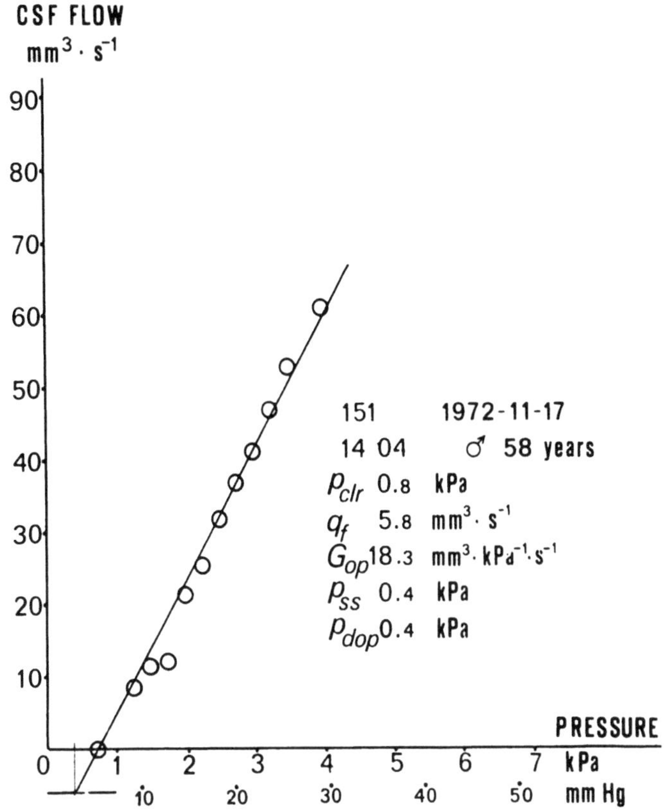

Fig. 2. Normal investigation of pressure-flow relationship. Each CSF pressure and corresponding inflow of artificial CSF is measured when system is in dynamic equilibrium. Slope of regression line is *conductance* of CSF outflow pathways (G_{op}) ("facility of outflow"). Horizontal line under abscissa represents CSF formation rate, q_f, determined by drainage of CSF at a pressure of 0.25 kPa. Intersection between this line and extension of regression line represents sagittal sinus pressure (P_{ss}) which would be equal to CSF pressure that should have been found if there were no CSF formation. 1 kPa = 7.5 mm Hg.

$P_{dop} = P_{clr} - P_{ss} = q_f/G_{op}$

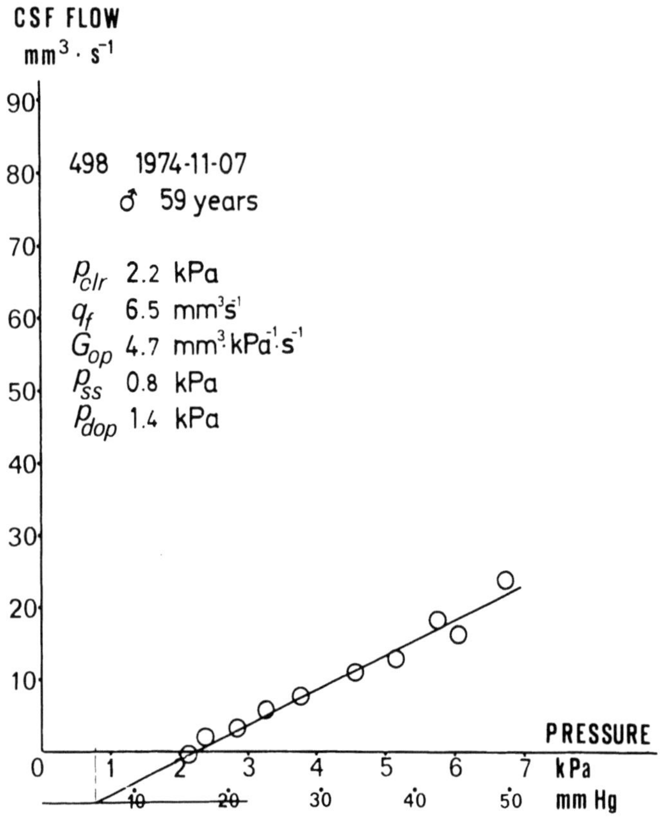

Fig. 3. CSF hydrodynamics of type considered typical for adult hydrocephalus syndrome. Resting pressure is increased due to an increase in pressure difference across outflow pathways (p_{dop}), which is in turn due to a decreased conductance (G_{op}). 1 kPa = 7.5 mm Hg

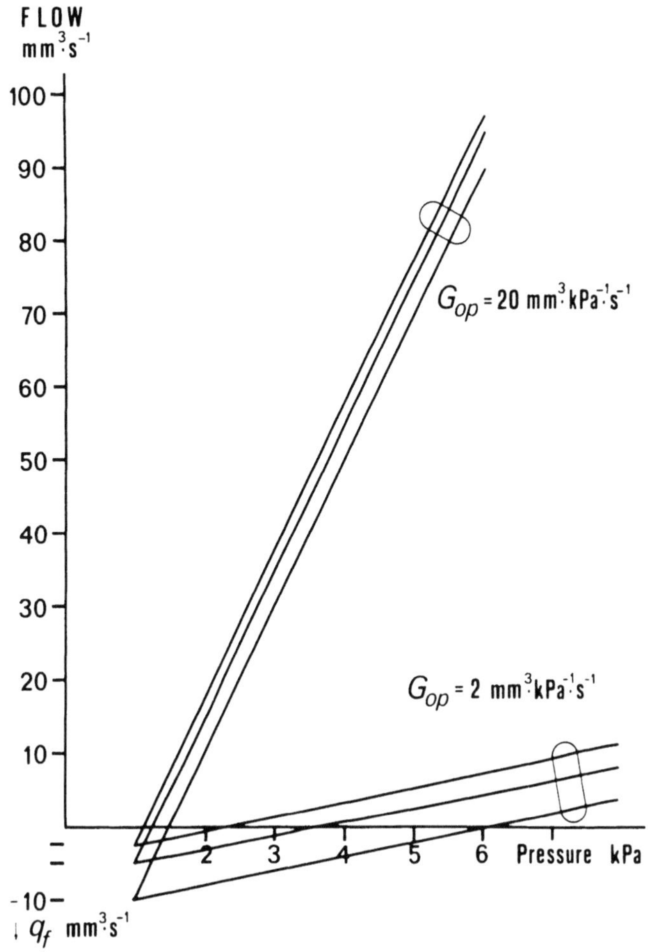

Fig. 4. Schematic illustration of dependence of conductance and CSF formation rate on CSF pressure. Sagittal sinus pressure (P_{ss}) of 1.0 kPa is assumed. If CSF formation rate (q_f) is changed and conductance is high, the resulting change in pressure is small. If, however, conductance is low, the influence of q_f on CSF pressure is considerable. 1 kPa = 7.5 mm Hg

Ventriculo-Lumbar Perfusion in Adult Communicating Hydrocephalus[1]

A. Stevenaert, D. Godin, and J.C. Depresseux

Introduction

The recognition of normal pressure hydrocephalus (NPH) as a treatable form of dementia (2, 5) was followed by an early period of enthusiasm; but afterward, disappointing results of surgical therapy in some cases (3) and shunt-related complications (18) were more and more frequently reported. For these reasons, re-evaluation of the diagnostic criteria (13) is needed and new criteria (7, 8, 11, 17) are proposed.

Under such circumstances, we used the ventriculosubarachnoid perfusion technique to determine a better selection of cases. This method introduced in 1938 by ADAM et al. (1) was first systematically used by LEUSEN in anesthetized dogs (9, 10) and by PAPPENHEIMER and co-workers in unanesthetized goats (6, 15).

Methods

Our method is similar to that applied by other workers (4, 11, 12, 14, 16) in man. Each patient was premedicated with an intramuscular injection of 10 mg of Valium; additional injections could be given during perfusion. Constant monitoring was carried out with surface electrodes for ECG and for respiration and signals were recorded on a polygraph. Blood pressure was measured by sphigmomanometry. Neither of these parameters changed during perfusion. The patients were apparently not disturbed by the procedure.

Artificial CSF (Elliott's B-solution prepared by our hospital chemist) containing tracer quantities (50 μCi/l) of ^{131}I human serum albumin ^{131}I HSA) was introduced with a constant infusion pump into the frontal horn of the left lateral ventricle via a Holter catheter and was collected from a 20-g spinal needle inserted in the lumbar subarachnoid space (Fig. 1). Several infusion rates were used from 1.6 to 3.75 ml/min; perfusion time varied from 7 to 11.5 h. The outflow or perfusion pressure was regulated by adjusting the height of the opening of the tube connected with the spinal needle. Pressure transducers were used to monitor ventricular and lumbar pressures. The reference level for both being the midline of the patient lying on his left side, there was a pressure gradient between the ventricle and the lumbar spaces related to the intrinsic resistance of the system. Effluent was collected fractionally at 10 min intervals and determined by gravimetry; by calculation, it was expressed in ml/min. Radioactivity in 1 ml samples was assayed in triplicate in a scintillation well-counter. Steady state was attained when counting indicated a constant level of activity in five consecutive fractions. The rates of CSF formation (V_f) and absorption (V_a) and the volume of distribution of ^{131}I HSA (VDx) were calculated from the equations of HEISEY et al. (6).

[1] This work was supported by Fonds National Belge de la Recherche Scientifique.

$$V_f = V_i \frac{C_i - C_o}{C_o},$$

$$V_a = V_i + V_f - V_o,$$

$$VDx = \sum_{1}^{n} \left[\frac{V_i C_i - (V_o + V_a) C_o}{\bar{C}_{ss}} \right] \Delta t - DS.$$

Results of the equations were written on a pressure-flow diagram and the regression lines of formation and absorption rates as a function of pressure were calculated by the method of least squares.

Data from representative perfusions are shown in Figure 2. As the endogenous CSF was mixed with the perfusate, the outflow activity of ^{131}I HSA increased gradually until a plateau was reached after 2,5 h, remaining more or less constant during perfusion. On the other hand, the outflow itself reached a plateau more rapidly but fluctuated inversely with pressure changes. Such a steady state was obtained in eight patients while it was impossible in a ninth one, despite an 8-h period of perfusion. That was probably due to the very large volume of CSF in this patient who had suffered from hydrocephalus for a very long time and had an enormous ventricular dilatation. In fact, calculation showed that with the chosen inflow rate (3.75 ml/min), the time necessary to reach steady state in this particular case should have been approx. 30 h.

Material

The essential data for clinical state, radiologic examinations, and intraventricular pressure (IVP) measurements for each patient are presented in Tables 1 and 2. Four patients had suffered from proven subarachnoid hemorrhages and three of them had shown akinetic mutism, while the last one had a triad of dementia, gait disturbance, and incontinence, although finally complicated by brain softening. The four other cases were idiopathic and had incomplete or atypical clinical pictures. Brain softening was present in four cases in this series while patient no. 8 suffered from chronic brain ischemia.

Isotope cisternography was performed in seven cases. In two patients (cases 1 and 7), there was lasting (more than 48 h) ventricular reflux of the isotope with block in the basal cisterns. Two other cases (cases 5 and 6) with lasting reflux showed filling of their sylvian fissures, while the last three showed partial or asymmetrical activity over the convexity or in the interhemispheric subarachnoid spaces.

In all patients, pneumoencephalography demonstrated total ventricular dilatation. Only two cases showed cisternal blocks, three had convexity blocks and the last three had some open and nondilated sulci over the convexity.

IVP was monitored in all patients by means of a method according to LUNDBERG, with a mean time of approx. 27.5 h, including nocturnal measurements. The mean pressure was less than 15 mm Hg but only two patients showed normal patterns while six had B waves, one of them also having plateau waves.

Results

The average formation rate was 0.256 ± 0.073 ml/min, but in patients suffering from posthemorrhagic hydrocephalus it was only 0.133 ± 0.046 ml/min, while in the other patients it was 0.315 ± 0.119 ml/min (Fig. 3). When the formation rate was plotted against the opening pressure, there was a decline in formation of 0.1 µl/min/mm of pressure. This decline, however, was well within the standard error as calculated.

Table 1. Summary of patients clinical data

Case	Age	Etiology	Clinical Syndrom	Associated diseases
1.V.G.	46	SAH, ruptured aneurysm	Akinetic mutism	Brain softening
2.T.M.	46	SAH, ruptured aneurysm	Akinetic mutism	Brain softening
3.W.P.	69	SAH, arteriosclerosis	N.P.H. syndrom	Brain softening
4.M.D.	42	SAH, head trauma	Akinetic mutism	-
5.V.C.	59	Unknown	Atypical	Brain softening
6.O.J.	53	Unknown	Atypical	-
7.D.M.	57	Unknown	Atypical	-
8.B.V.	55	Unknown	Atypical	Brain ischemia

Table 2. Summary of patients diagnostic data

Case	Cisternogram	Pneumoencephalogram	IVP Mean	mm Hg Waves
1	Cisternal block	Cisternal block	10	B
2	Not performed	Cisternal block	8-12	A,B
3	Atypical	Convexity block	7- 8	B
4	Atypical	No block	2- 3	-
5	Convexity block	No block	3- 4	B
6	Convexity block	Convexity block	5	-
7	Cisternal block	No block	10-12	B
8	Atypical	Convexity block	10-15	B

The average volume of distribution of ^{131}I HSA was 250 ± 83 ml. When the volume of distribution was plotted against the EVANS index as measured on the pneumoencephalogram, there was a linear relationship but further studies are needed to establish this point firmly.

The rate of turnover of the CSF compartment is calculated on the basis of the hourly rate of CSF production expressed as a percentage of the total CSF volume. In this series, it was 6.2 %/h. However, since the calculation is based solely on the formation rate, the rate of turnover was quite different in the group of patients suffering from posthemorrhagic hydrocephalus (3.5 %/h) as compared with the other group (7 %/h).

The absorption rate (Fig. 4) varied from 2.2 to 6.1 µl/min/mm H_2O in seven cases while it was 8.8 µl/min/mm H_2O in the last one, who was considered as having normal absorption. The other patients could be divided into three groups on the basis of CSF absorption, according to the three types described by LORENZO and co-workers (11, 14). In five patients, absorption began at a pressure of approx. 68 mm H_2O and in two of them the absorption rate was slow from the start (type II). In the three others, the rate increased normally from a pressure of 68 mm H_2O to a level ranging between 100 and 120 mm H_2O; but above this pressure range there was a decline and the absorption rate was located to be between 2.8 and 4.9 µl/min/mm H_2O (type III). Finally, in the two remaining patients, absorption began at a level considerably higher than 68 mm H_2O and then it increased at a mean rate of 5.7 µl/min/mm H_2O (type I).

Discussion

In our series, the average formation rate of CSF (0.256 ± 0.073 ml/min) is slower than that measured in children (0.35 ± 0.02 ml/min) (4) or adults (0.37 ± 0.10 ml/min) (16) and even in patients suffering from NPH (0.31 ± 0.02 ml/min) (11). However, there is a difference between the two etiologic groups of patients. In the posthemorrhagic hydrocephalus cases, the formation rate is more considerably diminished (0.133 ± 0.046 ml/min); this could be explained by alterations in CSF secreting structures due to hemoglobin metabolites. In the remaining cases, the formation rate (0.315 ± 0.119 ml/min) is quite similar to that observed in NPH cases. Therefore, CSF formation does not seem to be much influenced by pressure, since transient elevations of CSF pressure have been observed even in cases of so-called NPH (17).

The three types of absorption patterns, as described by LORENZO et al. (11, 12, 14) in hydrocephalic patients, we also observed. The disturbance of absorption in types I and II is evident. In type III, the absorption rate is at first normal and then decreases after reaching a pressure threshold. In this short series, no correlation is evident between either the absorption patterns or etiology of hydrocephalus, clinical state, cisternal, or convexity block. Nevertheless, it seems interesting to point out that in two patients with type III, the cisternograms had shown ventricular reflux of the isotope during the 48 h period, although the isotope was present also in the subarachnoid spaces of the convexity despite the fact that no air was seen in these spaces on the pneumoencephalograms. Perhaps this type III represents a partially compensated trouble in CSF circulation.

In one case, the absorption rate was normal; however, there was a 24-h isotope ventricular reflux on the cisternogram, there was air in nondilated sulci of the convexity on the pneumoencephalogram, and IVP was quite normal. This patient probably suffered from posttraumatic cerebral atrophy.

Five patients received ventriculoatrial shunts. The best results were seen in two patients with type II deficit (cases 2 and 7) while a third patient with type III deficit (case 8) improved slightly. Two nonresponding patients (cases 1 and 5) had type I deficit, although complicated by brain softening. These cases illustrate the importance of associated intrinsic brain disease.

Summary

Ventriculolumbar perfusions were performed in eight adults. Average CSF formation rate in patients with idiopathic hydrocephalus (0.315 ± 0.119 ml/min) was approximately the same as in patients without obstruction of CSF pathways and it did not seem to be influenced by pressure changes. On the other hand, formation rate was considerably slower in patients suffering from posthemorrhagic hydrocephalus (0.133 ± 0.046 ml/min). CSF turnover rate was diminished, depending on the increased CSF volume and the decreased formation rate.

Three different patterns of absorption disturbance were observed in seven patients; the absorption rate varied from 1.2 to 6.1 µl/min/mm H_2O. No trouble in CSF dynamics could be found in the eighth patient who probably had white matter atrophy.

References

1. ADAM, H.M., Mc KAIL, R.A., OBRADOR, S., WILSON, W.C.: Acetylcholine in the cerebrospinal fluid. J. Physiol. 93, 45-46 (1938).

2. ADAMS, R.D., FISHER, C.M., HAKIM, S., OJEMANN, R.G., SWEET, H.H.: Symptomatic occult hydrocephalus and normal cerebrospinal fluid pressure. Treatable syndrome. New England J. Med. 273, 117-126 (1965).

3. BANNISTER, C.M.: A report of eight patients with low pressure hydrocephalus treated by C.S.F. diversion with disappointing results. Acta Neurochir. 27, 11-15 (1972).

4. CUTLER, R.W.P., PAGE, L.K., GALICICH, J., WATTERS, G.V.: Formation and absorption of cerebrospinal fluid in man. Brain 91, 707-720 (1968).

5. HAKIM, S., ADAMS, R.D.: The special clinical problem of symptomatic hydrocephalus with normal cerebrospinal fluid pressure. J. Neurol. Sci. 2, 307-327 (1965).

6. HEISEY, S.R., HELD, D., PAPPENHEIMER, J.R.: Bulk flow and diffusion in the cerebrospinal fluid system of the goat. Am. J. Physiol. 203, 775-781 (1962).

7. HUSSEY, F., SCHANZER, B., KATZMAN, R.: A simple constant infusion manometric test for CSF absorption. II. Clinical studies. Neurol. 20, 665-680 (1970).

8. KATZMAN, R., HUSSEY, F.: A simple constant-infusion test for measurement of CSF absorption. I. Rationale and method. Neurol. 20, 534-554 (1970).

9. LEUSEN, I.: Influence de la teneur en calcium et en potassium du liquide céphalo-rachidien sur le système vasomoteur. Archs. int. Pharmacodyn. Thér. 75, 422-424 (1948).

10. LEUSEN, I.: The influence of calcium, potassium and magnesium ions in cerebrospinal fluid on vasomotor system. J. Physiol 110, 319-329 (1950).

11. LORENZO, A.V., BRESNAN, M.J., BARLOW, C.F.: Cerebrospinal fluid absorption deficit in normal pressure hydrocephalus. Arch. Neurol. 30, 387-393 (1974).

12. LORENZO, A.V., PAGE, L.K., WATTERS, G.V.: Relationship between cerebrospinal fluid formation, absorption and pressure in human hydrocephalus. Brain 93, 679-692 (1970).

13. MESSERT, B., WANNAMAKER, B.B.: Reappraisal of the adult occult hydrocephalus syndrome. Neurol. 24, 224-231 (1974).

14. PAGE, L.K., BRESNAN, M.J., LORENZO, A.V.: Cerebrospinal fluid perfusion studies in childhood hydrocephalus. Surg. Neurol. 1, 317-320 (1973).

15. PAPPENHEIMER, J.R., HEISEY, S.R., JORDAN, E.F., DOWNER, J. De C.: Perfusion of the cerebral ventricular system in unanesthetized goats. Amer. J. Physiol. 203, 763-774 (1962).

16. RUBIN, R.C., HENDERSON, E.S., OMMAYA, A.K., WALKER, M.D., RALL, D. P.: The production of cerebrospinal fluid in man and its modification by acetazolamide. J. Neurosurg. 25, 430-436 (1966).

17. SYMON. L., DORSCH, N.W.C., STEPHENS, R.J.: Pressure waves in so-called low-pressure hydrocephalus. Lancet 1972 II, 1291-1292.

18. UDVARHELYI, G.B., WOOD, J.H., JAMES, Jr., E.J., BARTELT, D.: Results and complications in 55 shunted patients with normal pressure hydrocephalus. Surg. Neurol. 3, 271-275 (1975).

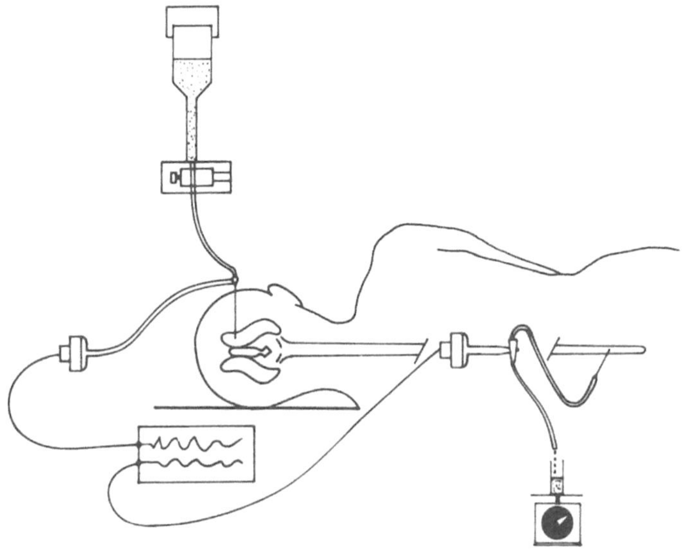

Fig. 1. Ventriculolumbar perfusion system

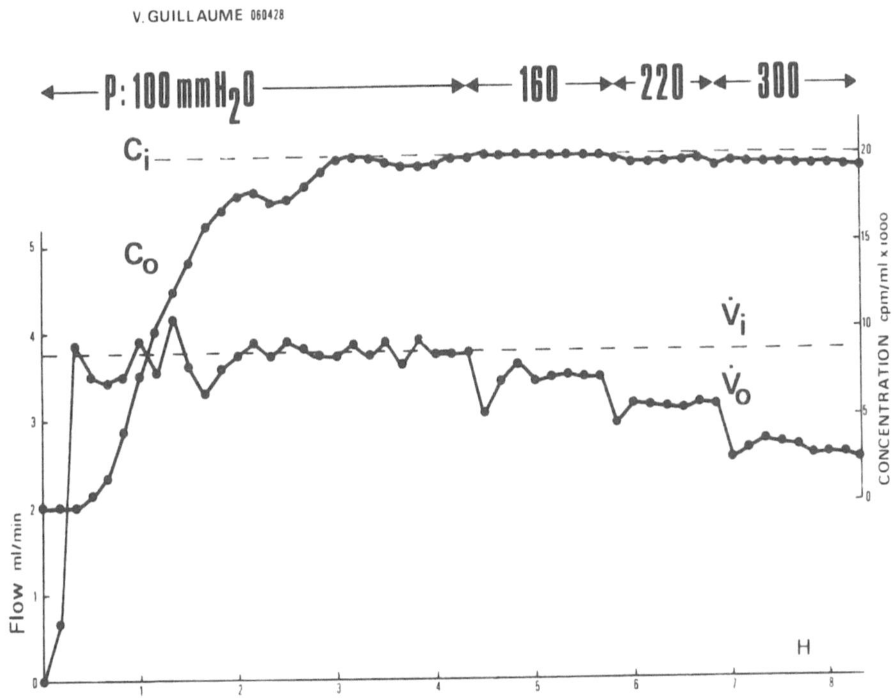

Fig. 2. Primary data from representative perfusions. Outflow rate (Vo) and ^{131}I HSA activity in effluent (Co) are plotted as a function of time. Interrupted lines represent the ^{131}I activity in perfusate (Ci) and inflow rate (Vi). Perfusion pressures are indicated above plots

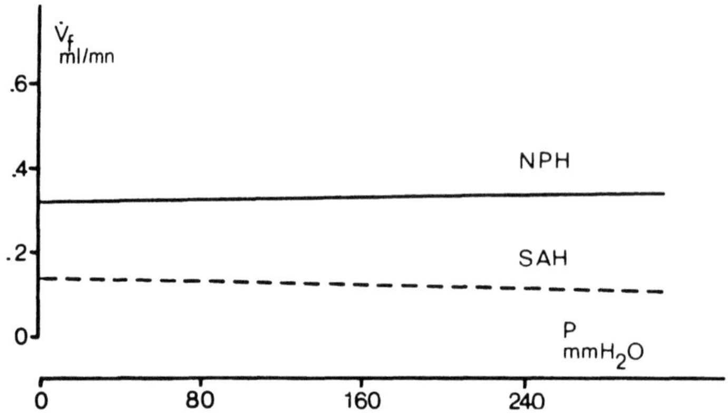

Fig. 3. Relationship between CSF formation rate and perfusion pressure in patients with signs of normal pressure hydrocephalus (NPH) and in others suffering from hydrocephalus following subarachnoid hemorrhage (SAH). Regression lines

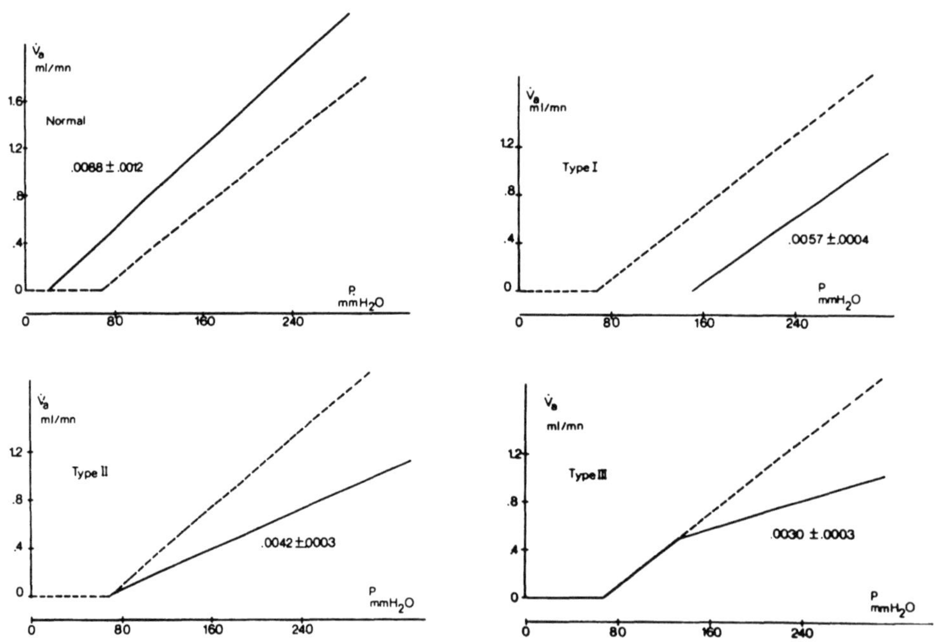

Fig. 4. Pressure-absorption relationships. Regression lines for normal absorption (case 4), type I deficit (averaging out cases 1 and 5), type II deficit (averaging out cases 2 and 7), type III deficit (averaging out cases 3, 6, and 8)

Subarachnoid Infusion Test. Its Value in the Prognosis of Shunted Normal Pressure Hydrocephalus

J. Philippon, B. George, A. Levante, C. Thurel, A. Visot, and J. Cophignon

Introduction

The main problem in the presence of clinical signs suggesting normal pressure hydrocephalus (NPH) is to demonstrate their possible relation to an impairment of cerebrospinal fluid absorption. It is then logical to propose a CSF diversion in expectation of an improvement in the patient's condition.

However, numerous studies have laid great emphasis upon the variability of the clinical picture (7, 8). More precise information may be found through radiologic studies and even more so by isotopic cisternography (7, 8). Contradictory results have been published concerning the value of these different techniques.

The subarachnoid infusion test (SIT), theoretically more valid in that it measures CSF absorption capacity, has met with controversial acceptance (1, 4, 5, 6, 9).

In order to evaluate the value of SIT, we decided to compare the results of this test to other criteria (mainly clinical signs, pneumoencephalographic, and isotopic studies). Postoperative improvement, which may be considered as the most reliable sign of the NPH syndrome (therefore offering an evaluation "a posteriori" of the different diagnostic techniques), has also been evaluated in relation to the preceding results. The test was performed in 63 patients using a technique derived from that of HUSSEY et al. (3).

Ringer solution was infused at a rate of 1 cc/min either in the subarachnoid lumbar space or through a ventricular catheter in a patient without anesthesia. CSF pressure was recorded for 10 min before infusion (the opening pressure was always inferior to 10 mm Hg) and then every minute. The infusion was stopped when a new steady-state pressure (plateau) was reached or when the CSF pressure rose to above 40 mm Hg.

An abnormal or positive test was defined by the increase in resistance to drainage, determined by using the same methods as MARTINS (5) and JANNY et al. (4), following a proposal by DAVSON et al. (2).

$$\text{Flow} = \frac{\text{Pressure gradient}}{\text{resistance}}.$$

The resistance is measured by the change in pressure versus the change in flow, or drainage rate. The normal value was considered as being between 10 and 13 mm Hg/ml/min (4, 5). The resistance of the tubing system, when measured, was found to be negligible.

Our interest in studying resistance to drainage concerns more its value in predicting CSF shunting results, rather than its theoretical aspects, which will not be discussed here. In order to eliminate tests with technical artifacts, we have used the same criteria as TROTTER et al. (9). Initial pressure must not be inferior to 4 mm Hg, the rise in pressure during the infusion should be equal or superior to 4 mm Hg, and the pressure curve should not be discontinuous.

Few complications directly related to the test have been observed. One patient developed an aseptic cellular reaction in the CSF (30 elements) for a few days. Another presented a transitory worsening of his mental symptoms (memory impairment beginning with the test and lasting for 36 h).

Postoperative surveys of 37 shunted patients were carried out. Only patients followed for more than 3 months (with an average of 1 year) have been considered, with the exception of eight recent cases. The latest, although shunted for a less lengthy period, showed an immediate marked improvement which left no doubt as to the success of the shunting.

The results of surgical treatment, based mainly on clinical examination of the patient and the impression of the family, were divided into three groups: marked improvement, slight improvement, and no modification.

Results

SIT positive results have been observed in 29 cases, negative in 34 cases. The etiology of hydrocephalus does not permit the prediction of a positive or negative SIT result, as one might presume. However, it is interesting to note that ventricular dilatation following precise causes (subarachnoid hemorrhage, traumatism, meningitis) has been encountered in 72% of the positive tests and in 35% of the negative. Idiopathic hydrocephalus shows an inverse proportion (28% positive test, 65% negative).

If one compares the results of SIT to the clinical picture (Fig. 1), no precise correlation can be drawn as above. It is interesting, however, to point out that the classical triad of mental deterioration, motor symptoms, and urinary incontinence is more frequently encountered (48%) with a positive SIT than with a negative one (12%). On the contrary, patients showing isolated mental symptoms are observed in 21% of negative tests, and those with focal signs in 30%. No other significant relation could be drawn with the other clinical aspects.

Pneumoencephalographic findings (Table 1) have been obtained in 27 patients. One may note that positive SIT is frequently associated with two basic radiologic signs of normal pressure hydrocephalus, namely dilatation of temporal horns and absence of air over the convexity. No conclusive statement can be made concerning the negative results.

Comparison of SIT and radioisotopic studies (Fig. 2) shows that normal cisternograms are as rare with negative as with positive tests (6.25% versus 4.1%). However, permanent ventricular filling (V.F.) is encountered in one half of the positive tests and only in 25% of the negative ones. The percentage of delayed clearance with or without transient V.F. presents a slight difference (45% of positive tests, 68% of negative).

Postoperative evolution provides the most interesting point of comparison (Table 2). Of the patients with a positive SIT, 78% presented a marked or slight improvement following CSF diversion: on the other hand, only 3 out of 10 had similar results with a negative test. The number of patients with no modification of their clinical status shows an inverse proportion.

A relatively small number of patients in each category of positive and negative tests gives contradictory results. Three out of nine (with negative SIT) had a postoperative improvement, one of which developed peaks of high pressure during a 24-h recording. Three patients with

Table 1. Correlation of SIT to pneumoencephalography

	Pneumo E°	Dilated temp. horns	C.C. angle<110°	Absence of air over convexity
Positive SIT	13	13	4 (7 measurable)	11
		100%	57%	84%
Negative SIT	14	5	3 (11measurable)	5
		36%	27%	36%

Table 2. Postoperative studies

		Marked improvement	Slight improvement	no modification	Unknown
Positive SIT 27 shunts	No. cases	18	3	3	3
	%	67	11	11	11
Negative SIT 10 shunts	No. cases	2	1	6	1
	%	20	10	60	10

Table 3. Postoperative improvement correlated to SIT and isotope cisternography

	No. of shunt	No. patients improved	%
Positive SIT	24[a]	21	87
Isotope – Permanent V.F.	15	10	66
Isotope – Delayed clearance convexity	12	8	66

[a]Patients without follow-up not included.

a positive test showed no modifications: one was related to a severe head injury with possible diffuse brain lesions; the second had a removal of his shunt because of an infection. In the third case, the preoperative evolution was exceptionally long (12 years).

If the decision for CSF shunting is based upon positive SIT alone (Table 3), one may predict a good result in 87% of the cases. On the other hand, an abnormal cisternogram will lead to a favorable evolution in 66% of the cases (considering either permanent ventricular filling or delayed clearance over convexity).

Discussion

The high percentage (78%) of postshunting improvement in hydrocephalus following a positive SIT has convinced us of its value as a test for predicting the eventual results of CSF diversion. This seems logical if one admits that this test is a reliable means of measuring CSF absorption capacity (4, 5, 6). This impairment of CSF circulation has been classically demonstrated through radiologic and isotopic data: absence of air over the convexity and dilatation of temporal horns during encephalography; permanent ventricular filling with stasis at cisternography. The parallelism, even if not absolute, between these signs and the results of SIT is worth noting.

Nevertheless, SIT cannot be considered as the answer to all diagnostic problems (1, 8). The presence of contradictory results in certain patients raises the problem of "false positive" or "false negative" tests. Even after eliminating technically imperfect tests, some cases still escape absolute analysis.

We have observed three positive SIT's with no clinical modification. As mentioned above, a possible explanation could be put forward in these cases. Despite its relative value, we would consider a positive test with a ventricular dilatation, even associated with an incomplete clinical picture and an equivocal isotope cisternogram, as an indication for CSF shunting.

We would not be so certain with a negative test. False negative results have been frequently recognized (4, 5, 6, 9) even if CSF leak cannot always be detected. The slight possibility of improvement in our opinion is not sufficient to recommend a shunt. In these doubtful cases, it seems reasonable to propose a continuous 24-h pressure recording, especially if other elements are strongly in favor of NPH (mainly hydrocephalus secondary to a precise etiology, ventricular enlargement with dilated temporal horns, ventricular stasis). This procedure is in our hands not a routine test, because of occasional technical difficulties with these restless patients.

Once these tests have been carried out, only very few contradictory cases will persist. However, one should keep in mind that no test is of absolute value, and that finally the decision for surgery must take into account all the clinical and laboratory data.

References

1. BELLONI, G., Di ROCCO, C., FOCACCI, C., GALLI, G., MAIRA, G., ROSSI, F.G.: Surgical indications in normotensive hydrocephalus. A retrospective analysis of the relation of some diagnostic findings to the results of surgical treatment. Acta Neurochir. 33, 1-21 (1976).
2. DAVSON, H., HOLLINGSWORTH, G., SEGAL, M.B.: The mechanism of drainage of the cerebrospinal fluid. Brain 93, 665-678 (1970).
3. HUSSEY, F., SCHANZER, B., KATZMAN, R.: A simple constant infusion manometric test for measurement of CSF absorption. Neurol. 20, 665-680 (1970).
4. JANNY, P., GODENECHE, P., FLORI, B., RAYNAUD, E.J.: La résistance :a l'écoulement du LCR. Méthode de mesure et application clinique. Revue Neurol. 128, 161-170 (1973).
5. MARTINS, A.N.: Resistance to drainage of cerebrospinal fluid; clinical measurement and significance. J. Neurol. Neurosurg. Psychiat. 36, 313-318 (1973).
6. NELSON, J.R., GOODMAN, S.J.: An evaluation of the cerebrospinal fluid infusion test for hydrocephalus. Neurol. 21, 1037-1053 (1971).
7. PHILIPPON, J., ANCRI, D.: Chronic adult hydrocephalus. In: Advances and technical standards in neurosurgery (Vol. I) (H. KRAYENBÜHL, ed.), pp. 61-92. Vienna, New York: Springer 1974.
8. STEIN, S., LANGFITT, T.W.: Normal pressure hydrocephalus. Predicting the results of cerebrospinal fluid shunting. J. Neurosurg. 41, 463-470 (1974).

9. TROTTER, J., LUZECKY, M., SIEGER, B.A., GADO, M.: Cerebrospinal fluid infusion test. Identifications of artifacts and correlation with cisternography and pneumoencephalography. Neurol. 24, 181-186 (1974).

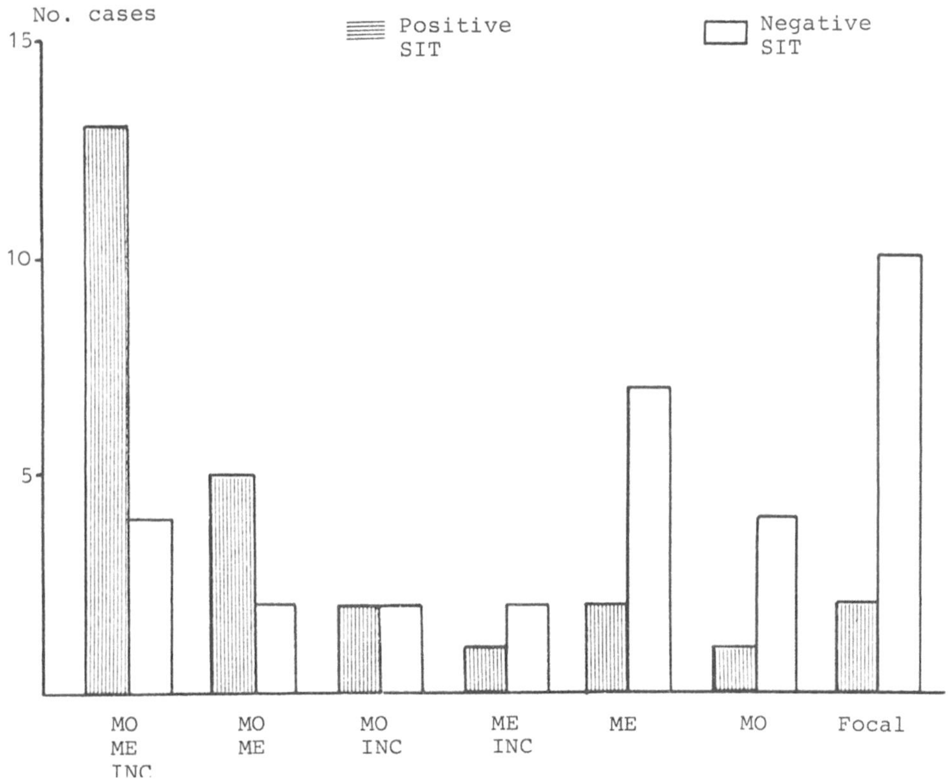

Fig. 1. Correlation of clinical signs with positive or negative SIT. Mo motor, Me mental, Inc urinary incontinence. Focal indicates a localized sign regardless of its significance

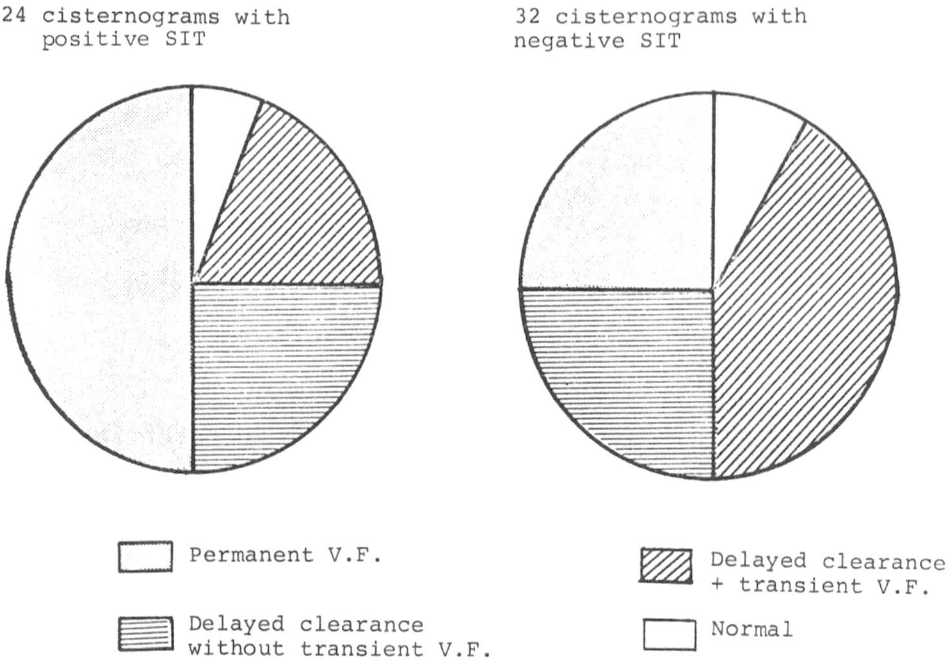

Fig. 2. Correlation fo radioisotopic studies with positive or negative SIT

Low Output and Low Pressure Failure of Valve Revealed by Shunt Perfusion

G. Martin and R. Worth

Introduction

All neurosurgeons have faced the problem of patients who have been shunted for hydrocephalus and in whom it seems doubtful if the valve is working properly. Usually the doubt is resolved by observing the patient, since surgeons are reluctant to operate because of the steep rise in morbidity that goes with multiple operations on valves.

The introduction of the Braden twin reservoir valve provided the opportunity to test the upper and lower ends of the shunts separately, quantitatively as well as qualitatively. Sometimes shunts appear to be working yet there are symptoms suggestive of hydrocephalus.

The technique of testing twin reservoir shunts by infusion and pressure measurement and some results are described.

The work is presented not because it is complete, but because the results are interesting and the technique needs to be used more widely for a fuller understanding of how shunts function after being inserted in the patient.

Methods

The reservoirs of the Braden twin reservoir valve (Heyer Schulte) are punctured by a fine 25-gauge infant scalp vein needle (Butterfly short 25, paediatric infusion set - Abbott) after the scalp over the valve has been shaved.

Attached to the scalp vein needle is an intravenous drip set with a micro drip burette (Metriset, McGaw) in the system. An intramuscular needle attached to a pressure transfuser (Ailtech M.S. 10B) is inserted into the lumen of the intravenous set through the rubber near the distal end. This transfuser is kept at the same level as the valve and the pressure recorded on a Hewlett Packard Moseley 7100BM strip chart two channel recorder.

First the ventricular pressure is measured by punturing the ventricular end dome and occluding with the finger the other dome. Then the distal end dome is punctured and the ventricular end occluded. The pressure is recorded, then the flow recorded at several different pressures.

Results

This has been done only when there has been real difficulty in reaching a decision about shunt function by any other means. It was felt that the hazards of infection from the valves precluded investigation of those valves where the shunt was clearly functioning, and also those where a decision could clearly be made that it was not functioning. Hence, it has only been done on four patients, three of whom are described below. The fourth was done on a ventriculoperitoneal shunt while lying down and anesthetized and showed the sort of flow characteristics one would expect.

The first patient was a 4-year-old girl (C.B.) with hydrocephalus and a closed meningomyelocele. A ventriculoatrial single chamber shunt had been put first on the right, then removed to the left at 8 weeks. This controlled her hydrocephalus until she was 4.5 years when a urinary tract and middle ear was associated with a recurrence of the hydrocephalus. The shunt was replaced with a Braden twin reservoir ventriculosagittal sinus shunt, using a low pressure rat's tail catheter (Heyer Schulte) with infant tip, measured to open at 30 mm H_2O. A postoperative skull x-ray showed that the tip of the catheter lay in the lateral sinus.

The symptoms and signs of her hydrocephalus subsided for a few days then recurred.

When radioiodinated human serum albumin (RIHSA) was put into the shunt and the valve pumped, the RIHSA could be clearly seen on the gamma camera passing from the tip of the catheter into the sigmoid sinus and down the internal jugular. Yet equally clearly the shunt did not seem to be controlling the symptoms of the hydrocephalus.

The ventricular dome was punctured and a pressure trace made which showed an intraventricular pressure fluctuating between 30 and 50 mg of mercury in a series of B waves. It was concluded that the valve might be passing C.S.F. but not enough to keep the pressure down. It was perfused and it appeared that at a constant pressure of 30 mm of mercury it passed 0.25 ml/min. The valve was removed and tested in vitro when it was found to pass 14 ml/min at 30 mm Hg. It was found to have a "popping pressure", a term introduced by HAKIM (8) to denote the pressure at which a valve first permits flow, varying between 2 and 7 mm Hg in vitro.

Another distal end was inserted, a standard medium pressure valve which passed 10 ml/min at 17 mm Hg. Her condition did not improve, the ventricular pressure remained high despite a further revision of the valve to eliminate kinking. For a number of reasons related to the child's ultimate prognosis, no further surgery was undertaken, she was digitalized to try and reduce C.S.F. production and had a short remission of a fortnight before she died.

A second patient was a 3-week-old infant (A.N.) who had a severe hydrocephalus with a single common ventricle and a 1 cm cortical mantle. As the child's head circumference was 54 cm at 3 weeks it was decided to put in a ventriculoperitoneal shunt for cosmetic reasons alone; a low pressure Ramondi catheter was used. The head circumference declined to 51.5 cm but returned to 55 within 5 days and stayed there. At this stage measurements of intraventricular pressure were made and they were found to be atmospheric while the Ramondi valve opened at 20 mm Hg (270 mm H_2O). Attempts to bind the head were ineffective in reducing the size and the situation was considered hopeless.

The third patient was a 64-year-old female who had a ventriculosagittal sinus shunt inserted for low pressure hydrocephalus, demonstrated by pneumoencephalogram and RIHSA ventriculogram.

After two good years following a shunt she began to deteriorate, apparently due to Parkinsonism. Shunt testing was undertaken to exclude a recurrence of low pressure hydrocephalus as a cause of the deterioration.

This demonstrated a good flow of fluid with a popping pressure of 5 mm Hg and a flow of 2 ml/min at 5 mm Hg. More interestingly it showed that the intraventricular pressure was between 0 and 2 mm Hg (0 to 30 mm H_2O) lying down and minus 4 to minus 6 mm Hg (50 to 75 mm H_2O) while sitting up. The pressure in the outflow tract of the valve while sitting up was zero.

Discussion

Because of the hazards of infection, this series is necessarily small, having been used only where there was real clinical doubts about the function of the shunt.

Two causes of shunt failure have been identified, low output failure and low pressure failure.

Firstly, the patient C.B. demonstrates a low output failure; though the shunt appears to be working to clinical and isotopic testing, it in fact passes less than the normal production per minute of C.S.F.

Also this shows that in vitro testing does not show how a valve will work in vivo. According to the in vitro test of the valve, after removal, it should have passed 14 ml/min but in vivo it passed only 0.25 ml/min at the intracranial pressure of 33 mm Hg. In addition it had a variable popping pressure in vivo of 2 to 7 mm Hg (25 to 100 mm H_2O). Perhaps this is related to varying venous pressures within the sinus.

Valves have been perfused before (10, 5) to examine their hydrodynamic characteristics, but only in vitro, there being no series of valves perfused in vivo. Even perfusion in vitro showed that valves vary widely from their nominal characteristics, but in vivo the variation may be even wider.

Moreover, this shows that neither pumping the dome of the valve nor demonstration of the passage of isotope are infallible tests of shunt function. The question of whether the outflow will permit an adequate volume flow may have to be considered at times.

This also raised the question again of whether an increase in the C.S.F. production may play a part in the production of hydrocephalus. While this valve passed less than the normal production of C.S.F. per minute (0.25 instead of 0.35 ml) other valves may be found whose output is limited but above the normal range of C.S.F. production. A patient who required two shunts to keep the pressure down was reported (10) and another in whom increased C.S.F. production was measured at 1.7 ml/min instead of the usual 0.35 ml/min (2). It seems likely that these patients will be detected by the presence of a raised ventricular pressure with a limited flow rate through the distal end of the valve.

Secondly, shunt failure has been shown to be due to too low a pressure in very large ventricles, i.e., a pressure below the "popping pressure."

It has been pointed out (7) that for ventricles which approach a spherical shape

$$P = \frac{2T}{R},$$

where P = intraventricular pressure, T = the tension in the walls, R = the radius of the sphere.

Thus as the skull is attenuated due to expansion of the cavity the tension T falls as R increases so the intraventricular pressure becomes smaller and smaller. We found it was virtually atmospheric and hence too low to operate any valve.

Binding the head to increase T is the logical answer but we found it ineffective presumably because we were not violent enough. Others have recorded serious complications from its use (9).

There seems to be still no answer to this problem except perhaps long continued negative pressure external drainage with its great risk of infection. Probably this situation is untreatable.

Finally, the question of whether ventriculosagittal sinus shunts will prevent siphoning has been raised.

The problem of siphoning has been well described by FOX (6); that is, that in the upright position the long descending limb of the shunt into the atrium or peritoneum, may produce low pressures and predispose to subdurals by siphoning off the ventricular fluid. He demonstrated negative pressures of about minus 220 mm H_2O (15 mm Hg) for ventriculoperitoneal shunts and minus 190 mm H_2O (minus 14 mm Hg) for ventriculoatrial shunts in adults. These pressures were lower than the normal range of minus 10 to minus 140 mm H_2O (minus 1 to minus 10 mm Hg). However, the prediction that ventriculosagittal sinus shunting would not eliminate the problem of siphoning does not appear to be true. It was predicted that the negative pressure of a column of blood from the sagittal sinus to the atrium would produce similar pressures. Our measurements in the third patient, who had a negative pressure of minus 50 to minus 70 mm H_2O (minus 14 to minus 15 mm Hg), lay within the normal range.

There do not seem to be any figures for venous pressure within the sagittal sinus. Probably it is not as low as the distance above the atrium would suggest because the neck veins in the erect position are well known to be collapsed and not a continuous column of fluid. Presumably flow through them is only intermittent. Indeed the figures for the normal range and the figures we observed are equal to the pressure exerted by a column of water (or blood) from vertex to the jugular foramen.

Once again shunt function needs to be measured in vivo instead of being predicted from in vitro results.

Summary

A technique of examining the pressure flow relationships of the outflow and the intraventricular pressure of shunts is described, using the Braden twin reservoir shunt, a pressure transducer and ordinary paediatric intravenous equipment.

It is shown that valves in vivo do not behave as in vitro experiments would suggest and that more work needs to be done on how shunt systems actually function after being inserted.

Two causes of shunt failure have been identified, namely low output failure and low pressure failure. It is suggested that ventriculosagittal sinus shunts may prevent siphoning.

References

1. BRISMAN, R., SCHNEIDER, S., CARTER, S.: Lumbar C.S.F. infusion test and shunt patency. Trans. Amer. Neurol. Assoc. 96, 212-213 (1971).
2. CUTLER, R.W.P., PAGE, L., GALICICH, J., WATTERS, G.V.: Formation and absorption of cerebrospinal fluid in man. Brain 91, 707-720 (1968).
3. CUTLER, R.W.P., MURRAY, J.E., MOODY, R.A.: Overproduction of cerebrospinal fluid in communicating hydrocephalus. A case report. Neurol. (Minneapolis), 23, 1-5 (1973).
4. DAVSON, H.: Physiology of the cerebrospinal fluid. London: Churchill 1967.

5. FOX, J.L., McCULLOUGH, D.C., GREEN, R.C.: Cerebrospinal fluid shunts: An experimental comparison of flow rates and pressure values in various commercial systems. J. Neurosurg. 37, 700-705 (1972).

6. FOX, J.L., McCULLOUGH, D.C., GREEN, R.C.: Effect of cerebrospinal fluid shunts on intracranial pressure and on cerebrospinal fluid dynamics.
2. A new technique of pressure measurements, results & concepts.
3. A concept of hydrocephalus. J. Neurol. Neurosurg. & Psychiatry 36, 302-312 (1973).

7. GESCHWIND, N.: The mechanism of normal pressure hydrocephalus. J. Neurol. Sci. 7, 481-493 (1968).

8. HAKIM, S., DURAN de la ROCHE, F., BURTON, J.D.: A critical analysis of valve shunts used in the treatment of hydrocephalus. Develop. Med. Child Neurol. 15, 230-254 (1973).

9. MEYER, H., PRICE, B.E., RUEBEL, C.D.: Complications arising from head wrapping for the treatment of hydrocephalus. Paediatrics 52, 867-868 (1973).

10. RAYPORT, M., REISS, J.: Hydrodynamic properties of certain shunt assemblies for the treatment of hydrocephalus. Part 1. Report of a case of communicating hydrocephalus with increased cerebrospinal fluid production treated by duplication of the shunting device. Part 2, Pressure flow characteristics of the Spitz Holter, Pudenz Heyer and Cordis Hakim shunt systems. J. Neurosurg. 30, 455-467 (1969).

Correlations Between Ventricular Fluid Pressure (VFP) and Computerized Tomography in Patients with Normal Pressure Hydrocephalus[1]

H.A. Crockard, K. Hanlon, and E. Duda

Introduction

While the concept of normal pressure hydrocephalus (NPH), being associated with periods of raised intracranial pressure (ICP) has received wide attention (1, 4, 9) the diagnosis and, more particularly, the clinical management of such patients, is far from clear.

To test the dynamic situation in this disease, RISA scans (3) have been used, as have tests of CSF absorption and formation (2). As many of the tests are complicated and not without risk to the patient, and as shunting procedure may not produce clinical improvement by may itself be associated with a high morbidity, there are many who feel that invasive testing in such patients is unjustifiable. On theoretical grounds it would seem more reasonable to perform a shunting procedure in those patients who had demonstrable elevations of pressure, regardless of ventricular size, RISA scan, etc.. SYMON and DORSCH (9) and CHAWLA et al. (1) have shown that in such patients there are rises of ICP. The discovery of such pressure changes would seem to be important in the diagnosis.

Computerized tomography has provided a noninvasive method for detecting ventricular enlargment, etc., and is an excellent screening procedure for demented patients. HUCKMAN et al. (5) have described various measurements on the computerized tomogram which they have related to neurologic conditions. Our study then was to discover how these measurements correlated with ICP in such patients and to determine if the two tests would be useful in the evaluation of this condition. This work is in a preliminary stage and requires further evaluation.

Materials and Methods

To date 19 patients have been studied: 14 patients were referred for evaluation of a variety of symptoms and signs, the predominant one being progressive dementia. The other 5 patients were investigated during their readmission for malfunction of their previously inserted shunt. VFP was measured in all patients for at least 2 days, (range 2 - 5 days). The decision to insert or revise a shunt was based on clinical grounds and the VFP measurements to be described. Preoperative computerized tomogram was performed in 14 patients and postoperative in all; serial studies over months were performed in 6 patients. The CT measurements to be described and the classification were performed without the knowledge of the intended surgical procedure.

[1] Supported by grants FO5-2144 and NS 7834-08.

VFP Measurements

The following information was determined from the VFP record:

1. The *resting pressure*, i.e., the pressure which was noted when the patient was awake and alert, and during the absence of any waves.
2. The presence or absence of *waves*, particularly B waves. Only those waves that were at least 10 mm Hg higher than resting pressure were considered to constitute a pressure problem.
3. The *percentage of time that the record was abnormal* was also measured. It was considered to be significantly abnormal if there were more than two hours during a 24-h period when there was extensive significant wave activity, i.e., 8-10% wave time.

CT Measurements

The following measurements were made on the CT scan (Fig. 1).

(A) The width at most lateral portion of each of the frontal horns.
(B) The width of the lateral ventricles at the cauda nuclei.
(C) The sum of (A) and (B) - an index of ventricular size.
(D) The total width of the four largest cortical sulci seen in the three highest tomographic cuts.

Using these measurements HUCKMAN et al. graded the CT scans into five categories, as shown in Table 1.

Table 1. Clinical classification of ventricular size by computed tomography [Method of HUCKMAN (Radiology 116, 85-92 (1975)]

Clinical category	Relative ventricular size (mm)	Sum of 4 largest sulci (mm)
1 Normal	15 or less	5 or less
2 Questionable	16-20	<6
atrophy	<16	6-9
3 Mild atrophy	16-20	6-9
4 Moderate to	>20	>5
severe atrophy	16-20	>9
5 Enlarged ventricles only	>20	<5

Both the individual CT measurements and the clinical categories were compared to the VFP in each patient. A diagnosis of NPH was made in those who had evidence of ventricular enlargment without significant elevation in the resting VFP, but who had a significant elevation during waves which were present for at least 10% of the time. If the resting pressure was higher than 20 mm Hg they were considered to have raised pressure hydrocephalus. Cerebral atrophy was diagnosed in those who had ventricular enlargment and extensive cortical sulci with no pressure rise.

Results

Of the 14 patients investigated with dementia, 8 were considered to have NPH, 2 had raised pressure hydrocephalus, 3 had cerebral atrophy, and 1 was considered to have vascular insufficiency as the basic pathology of the dementia.

ICP Results

In those with NPH the resting VFP was 11.7 ± 6.7 mm Hg (a range of 6-20 mm Hg) (mean + SD). The ICP waves rose above the resting ICP by an average of 17.1 ± 8.9 (range 10-30 mm Hg), and there was 41.5% ± 28.1% of the time monitored during which there were abnormal patterns (range 17-91%). This group was compared to the five patients who had shunt malfunction; their resting VFP was 17.4 ± 11.1 mm Hg (range 4-30 mm Hg), and the waves were 22.8 ± 12.1 mm Hg (range 10-40 mm Hg) above the resting VFP. There were waves for 63 ± 35.5% of the time monitored (range 13-100%). In the three patients considered to have cerebral atrophy, the VFP measurements were as follows: Resting pressure 8.3 ± 3.2 mm Hg (range 5-10 mm Hg) with a wave height of 5.3 ± 4 mm Hg (range 3-10 mm Hg). The record was abnormal 1.7 ± 2.9% (range 0-5%) of the time. Two patients discovered with high pressure showed a mean resting VFP of 25.7 mm Hg. Waves were 29.3 mm Hg above resting pressures and the record was abnormal for 89 and 100% of the time monitored.

Table 2. Pressure profiles of three conditions

Condition	Resting VFP mm Hg	Wave amp. mm Hg	% Time - abnormal
NPH (n = 8)	11.7 ± 6.7	17.1 ± 8.9	41.5 ± 28.1
Blocked shunt (n = 5)	17.4 ± 11.1	22.8 ± 12.1	63.6 ± 35.5
Cerebral atrophy (n = 3)	8.3 ± 2.4	5.3 ± 4.0	1.7 ± 2.9

Results are (mean ± SD)

When the groups were compared statistically, those with cerebral atrophy were significantly different from the NPH group and those requiring shunt revision, in the resting pressures and the percentage of time with abnormal record. There was no statistical difference between the NPH group and those who had a shunt revision, although in the latter the percentage time with abnormal record was higher, and the ICP waves were also higher. The insertion of a shunt abolished the waves (Fig. 2).

CT Results

The patients with NPH were placed in categories 2 or 5 and those with no rise in pressure were placed in categories 3 or 4. The patients investigated for blocked shunt had CT scans in groups 1, 2, or 5. To date the number of patients is too small to pass any comment on these clinical categories. The individual measurements from the CT scans were compared in the group who were shunted (NPH plus shunt revision), with those who did not have a shunt inserted (cerebral atrophy). In the nonshunted group there was a slightly bigger ventricular measurement (22.5 mm) as compared to those who were shunted (18.6 mm), but these were not statistically different. Measurements of the sulci, however, were significantly different. Those who were not shunted had a mean sulcal measurement of 6 mm as compared to the 3.1 mm in the shunted group (Table 3).

Table 3. Comparison of CT measurement in those with raised and normal ICP (CT measurements (mm))

	A	B	C	D
Shunted (n = 11)	11.5 (2.2)	7.1 (1.6)	18.6 (3.4)	3.1 (0.3)
Nonshunted (n = 3)	14.0 (3.0)	8.5 (2.8)	22.5 (5.6)	6.0 (0.0)
	n.s.	n.s.	n.s.	P<0.05

Results are (mean ± SD)

Discussion

The pressure profile of the group with NPH and the five who had their shunts revised were remarkably similar in resting pressures, height of waves, and percentages of time investigated when abnormal waves were present, a fact reported by others (1, 9). The VFP records of the three patients not shunted showed no rise in pressure, no waves and no significant abnormal record time, and so it was not considered justified to insert a shunt in these patients. If the basic pathology in NPH is obstruction of or a failure to absorb CSF (4), then a stress test, such as saline infusion test or estimation of CSF absorption, would display the condition. However, these tests are technically difficult and often the results may be difficult to interpret due to leakage around the lumbar needle and, if an anesthetic is given, modified by anesthesia. It is our opinion that continuous ICP measurement will infer the same as the stress tests and, while it may not point to the exact cause, will decide whether or not the patient needs a shunt. When the computerized tomograms were divided into categories, there was a suggestion that those with cerebral atrophy were predominantly from group 4, and those with NPH in groups 2 and 5. However, our numbers are too small to be any more specific at this time. When the individual CT measurements are compared for each group, the width of the cortical sulci, (D), was most significant, and would seem to be a useful point to work for when screening demented patients.

While it has been clearly shown that there are some demented patients who have raised ICP at times and this may be the etiologic cause in part or on whole for their symptomatology, there are, as yet, no good studies showing the beneficial effects of shunting. The problem has been the method of assessing improvement. Many of the psychological tests are too complicated for many of these demented patients (2), and there is, too, the problem of irreversibility. RUBIN et al. (7) have shown experimentally that if hydrocephalus is prolonged and severe there are permanent changes in the white matter surrounding the ventricles. The prolonged follow-up (18.8 years) of LÖNNUM and KORNSTAD (6) shows the overall poor prognosis of patients with ventricular enlargment. It is all the more important then that in such patients the investigation be curtailed to the minimum, and surgical intervention be considered only in cases where there is an undoubted pressure problem. STEIN and LANGFITT (8) reviewing 43 patients after a shunting procedure with NPH, showed that, in those with a definite etiology, 80% improved following shunting, whereas there was only a 24% chance of success in those where no cause for their enlarged ventricles was determined.

It is our suggestion then, that patients with dementia should be screened noninvasively by computerized tomography; and, if there are significant cerebral sulci, then little else need be done. On the other hand, those patients with small sulci and enlarged ventricles, with a suggestive history, should be investigated for the possible occurrence of NPH. In our experience the least traumatic and most reliable investigation is continuous ICP measurement for 48 h.

Summary

A total of 19 patients, whose ICP and computerized tomograms were measured, are presented. There were 8 patients who had NPH characterized by a normal resting pressure but with periods of wave activity exceeding 10% of the time monitored, and the pressure during the waves exceeding the resting pressure by 10 mm Hg. These pressure results were similar to those obtained from patients with blocked shunts. The computerized tomograms of such patients showed enlarged ventricles and small sulci. Three other patients who had no raised ICP showed enlarged ventricles and significant cortical sulci on CT scan. It is suggested that an ideal method of investigating such patients is firstly by noninvasive computerized tomography, followed by 48 h of ICP monitoring in those with no small cortical sulci and large ventricles.

References

1. CHAWLA, J.C., HULME, A., COOPER, R.: Intracranial pressure in patients with dementia and communicating hydrocephalus. J. Neurosurg. 40, 376-380 (1974).
2. COBLENTZ, J.M., MATTIS, S., ZINGESSER, L.H., KASOFF, S.S., WISNIEWSKI, H.M., KATZMAN, R.: Presenile dementia: Clinical aspects and evaluation of cerebrospinal fluid dynamics. Arch. Neurol. 29, 299-308 (1973).
3. FORSLO, H., FORSSMAN, B., JARPE, S., RADBERG, C.: RISA cisternography in possible hydrocephalus. Acta Radiolog. Diagnosis 13, 531-545 (1972).
4. HAKIM, S., VENEGAS, J.G., BURTON, J.D.: The physics of the cranial cavity, hydrocephalus and normal pressure hydrocephalus. Surg. Neurol. 5, 187-210 (1976).
5. HUCKMAN, M.S., FOX, J., TOPEL, J.: The validity of criteria for the evaluation of cerebral atrophy by computed tomography. Radiol. 116, 85-92 (1975).
6. LONNUM, A., KORNSTAD, S.: Long-term prognosis of patients with central cerebral ventricular enlargment. Acta Neurol. Scand. 50, 409-433 (1974).
7. RUBIN, R.C., HOCHWALD, G.M., TIELL, M., MIZUTANI, H., GHATAK, N.: Hydrocephalus: Histological and ultrastructural changes in the pre-shunted cortical mantle. Surg. Neurol. 5, 109-114 (1976).
8. STEIN, S.C., LANGFITT, T.W.: Normal pressure hydrocephalus: Predicting the results of cerebrospinal fluid shunting. J. Neurosurg. 41, 463-470 (1974).
9. SYMON. L., DORSCH, N.W.C.: Use of long-term intracranial pressure measurement to assess hydrocephalic patients prior to shunt-surgery. J. Neurosurg. 42, 258-273 (1975).

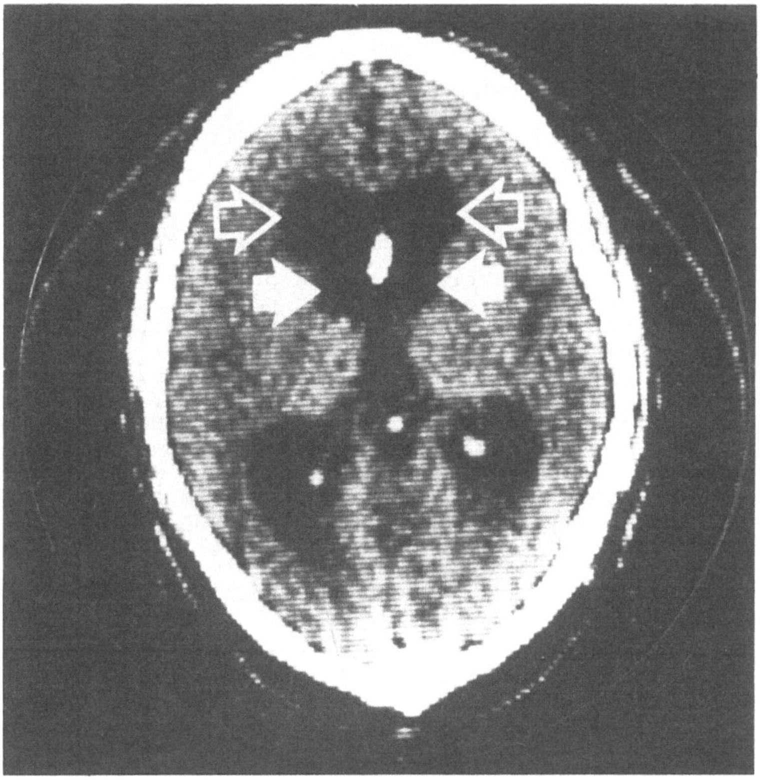

Fig. 1. A computerized tomogram showing (A) (*open arrows*) and (B) (*closed arrows*) measurements. Relative ventricular size (C) is sum of these two measurements

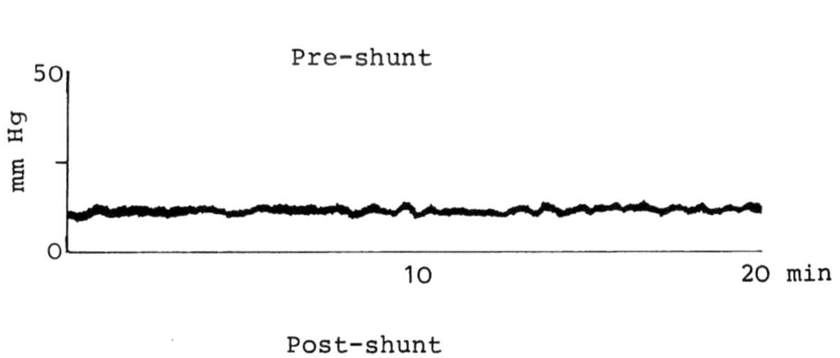

Fig. 2. Effect of a shunt procedure in a patient with NPH is shown here. Waves are abolished and there is little or no decrease in resting ICP

Summary

U. Pontén and G.M. Hochwald

"To shunt or not to shunt" - that is the question!

This was the scenario for the papers presented in this session. The effects of ventricular dilatation on periventricular white matter water content and microcirculation was thought to be a possible mechanism for memory defects in patients with chronic or so-called normal pressure hydrocephalus. Periventricular structures, such as fornix and hippocampal formation in the limbic system, are most vulnerable to this disease. This hypothesis was suggested by GRANHOLM (pp.173-176) to explain the reversibility of memory defects after shunting. He was able to demonstrate edema around these structures with computerized tomography (CT) scans with metrizamide in the ventricles. His preliminary results from several patients after shunting demonstrated marked decrease in periventricular edema, which was visible in the CT scan. However, an improvement of microcirculation will have to be inferred as techniques for measuring blood flow in this discrete region are not yet available.

Various tests have been devised to determine which patients with enlarged ventricles will benefit from cerebrospinal fluid (CSF) shunts. These tests are primarily concerned with CSF hydrodynamics to determine whether ventriculomegaly is a result of abnormal CSF circulation or secondary to brain atrophy.

PHILIPPON et al. (pp.193-198) compared the accuracy of the subarachnoid infusion test (SIT) of KATZMAN and HUSSEY with that of isotope cisternography and pneumoencephalography on the prognosis of shunting normal pressure hydrocephalic patients. Shunting improved the "clinical status" in 80% of the patients with a positive SIT. This prediction was better than that obtained with the other diagnostic techniques. These results are still somewhat difficult to evaluate as no comparison was made with results of similar tests available in the literature. Moreover, a definition of "clinical status" and follow-up data would enhance the value of prognostications.

EKSTEDT (pp.177-185) presented his results on CSF hydrodynamics obtained with the constant pressure infusion method, a technique described in the last symposium on ICP. Adult hydrocephalic patients with an elevated resting CSF pressure due to an increased pressure difference across the arachnoid villi were shunted. Only half (7 patients) showed improvement. The 12 other patients with enlarged ventricles but with both normal CSF resting pressures and CSF hydrodynamics were also shunted. None of these patients with presumed brain atrophy showed any improvement.

In their studies on ventricle to lumbar perfusion, STEVENAERT et al. (pp.186-192) verified conclusions previously made by others that, in patients with communicating hydrocephalus, there is an abnormal relationship between perfusion pressure and CSF absorption. An increase in the absorption threshold, a decrease in the absorption capacity, or both were found. In three patients with subarachnoid hemorrhage, the marked decrease in CSF formation rate was attributed to the effects of extravasated blood on the CSF-forming organs. The authors suggested the use of this technique as an aid in diagnosing communicating hydrocephalus. The use of this method, however, is limited by its complexities and need for experience.

A different method to determine the efficacy of shunting patients with normal pressure hydrocephalus was described by CROCKARD et al. (pp. 204-209). The width of sulci and ventricular size were measured in the CT scan and results were correlated with ventricular fluid pressure. Patients with sulci wider than 9 mm and normal intraventricular pressure were classified senile dements. When the sulci were less than 5 mm and the intraventricular pressure was elevated the patients were classified normal pressure hydrocephalics. Since ventriculomegaly was similar in both groups of patients, the important criterion for the diagnosis of normal pressure hydrocephalus was the width of the sulci. This measurement provides the basis for a screening test to limit the number of needless ICP measurements in demented patients. Should this method prove successful, it would also benefit patients to be shunted.

In conclusion: "To shunt or not to shunt" - that is still the question!

Session G

Drugs and Anaesthetica

Chairman: J. D. Miller
Co-chairman: H. J. Reulen

Effects of Depolarizing, Non-Depolarizing Muscle Relaxants and Intubation on the Ventricular Fluid Pressure

W. Lewelt, K. Moszyński, and H. Koźniewska

Introduction

Induction of anesthesia may cause an increase in ventricular fluid pressure (VFP), espcecially in patients with intracranial space-occupying lesions. This is related to fasciculations caused by depolarizing muscle relaxants (3) as well as to intubation (1, 2). It seems, therefore, that prevention of fasciculations should minimize the increase in VFP during the induction. The purpose of this paper is to compare the influence of two methods of induction, one based on depolarizing and the other on nondepolarizing muscle relaxants, on VFP.

Materials and Methods

In 24 patients, aged from 31 to 65, undergoing a craniotomy for a supratentorial neoplasm or a hematoma, VFP was measured continuously, starting prior to the induction of anesthesia. 7 patients (Group I) received an injection of a barbiturate in an anesthetic dose, followed respectively by suxamethonium chloride (100 mg) and intubation. 17 patients (Group II) received pancuronium bromide and after about 2 min of oxygenation they were inducted with a barbiturate and intubated.

Results

In group I, the administration of a barbiturate caused a fall in VFP in all the cases. VFP rose again during the period of fasciculations due to the suxamethonium and reached the highest value during intubation (Fig. 1): raising on the average 9.14 mm Hg, i.e., 27.5% as compared with the value before the application of the barbiturate. The course of one of these inductions is shown in Figure 2.

In group II the induction was reflected in a small decrease in VFP with an average of 0.06 mm Hg, i.e., 0.24% as compared to the value before the injection of the barbiturate, and an average of 0.7 mm Hg, i.e., 2.8% as compared to the value before the administration of pancuronium. We observed a slight fall of VFP after the injection of pancuronium and a more distinct one following the administration of the barbiturate. The intubation in most of the cases was smooth and without the evident rise of VFP as seen in group I (Fig. 3). In 5 cases, however, the increase of VFP was marked, this being the effect of insufficient relaxation, or difficulty with the intubation.

In all the cases of both groups, barbiturates gave an evident decrease of VFP, with an average of 14.04 mm Hg, i.e., 51.92% as compared to the initial value.

Discussion

Fasciculations, reflexes from the respiratory tract and difficulties with intubation can evoke a rise in venous pressure that is reflected in an increase in cerebral blood volume. This, in patients with exhausted intracranial compensatory mechanisms will result in a marked increase in VFP. HULME (2) observed intracranial pressure values of 60 - 80 mm Hg during intubation. ADAMS et al. (1) stated that the increase in intracranial pressure depends on the degree of narcosis and of muscle relaxation and on the difficulty in intubation.

The introduction of pancuronium, which proved to be a quickly acting agent, and without causing fasciculations, allows to depart from the classical method of induction based on suxamethonium. It seems, that the extention of time to about 5 min between the injection of pancuronium and intubation in all the cases is sufficient to achieve an adequate relaxation and to prevent an increase in VFP during this period.

Summary

In 24 patients operated for supratentorial processes, the influence of two methods of induction of anesthesia on ventricular fluid pressure was compared.

Induction with suxamethonium chloride, a depolarizing muscle relaxant, was followed by an increase in VFP (average of 9.14 mm Hg, i.e., 27.5%), while the induction with pancuronium bromide, a nondepolarizing agent, was reflected in a small decrease in this pressure (average of 0.7 mm Hg, i.e., 2.8%) as compared to the initial value.

References

1. ADAMS, R.W., GRONERT, G.A., SUNDT, T.M., MICHENFELDER, J.D.: Halothane, hypocapnia, and cerebrospinal fluid pressure in neurosurgery. In: Intracranial Pressure (M. BROCK, H. DIETZ, eds.), pp. 320-325. Berlin-Heidelberg-New York: Springer 1972.
2. HULME, A.: Discussion on anesthetic drug effects. In: Intracranial Pressure II (N. LUNDBERG, U. PONTEN, M. BROCK, eds.), p. 330. Berlin-Heidelberg-New York: Springer 1975.
3. MOSZYNSKI, K., LEWELT, W., KOZNIEWSKA, H.: Effects of thiobarbiturates and scoline on the cerebrospinal fluid pressure. In: Proceedings. 6th Congress of Polish Society of Anesthesiologists, Gdańsk, June 7-9, 1973, pp. 126-131. Polish Society of Anesthesiologists, Gdańsk, 1973.

Fig. 2. Induction of anesthesia in case of a 65-year-old patient, operated for a glioblastoma multiforme in the left frontal lobe. VFP rose significantly when the patient became agitated (1). The injection of a barbiturate (Brevinarcon) 0.45 g reduced VFP from 52 mm Hg to 22 mm Hg. The administration of suxamethonium chloride Scoline 100 mg and the intubation caused an increase in VFP to 77 mm Hg. The beginning of hyperventilation (2) was reflected in an evident decrease in VFP

▷

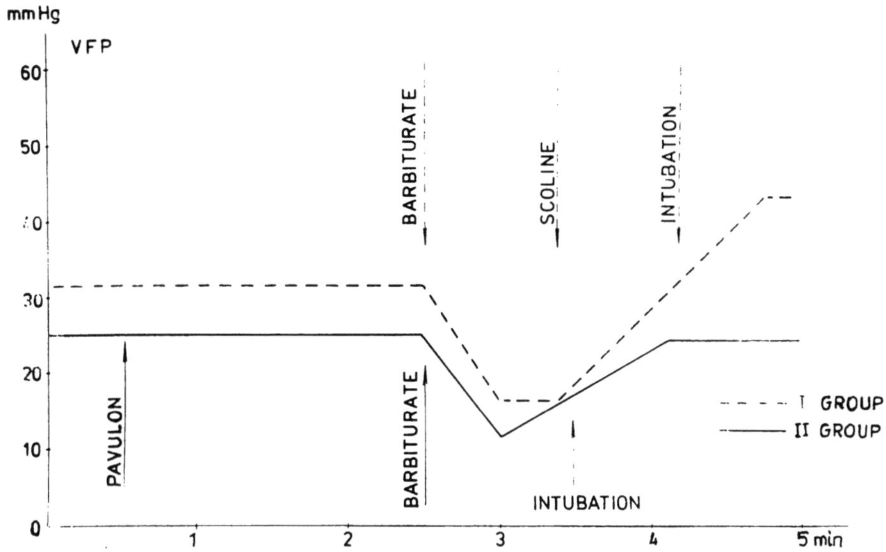

Fig. 1. Average values of VFP during the induction of anesthesia in group I (*dashed line*) and in group II (*solid line*)

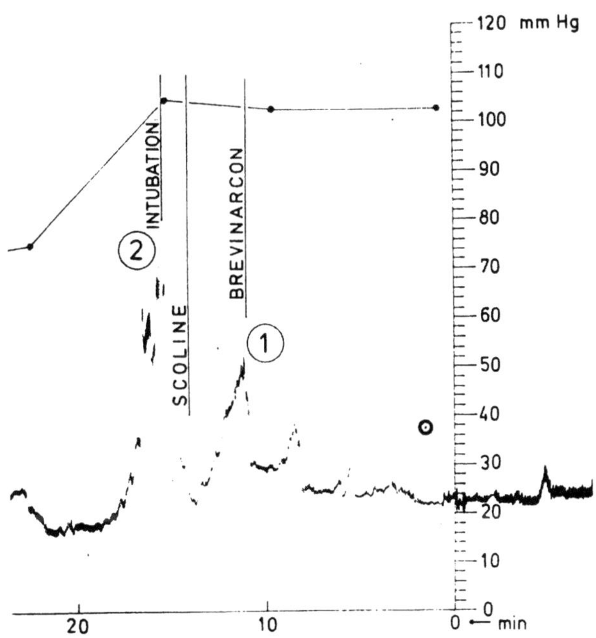

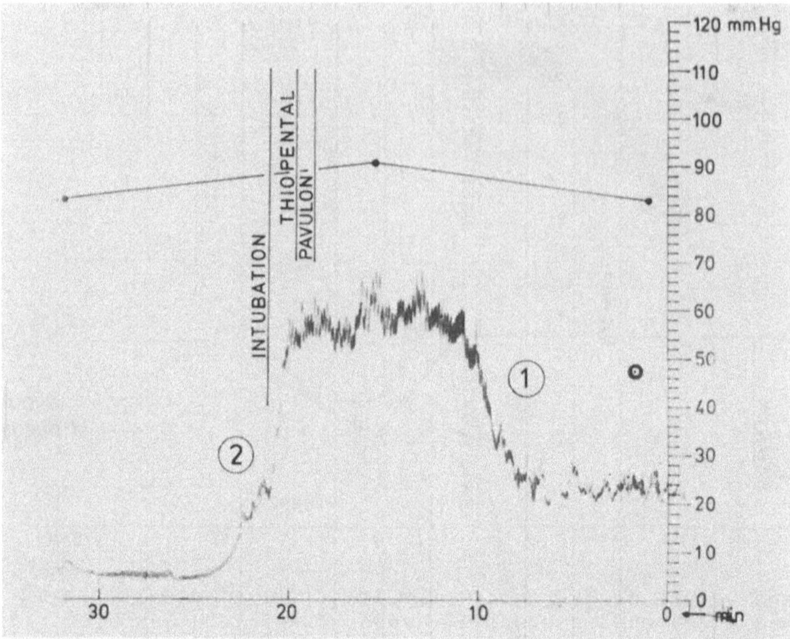

Fig. 3. Induction of anesthesia in the case of a 34-year-old patient operated for a glioblastoma multiforme in the left frontal lobe. Motor agitation provoked an increase in VFP to 64 mm Hg (1). The patient received 4 mg pancuronium bromide (Pavulon). Administration of a barbiturate (Thiopental) 0.3 g was reflected in a fall in VFP to 22 mm Hg and there was only an increase of 2 mm Hg during intubation. Hyperventilation (2) caused a further fall in VFP

The Effect of THAM on Acute Intracranial Hypertension. An Experimental and Clinical Study

T. Akioka, K. Ota, A. Matsumoto, K. Iwatsuki, A. Doi, S. Okao, K. Ninomiya, and A. Nishimoto

Introduction

Brain tissue acidosis due to hypoxia may exist in the case of intracranial hypertension. Increased hydrogen ion concentration produces reduction in the vasoconstrictor tone resulting in an enlarged vascular bed that increases intracranial pressure (ICP), which makes a vicious cycle. DOS and coworkers (2) reported that an adequate maintenance of pH with an alkalizing agent, Trishydroxymethylamino methane (THAM), helped to prevent elevation of ICP in cases of hypercapnia due to apneic oxygenation. In the present study, we investigated the effects of alkalizing agents, mainly THAM, on acute intracranial hypertension in experimental animals and clinical cases.

Materials and Methods

Experimental studies: Under light pentobarbital anesthesia, 11 adult mongrel dogs were paralyzed with succinyl choline chloride and ventilation was controlled to maintain normal arterial blood gas levels. To obtain intracranial hypertension, a rubber balloon was placed in the left frontal extradural space and was inflated intermittently. ICP was monitored by a small epidural balloon in the right frontal region, filled with water. Arterial blood pressure was recorded from the femoral artery. Intermittently, arterial blood was sampled from the femoral artery and pH, $PaCO_2$, and PaO_2 were determined by the use of a Radiometer. On occasions, the cerebral venous blood and cerebrospinal fluid (CSF) were also taken from the superior sagittal sinus and cisterna magna for the same purpose. Cortical pH was recorded using a microglass electrode attached to the brain surface. Cerebral blood flow (CBF) was determined by a heat clearance technique. Electroencephalogram (EEG) was recorded from the bilateral frontoparietal regions. ICP was increased by intermittent expansion of the compression balloon at the rate of 0.2 ml/min. After getting a Cushing response, ICP was dropped abruptly by deflation of the balloon. Then, within a few minutes ICP increased again spontaneously up to the systemic arterial pressure level. This situation is called "acute brain swelling" (4). To examine CO_2 reactivity, 10% CO_2 was given for inhalation. For the treatment of acute brain swelling, 0.3 mol THAM or 20% mannitol (15 ml/kg) was injected intravenously over a period of 20 min. Clinical studies: Six patients with increased ICP due to a brain tumor were investigated. All had a ventricular drainage. ICP was recorded continuously with a pressure gauge transducer connected to the ventricular drainage. CSF was collected from the lateral ventricle and the arterial blood was sampled from the femoral artery. pH, pCO_2, and pO_2 of CSF and arterial blood were determined with a Radiometer. To decrease ICP, 0.3 mol THAM, 7% sodium bicarbonate or 20% mannitol (120-200 ml) were infused intravenously for a couple of hours.

Results

In our experiment, after intravenous dripping of 0.3 mol THAM, ICP decreased in the dogs, as shown in Figure 1. Following the intravenous administration of 7% sodium bicarbonate (140 ml) in a patient with increased ICP, the ICP also decreased markedly (Fig. 2). We had the same results by using THAM in clinical cases. Table 1 shows for the experiment the data of pH, pCO_2, and pO_2 in arterial blood, cerebral venous blood, and CSF in the situation before the increase in ICP, the stage of acute brain swelling and after the treatment with THAM. pH in cerebral venous blood and CSF decreased during the stage of acute brain swelling, though the pH in arterial blood did not change significantly. After administration of THAM, pH had increased to even higher than normal levels. During the stage of acute brain swelling, the EEG was isoelectric before the THAM treatment. But after the infusion of THAM, ICP decreased and EEG and CO_2 reactivity were restored in 9 out of 11 animals (Fig. 3). In a comparative study between THAM and mannitol, we found that administration of mannitol significantly decreased ICP whereas administration of THAM also decreased ICP, but not as much as with mannitol. On the other hand, mannitol did not restore the CO_2 reactivity of cerebral vessels to normal though THAM could (Fig. 4).

Table 1. Changes of pH, pCO_2, and pO_2 in arterial blood, cerebral venous blood, and CSF in animal experiments

		Control	Acute brain swelling	After THAM
Arterial blood	pH	7.353±0.048	7.334±0.026	7.456±0.045[c]
	pCO_2	38±4	39±6	34±5
	pO_2	98±14	98±19	103±18
Cerebral venous blood	pH	7.272±0.043	7.178±0.083[b]	7.302±0.098[a]
	pCO_2	46±6	59±17[a]	47±7
	pO_2	40±8	23±4[c]	41±10[c]
CSF	pH	7.299±0.050	7.247±0.047[a]	7.343±0.053[c]
	pCO_2	45±4	53±6[b]	43±7[b]
	pO_2	44±8	30±5[c]	49±11[c]

Mean±SD (n=9), $^{a}p<0.05$, $^{b}p<0.01$, $^{c}p<0.001$.

Discussion

We reported earlier about the existence of occult cerebral acidosis in cases of intracranial hypertension as shown in our experiments using extracorporal CSF circuits (1). In this situation increased hydrogen ion concentration may produce a reduction in the vasoconstrictor tone resulting in an enlarged vascular bed (3) that may increase ICP, which makes a vicious cycle. In view of DOS's investigations (2), we tried to use an alkalizing agent for the treatment of acute brain swelling. At the stage of acute brain swelling, administration of THAM decreased ICP, but did not produce a decrease in ICP as much as mannitol. Furthermore, THAM could restore the CO_2 reactivity of cerebral vessels to normal, though mannitol did not. From these results we conclude that an alkalizing agent, as THAM, may act directly on the vascular wall, improve the vasoconstrictor tone and therefore may decrease the ICP. Is it possible to hypothesize that acute brain swelling is a situation of congestive shock? If so, we could, just as LILLEHEI (5) pointed out in general irreversible congestive shock, state that the vessels in the brain might lose their sensitivity to norepinephrine and/or epinephrine in a situation of acidosis that is caused by hypoxia. Namely, after THAM treatment the sensitivity to norepinephrine and/or epinephrine of the receptors in resistant vessels may be restored by the improvement of tissue pH. Accordingly, vasomotor tone may recover and then ICP may decrease. We would like to investigate these problems in a second phase of this research.

From these points of view, we'd like to emphasize that restoration of tissue pH is the most important and reasonable treatment in acute brain swelling.

Summary

The effects of alkalizing agents, mainly THAM, on acute intracranial hypertension were investigated in experimental animals and clinical cases. Administration of THAM in the stage of acute brain swelling decreased ICP and restored the CO_2 reactivity of cerebral vessels to normal. It is concluded that an alkalizing agent, as THAM, might act directly on the vascular wall, improve the vasoconstrictor tone, and therefore may decrease ICP.

References

1. DOI, A.: Studies on acid-base balance of the cerebrospinal fluid under acute intracranial hypertension (In Japanese). Okayama Igakkai Zasshi 82, 361-372 (1970).
2. DOS, S.J., NAHAS, G.G., PAPPEN, E.M.: Experimental correction of hypercapnic intracranial hypertension. Anesthesiology 23, 46-50 (1962).
3. IWATSUKI, K.: Cerebrovascular CO_2 reactivity under intracranial hypertension in dogs (In Japanese). Brain Nerve 27, 959-966 (1975).
4. LANGFITT, T.W., WEINSTEIN, J.D., KASSEL, N.F.: Cerebral vasomotor paralysis produced by intracranial hypertension. Neurology 15, 622-641 (1965).
5. LILLEHEI, R.C., LONGERBEAM, J.K., BLOCH, J.H., MANAX, W.G.: The nature of irreversible shock: Experimental and clinical observations. Ann. Surg. 160, 682-710 (1964).

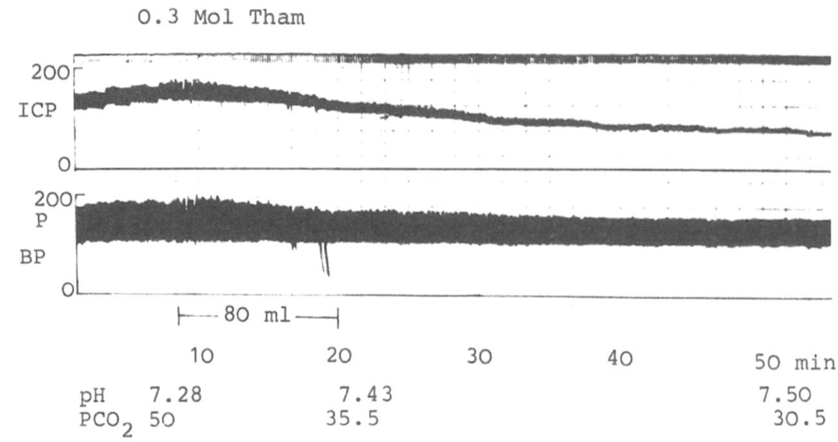

Fig. 1. Recordings from an experimental dog in which extradural balloon inflation was used to produce acute intracranial hypertension. After intravenous dripping of 0.3 mol THAM, ICP decreased. Changes of pH and $PaCO_2$ in arterial blood are also shown

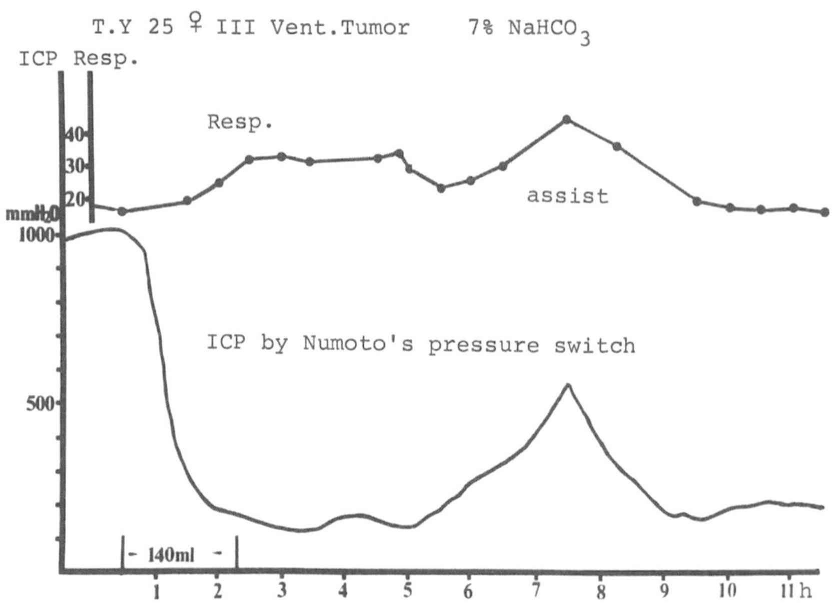

Fig. 2. Recordings from a patient with a third ventricle tumor. After administration of 7% sodium bicarbonate (140 ml), the ICP dropped from 1000 down to 150 mm water. However, ICP tended to increase again because of respiratory suppression. Therefore, assisted respiration was instituted. Consequently, ICP was kept under 500 mm water for more than 11 h

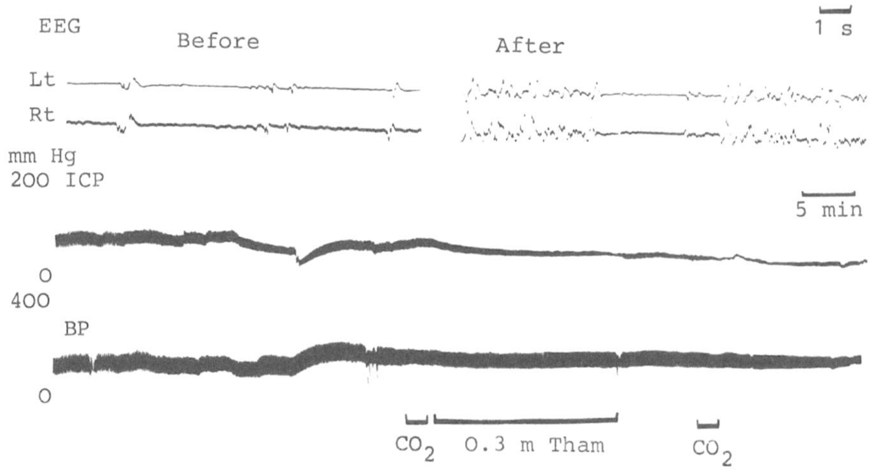

Fig. 3. At stage of acute brain swelling, EEG was isoelectric before THAM treatment. But after infusion of THAM, ICP decreased and EEG and CO_2 reactivity were restored

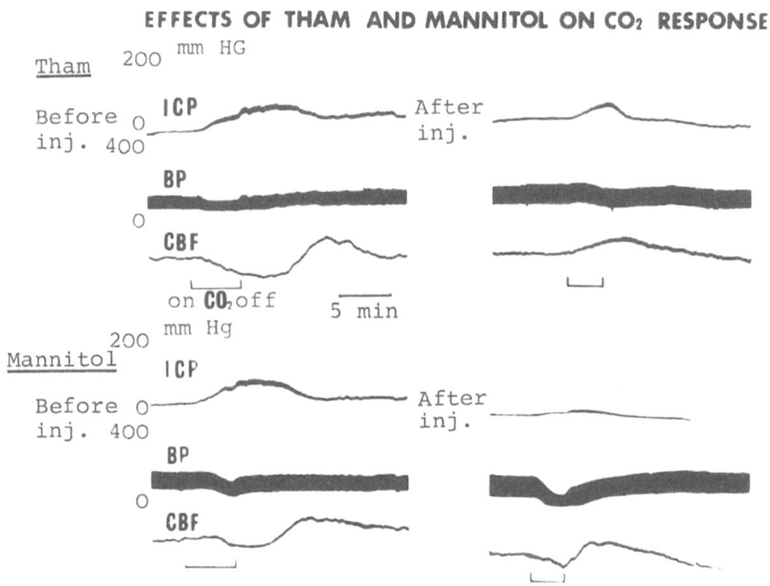

Fig. 4. A comparative study between THAM and mannitol: THAM could restore CO_2 reactivity of cerebral vessels to normal, but mannitol did not

Reduction of Raised Intracranial Pressure Following Infusion of Mannitol. A Review of Clinical Pressure Recordings

G. Kullberg and G. Sundbärg

Introduction

Administration of hypertonic solutions of mannitol as a means of reducing intracranial pressure (ICP) was introduced by WISE and CHATER in 1961 (7) and has since then been widely used in clinical practice for the purpose of temporary as well as long-term control of raised ICP. To what extent such treatment is effective is not clear, however. Several studies (2, 4-8) have demonstrated the temporary pressure fall produced by a single infusion of mannitol but doses varied and data on the effect are given for few patients only. Systematic studies on the value of protracted mannitol treatment are few and do not permit definite conclusions (1, 3). In order to obtain more information on the pressure reduction achieved with mannitol treatment, we started a review of the material of ventricular fluid pressure (VFP) recordings collected in the neurosurgical department in Lund over the years when mannitol has been in use. The results obtained so far are presented.

Methods

Fifty patients were selected, who had received mannitol on the usual clinical grounds during periods of VFP recording. On inspection of the records 234 infusions, given to 41 patients, were found acceptable for evaluation on the criterion that reasonably long and undisturbed pre- and postinfusion periods should be available. Although higher doses have been used in the clinic, all mannitol doses given to this group of patients were in the range of 0.5 g/kg body weight (30-40 g in adults), infused over approximately 1 h, although sometimes at faster or slower rates. Some of the patients had received mannitol on a regular basis, usually 6-hourly, others single or sporadic doses. A variety of diagnoses was represented in the group, with dominance of malignant glioma, metastases (15 patients) and head injuries (11 patients).

The majority of the pressure curves showed a considerable amount of "spontaneous" irregular fluctuations, which made separation of mannitol effects from other pressure variations difficult. The decrease in pressure produced by each individual mannitol infusion could not be exactly defined in terms of duration or magnitude in the absence of preceding steady state level and clear beginning and end of the change. For quantification of the effects a comparison of the mean pressure over a 2 h period preceding the infusion with the mean pressure for each following hour seemed best suitable. Numerical evaluation according to this principle was carried out for part of the material by manual extraction of the necessary pressure data from the curves. In some of the cases of serial mannitol treatment the effects were assessed by calculating the mean pressure for consecutive 3 h periods over the whole period of treatment.

Results

On inspection of the pressure records it was found that about one-third of the mannitol infusions were accompanied by a visible decrease in pressure, generally small but conceived as a significant change, with an approximate duration ranging from 1 to 3-4 hours. This type of "good response" is illustrated by the top curve in Figure 1. In the remainder of the infusions there was only a barely detectable, somewhat questionable change in pressure or no visible reduction at all (Fig. 2 exemplifies effects which were difficult to assess). The results varied between different patients but also between different infusions given to the same patient.

There were never any dramatic changes with these doses of mannitol like those regularly obtained with ordinary doses of urea, as would be expected in view of the greater osmotic gradients created by this agent. (Fig. 1, second and third curve from the top show the contrasting effects of mannitol and urea given to the same patient). Continually high pressure (above 50 mm Hg) was never brought down towards normal levels. Plateau waves and other pressure peaks were sometimes modified for a few hours. (Fig. 1, bottom curves). On other occasions, however, plateau waves continued totally unaffected by mannitol infusion. Neither would mannitol always influence high amplitude rapid variations (Fig. 3).

The result of quantitative assessment by comparing the mean pressure of the 2-h pre-infusion period with the mean pressure for each following hour is shown in Table 1. Data from 52 mannitol infusions given to nine patients have been grouped and averaged. Groups 1-3 each represent one patient on serial mannitol. In groups 4 and 5 several patients with comparable ICP levels have been lumped together. The individual data (not shown in the table) for the 52 infusions varied considerably, partly due to the disturbing influence of "spontaneous" pressure variations. When this influence was levelled out by the averaging procedure, a small effect of mannitol emerged, as shown by the figures in the table. The change in pressure varied in the different patients (groups) from practically nil to some 5 mm Hg lower pressure during 2-3 h, whereafter the effect wears off.

Table 1.

Group	Patients diagnosis	n	Mannitol n	ICP mm Hg 2-h pre	Change in ICP mm Hg 1-h periods postinfusion 1st	2nd	3rd	4th	5th
1.	Contusion	1	21	21	-3.6	-2.9	-1.5	-0.3	-0.2
2.	Contusion	1	12	25	-4.0	-7.2	-3.8	-2.3	-0.9
3.	Contusion	1	5	40	+3.2	-4.0	+2.0	-1.5	+0.5
4.	Malignant tumor	3	10	30	-5.8	-7.4	-5.2	-2.0	
5.	H.I. SAH	3	4	17	-0.8	-1.2	-1.0	+2.3	
		9	52						

Figure 4 shows the mean pressure over consecutive 3-h periods in two patients on serial mannitol. Periods ushered in by a mannitol infusion show fairly consistently somewhat lower pressure than the immediately preceding period, but this effect does not outlast the interval till the next infusion. Whether the mannitol treatment contributes to a gradual decrease in pressure over the whole period cannot be decided. There is no evident tendency to diminished effect with repetition of dose.

Discussion

The small and short-lasting effect of mannitol in a dose of 0.5 g/kg found in the present review of a mixed group of patients agrees well with the results of JOHNSTON et al. (3), who studied the effect of serial mannitol infusions of similar doses in 20 patients following surgery for intracranial aneurysm. These authors, in addition, compared the mannitol-treated patients with untreated controls and found no differences in mean pressure levels over longer periods of time.

While MILLER and LEECH (4) noted a pressure fall of 34% following rapid infusion of 0.5 g/kg mannitol in a short-term study (45 min), other authors reporting marked decrease in ICP, lasting several hours, used larger doses, 1-2 g/kg (5, 7, 8). BECKER and VRIES, in a study of long-term osmotic treatment of patients with high ICP, administered mannitol in such amount as were required to keep the pressure below 25 mm Hg. This led to intolerably high serum osmolarity in some of the patients, but in others seemed therapeutically successful.

Thus, available evidence indicates that effective control of raised ICP by mannitol will usually require larger doses than those given to the present group of patients. Doses of this magnitude are clearly insufficient in emergency situations with signs of brain stem herniation. If mannitol is used for pressure reduction over longer periods of time it appears essential that dosage is adapted to actual requirements by ICP monitoring. A schedule of mannitol, 0.5 g/kg 6-hourly, in many places routine treatment for patients with verified or suspected increase of ICP, seems little motivated.

Further, controlled, studies are required to solve the problem whether mannitol treatment contributes to final normalization of ICP and recovery of the patient.

Summary

The effect of hypertonic mannitol on raised ICP was studied by reviewing a series of ventricular fluid pressure recordings covering 236 infusions of mannitol in a dose of 0.5 g/kg given to 41 patients on usual clinical indications. One-third of the infusions were accompanied by clearly visible, although usually small, decrease in pressure, lasting some hours. Marked pressure falls were not seen. Fifty-two infusions given to 9 patients were assessed by comparing the mean ICP of the 2-h period preceding infusion with a mean ICP for each following hour. The average individual response varied from nil to about 5 mm Hg lower pressure during 2-3 h.

Key Words

Mannitol, Osmotherapy, Intracranial pressure.

References

1. BECKER, D.P., VRIES, J.K.: The Alleviation of Increased Intracranial Pressure by the Chronic Administration of Osmotic Agents. Intracranial Pressure (M. BROCK, H. DIETZ, eds.), pp. 309-315. Berlin-Heidelberg-New York: Springer 1972.

2. BRUCE, D.A., LANGFITT, T.W., MILLER, J.D., SCHUTZ, H., VAPALAHTI, M.P., STANEK, A., GOLDBERG, H.I.: Regional cerebral blood flow, intracranial pressure and brain metabolism in comatose patients. J. Neurosurg. 38, 131-144 (1973).

3. JOHNSTON, H.J., PATERSON, A., HARPER, A.M., JENNETT, W.B.: The Effect of Mannitol on Intracranial Pressure and Cerebral Blood Flow. Intracranial Pressure (M. BROCK, H. DIETZ, eds.), pp. 176-180. Berlin-Heidelberg-New York: Springer 1972.

4. MILLER, J.D., LEECH, P.: Effects of mannitol and steroid therapy on intracranial volume-pressure relationships in patients. J. Neurosurg. 42, 274-281 (1975).

5. SHENKIN, H.A., GOLUBOFF, B., HAFT, H.: The use of mannitol for the reduction of intracranial pressure in intracranial surgery. J. Neurosurg. 19, 897-901 (1962).

6. TINDALL, G.T., McGRAW, C.P., IWATA, K.: Subdural pressure monitoring in head injured patients. Intracranial Pressure (M. BROCK, H. DIETZ, eds.), pp. 9-13. Berlin-Heidelberg-New York: Springer 1972.

7. WISE, B.L., CHATER, N.: Use of hypertonic mannitol solutions to lower cerebrospinal fluid pressure and decrease brain bulk in man. Surg. Forum 12, 398-399 (1961).

8. WISE, B.L., CHATER, N.: The value of hypertonic mannitol solution in decreasing brain mass and lowering cerebrospinal fluid pressure. J. Neurosurg. 19, 1038-1043 (1962).

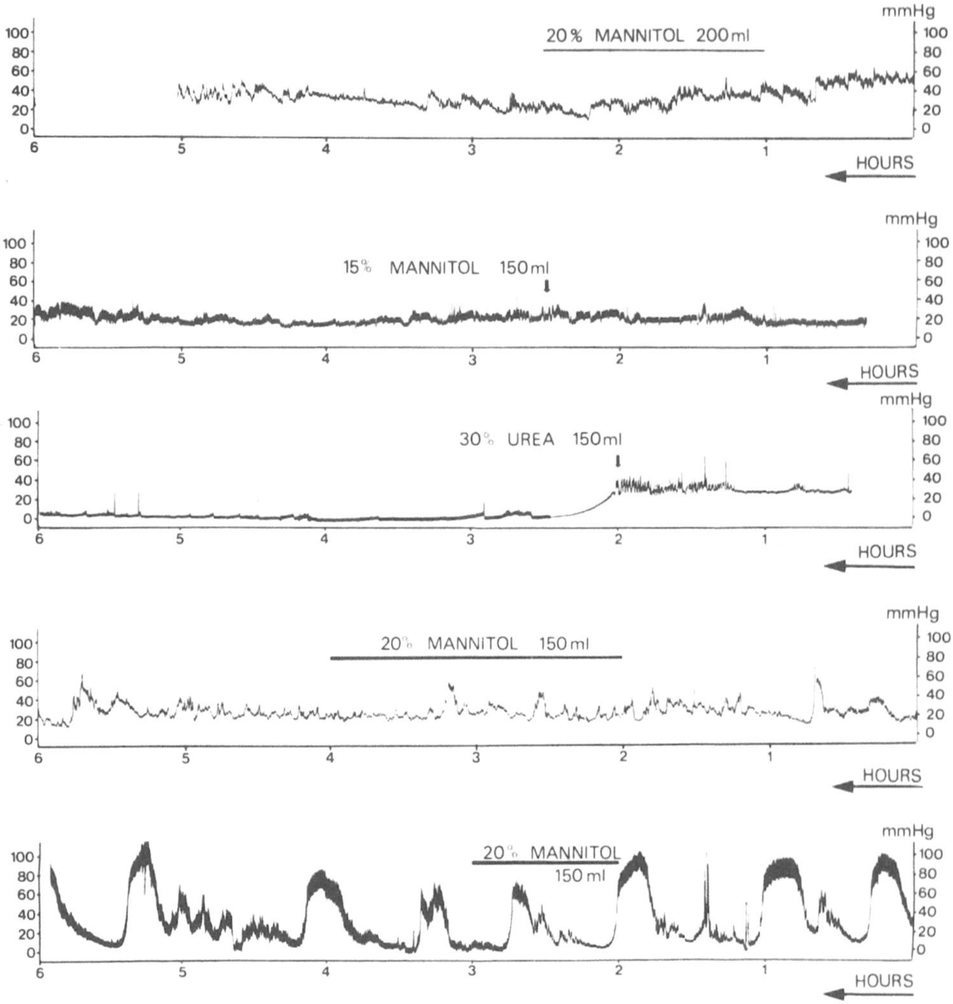

Fig. 1. VFP records illustrating effect of infusions of mannitol. Horizontal lines indicate periods of infusion, arrows start of infusion. Note that curves go from right to left.
Top curve: Exemplifies "good effect" of mannitol. (Record from patient with malignant glioma)
2nd and 3rd curve: Small pressure decrease following mannitol contrasting to marked and long-lasting pressure fall after urea in same patient (aneurysmal bleeding)
4th curve: Suppression of high pressure peaks during last part of infusion and following hour (head injury)
5th curve: Plateau waves lowered for 2-3 h (metastase)

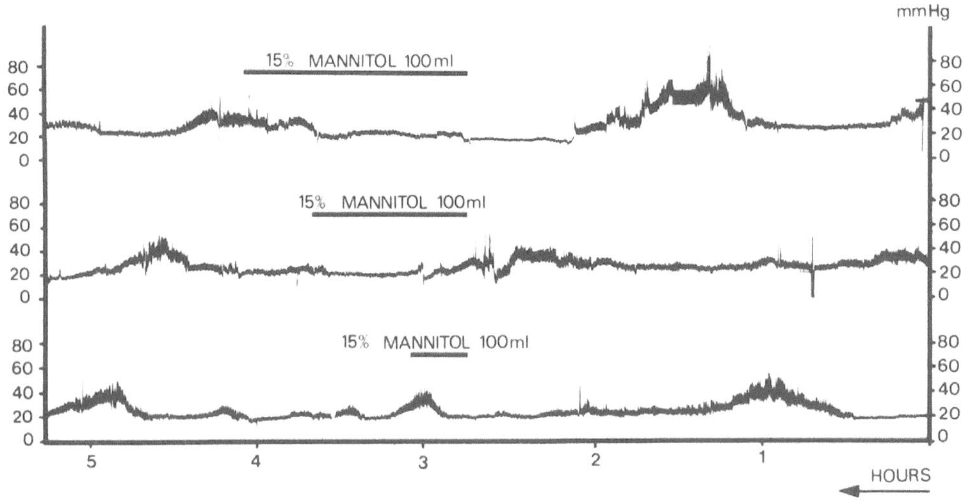

Fig. 2. VFP records showing three infusions of mannitol in one patient. The effects are difficult to evaluate in these fluctuating curves. Horizontal lines indicate periods of infusion. Curve goes from right to left (child, aged 12, with head injury)

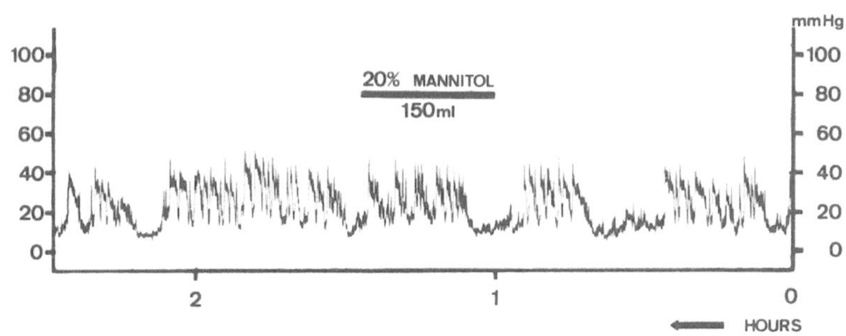

Fig. 3. VFP record with high-amplitude rapid variations; no effect of mannitol in spite of rapid infusion (denoted by horizontal line). Note that curve goes from right to left. (Head injury. Contusion evacuated. Unconscious, in respirator at the time of recording. Later complete recovery)

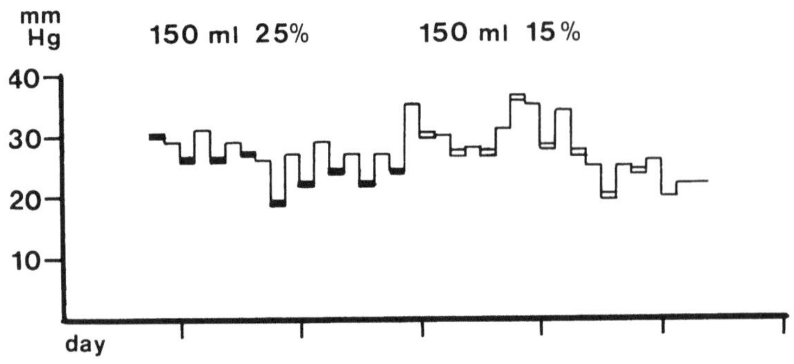

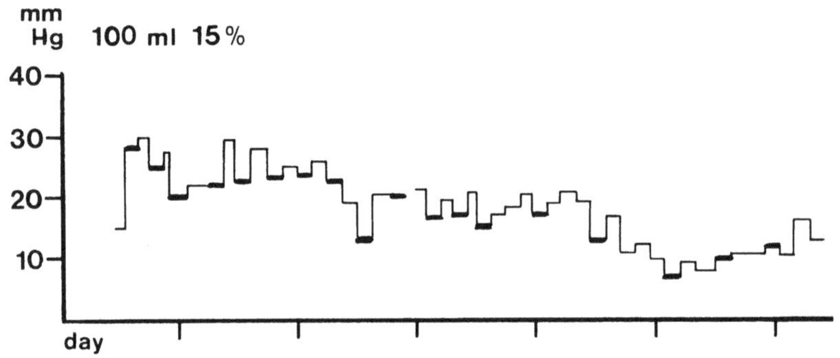

Fig. 4. Mean ICP for consecutive 3-h periods in two patients given serial mannitol infusions.
Upper diagram represents a patient with malignant glioma, partially removed 2 days earlier, on steroid treatment. Mannitol was given every 6 h in doses as shown in the figure. Mean ICP for periods ushered in by a mannitol infusion are denoted by thick bars, filled for 25% mannitol, unfilled for 15% mannitol
Lower diagram represents a 12-year-old boy, comatose after head injury 2 days earlier, temporal contusion evacuated. Mannitol (denoted by thick bars) was given approximately every 6 h the first three days, then at 12-h intervals. During the whole course also treated with artificial hyperventilation and steroids. Gradually recovered

Treatment of Acute Cerebral Edema with High Dose of Dexamethasone

W. Gobiet, W.J. Bock, J. Liesegang, and W. Grote

Introduction

In cases of traumatic cerebral edema most authors at present recommend as basic therapy hyperventilation and administration of saluretics or osmodiuretics (4). In considering the favorable experiences with dexamethasone in the treatment of perifocal edema in cases of brain tumors (5, 6), the objective of our study was to prove the use of steroids in varying doses to prevent and treat post-traumatic cerebral edema.

Materials and Methods

Examinations were carried out in 93 patients with head injuries. Patients were divided into three groups:

Group I: 35 patients without dexamethasone.
Group II: 24 patients who had received dexamethasone in normal doses.
Group III: 34 patients with dexamethasone in high doses (Table 1).

Table 1. Schedule for dexamethasone therapy in very high and low dosage. Children between 10 and 14 years received one-half, children below 10 years one-fourth of this dose

	day after trauma					
	initial	1	2	3	4	5 -8
high dose (mg)	48	8/2h	4/2h	8/2h	4/2h	4/4h
normal dose (mg)	16	4 x 4 daily				

The following parameters were established for all patients: 1. Intracranial pressure by an epidural pressure device, 2. laboratory data: daily - electrolytes, hemoglobin, hematocrit, blood gases and blood sugar profile; twice weekly - electrophoresis and transaminases (1). Only those patients were included in the study who at the time of admittance showed all our criteria for direct measurement of intracranial pressure, i.e., no responsiveness to command, defense reaction to pain stimulation in at least one extremity, signs of brain stem damage, presence of reaction to light in at least one pupil. A space-occupying lesion was either excluded or treated in all patients. Patients who were on admittance in a better condition or showed bilaterally widened fixed pupils were not included in this study.

We considered only those ICP increases which were of clinical significance and, therefore, treated by us. This is the case when ICP exceeds 50 mm Hg or when, due to increasing ICP the cerebral perfusion pressure decreases to less than 50 mm Hg. When this level was exceeded patients got hypertonic solutions (1 g/kg). Basic therapy was standardized in all patients. It consisted of moderate hyperventilation, parenteral high caloric feeding from day 1 to 3 after trauma, additional tube feeding starting on day 3 and maintenance of blood homostasis.

Results

Table 2 shows a classification of patients according to nature of lesion and age. It can be seen that the distribution of the patients within the groups is relatively homogeneous.

Table 2. Classification of patients according to nature of lesion, neurological symptoms and age

	Group I	Group II	Group III
Closed trauma (without mass lesion)	20	13	16
Subdural hematoma:			
acute	3	2	2
subacute	7	5	8
Epidural hematoma	3	3	4
Intracerebral hematoma	1	-	2
Open injuries	1	1	2
Adults/children	21/14	14/10	18/15
Brain stem symptoms (extension spasm, diabetes insipidus):			
adults	14	10	13
children	9	7	10

The doses of dexamethasone administered are listed in Table 1. When giving a normal dose we subdivided, for practical reasons, only adults and children under 10 years of age; in group III (high dose) we made a differentiation between adults, children above 10 years of age and children below the age of 10.

A classification of results with respect to mortality and complication rate is given in Table 3. The mortality in groups I and II (45.5% in group I as compared to 41.5% in group II) is almost the same. In group III (high dose of dexamethasone) mortality drops significantly to 22%. Under high doses of dexamethasone the decrease in complications (like pulmonary edema or gastrointestinal bleeding) is also very remarkable.

In order to obtain information regarding the incidence of increased ICP and, simultaneously, the extent of cerebral edema the total number of all ICP increases over 50 mm Hg per day after trauma was divided by the number of patients for each group. Table 4 shows the results. In groups I and II the frequencies of pathological ICP rises per day is almost the same whereas in group III this frequency is markedly lower.

Laboratory data like electrolytes, blood sugar, electrophoresis, transaminases or blood gases showed no significant differences for the various groups.

Table 3. Results of this study in respect of mortality and complication (group I = no dexamethasone, group II = normal dose, group III = very high dose). In group III mortality and complications were clearly lower than in the other groups

	Group I	Group II	Group III
number of patients	35	24	34
died	45.5%	41.5%	23%
pulmonary edema	7	4	0
gastric hemorrhage	5	3	0

Table 4. Frequency of pathological pressure rises over 50 mm Hg. Patients in group III (high dexamethasone) showed significantly less ICP increases

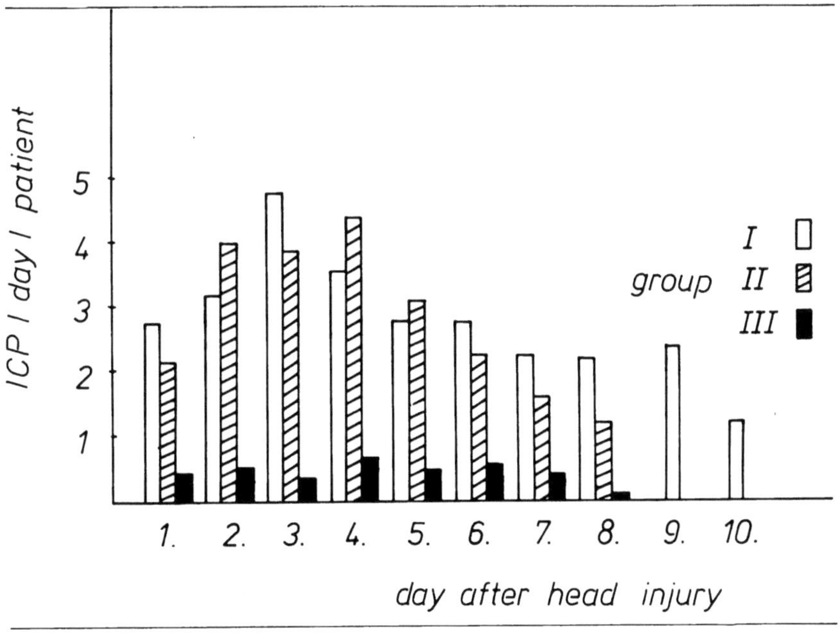

Discussion

Numerous investigations have shown the positive effect of steroids in the treatment of perifocal cerebral edema. Opinions as to treatment of post-traumatic cerebral edema are divergent. Most authors have denied the favorable effect of steroids in patients with head injury. So the administration of diuretics is preferred in treating post-traumatic cerebral edema (5).

The results of group I (no dexamethasone) demonstrate that such a therapy is not sufficient to serve as effective prophylaxis and treatment of cerebral edema. The mortality in this group was not lower than in the recent years, in which we did not monitor ICP (Table 5).

In comparing all parameters there were no significant differences between the groups that received either no or normal doses of dexamethasone. Marked improvement, however, could be demonstrated after administration of increased doses of dexamethasone.

Table 5. Results of a parallel study taken from 1973 to 1975. In 1975 all head-injured patients admitted to our clinic, received high steroid doses. In severely injured patients ICP was regularly monitored. Combined high steroid therapy and monitoring of ICP led to a reduction of mortality of 20% in adults and 24% in children

	adults>14 years		children<14 years	
	total	died(%)	total	died(%)
1973	85	51	28	46
1974	105	53	45	40
1975	102	33	50	16

In contrast to reports by other authors no increased gastrointestinal hemorrhage was seen when dexamethasone was administered in high doses. However, immediately after admission to the intensive care unit antacids are given and tube feeding is initiated early (7).

There are so little differences between the other parameters in the respective groups (e.g. electrolytes, blood sugar and delay in wound healing) that the medication of high doses of dexamethasone must be recommended as basic therapy to prevent traumatic brain edema even in younger patients (3). The indication for osmodiuretics is to lower pathological pressure rises which are found even when high doses of dexamethasone are given. In such cases continuous ICP monitoring is necessary in order to exactly recognize these increases and to differentiate them from the symptoms of primary brain stem lesions, like extension spasms, cardiac arrhythmias and hyperthermia.

Summary

Investigations in 93 patients with severe head injury have shown that successful prophylaxis and therapy of brain edema with only osmodiuretics or salidiuretics is in many cases not possible. After administration of high doses of dexamethasone, however, the frequency of pathological pressure rises, mortality and complication rate were significantly reduced. Therefore, it seems justified to give as a basic therapy high doses of dexamethasone for a period of several days following severe head injury.

References

1. GOBIET, W., BOCK, W.J., LIESEGANG, J., GROTE, W.: Experience with an intracranial pressure transducer, readjustable in vivo. J. Neurosurg. 40, 272 (1974).
2. GOBIET, W., GROTE, W., BOCK, W.J.: The relation between intracranial pressure, mean arterial pressure and cerebral blood flow in patients with severe head injury. Acta Neurochir. 32, 13 (1975).
3. GOBIET, W.: Die Behandlung des akuten traumatischen Hirnödems. Notfallmedizin 2, 98-103 (1976).
4. KÜHNER, A., et al.: The influence of high and low dosages of Mannitol 25% in the therapy of cerebral edema. Advances in Neurosurgery. Vol. 1, p. 81. Berlin-Heidelberg-New York: Springer 1973.
5. REULEN, H.J., HADJIMOS, A., HASE, U.: Steroids in the treatment of brain edema. Brain Edema. Berlin-Heidelberg-New York: Springer 1973.
6. REULEN, H.J., SCHÜRMANN, K.: Steroids and Brain Edema. Berlin-Heidelberg-New York: Springer 1972.

7. CANTU, R.C., AMIR-AHMADI, H., PRICTO, C.: Evaluation of the increased risk of gastrointestinal bleeding following intracranial surgery after high dosis of steroids. Int. Surg. Dig. 50, 325 (1968).

The Influence of Dexamethasone Therapy in ICP in Patients with Tumors of the Posterior Fossa

M. Brock, C. Zillig, H. Wiegand, C. Zywietz, and P. Mock[1]

Introduction

Only a few authors have studied the effect of dexamethasone on ICP in patients with brain tumor (5, 7, 22, 23), and none has reported specifically on tumors of the posterior fossa. This is due in part to the difficulties met with when trying to quantify ICP changes as slow as those expected under corticoid therapy. Although it has been a matter of general agreement that corticoids exert a beneficial clinical effect on patients with intracranial hypertension due to brain tumor (1, 10-12, 15, 16, 18, 22, 23, 28, 30, 33, 34, 36, 39), it is still a matter of controversy, if this is due to the action of corticoids on ICP itself (7, 22, 23), on the intracranial pressure/volume relationship (25, 30), on brain edema (17, 20, 26, 32), or on CSF production (13, 14, 29, 37, 38, 40).

In a previous study on the effect of dexamethasone on ICP in patients with supratentorial tumors (5) we suggested that the therapeutic benefit obtained with this drug might be due in part to a reduction of "intracranial tightness" and to an improved cerebral perfusion. Decreased CSF production should also play a role in this phenomenon. Since tumors of the posterior fossa usually cause intracranial hypertension mainly through blockage of CSF-pathways rather than through bulk increase due to edema, we decided to study the effects of dexamethasone on ICP in a series of patients with infratentorial tumors presenting ventricular dilatation.

Material and Methods

Eight patients with infratentorial tumors (Table 1) in whom ventricular catheterization was necessary for diagnostic and therapeutic reasons had continuous ventricular fluid pressure recording by means of a catheter introduced into the right frontal horn (27) and connected to a commercial pressure transducer (Statham P23Db) and to an electromanometer-recorder unit (Hellige, He 18). A 6-h period of frequency analysis (3, 6) took place in each patient prior to and on the 2nd day following the onset of dexamethasone treatment. The pressure histograms were compared graphically and submitted to statistical analysis (Mann-Whitney test). Further, the number and total duration of plateau waves (whenever present) recorded during the 6-h period of frequency analysis preceding therapy were compared to the number and total duration of plateau waves during a similar period on the 2nd day of therapy. The alterations in symptomatology during the study were also noted. The

[1] The authors are indebted to Miss E. Riechers, Miss I. Busche, Mrs. G. Wachholz and Mr. B. Akuskell for their valuable technical help. The equipment for frequency analysis was built with support of the Deutsche Forschungsgemeinschaft.

Table 1

Case No.	Age (years)	Sex	Diagnosis
240468 (POL)	7	M	Spongioblastoma of the IVth ventricle
150427 (FAL)	48	F	Meningioma of the clivus
270329 (DRU)	46	M	Medulloblastoma of the vermis
080868 (RAD)	7	F	Cerebellar angioblastoma (cystic)
070464 (ONN)	11	F	Medulloblastoma of the IVth ventricle
030831 (DIL)	44	F	Acustic neurinoma
051148 (TAS)	27	M	Cerebellar astrocytoma (cystic)
231057 (GAL)	17	M	Angioblastoma of the vermis (cystic)

periods of frequency analysis were at similar times of the day (either morning or afternoon) in order to avoid the influence of circadian ICP fluctuations. Following the control study all patients received a single intravenous dose of 12 mg of dexamethasone[2], complemented by subsequent intramuscular application of 4 mg every 6 h. No other agents known to alter ICP were administered during the entire study.

Results

Plateau waves were observed in four patients (Nos. 150427, 270329, 030833 and 231057) prior to treatment. Altogether, 20 plateau waves were observed in the four patients during the 6-h periods prior to therapy. These waves lasted a total of 190 min, corresponding to an average duration of 9.5 min per plateau wave. On the second day of treatment there were 6 plateau waves altogether, their total duration amounting to 34 min, which corresponds to an average duration of 5.7 min per plateau wave (Table 2). In two cases, plateau waves completely disappeared on the 2nd day of treatment (Fig. 1).

Table 2

	Number of plateau waves		Total duration (min)	
Case No.	before	after	before	after
150427	1	0	8	0
270329	9	4	80	22
030831	5	2	35	12
231057	5	0	67	0
Total	20	6	190	34

Intracranial pressure was reduced by at least one pressure class in 6 patients. As expected this effect was very evident in the four patients with plateau waves but it also occurred in two other cases. The joint histograms obtained by averaging the pressure-class values of all patients demonstrate this signigficant ($P<0.001$ Mann-Whitney Test) decrease in ICP under the influence of dexamethasone therapy.

[2]Decadron, Sharp & Dohme GmbH, Munich.

Barostabilization. Similar to what had been observed in patients with supratentorial tumors (5) the pressure-histograms in the present series were steeper, and their base narrower, on the 2nd day of therapy. This reduction in ICP fluctuations was observed both in patients with and without plateau waves (Fig. 3) and even when ICP as such did not shift toward a lower pressure class (case No. 080868). This homogenization of ICP was termed Barostabilization (5).

Comments

It has been shown previously that frequency analysis as used in the present study constitutes a practical and reliable method of detecting and analyzing quantitatively slow changes in ICP (6). This also explains the increasing interest in this type of data handling observed among those engaged in ICP monitoring (8, 21).

Reduction in Plateau Waves

The decrease in number and total duration of plateau waves under the effect of dexamethasone noticed in the present series is in agreement with the findings of previous authors (7, 22, 23). We believe that this beneficial effect of corticoids in general can be attributed to their influence on the intracranial pressure/volume relationship (25, 30), leading to an increase in the intracranial volume buffering capacity (9, 24, 35). Since the reduction in amount and duration of plateau waves was much more marked in patients with tumors of the posterior fossa as compared to those with hemispheric tumors, it is probable that the influence of dexamethasone on CSF production (13, 14, 29, 31, 37, 38, 40) rather than its effect on peritumoral edema (32, 34) plays an important role in this mechanism.

Intracranial Pressure

It remains unclear, through what mechanism(s) corticoids lead to a decrease in intracranial pressure. Our observations confirm the fact the ICP does decrease under dexamethasone therapy. They also confirm that this decrease is neither rapid nor necessarily marked. In our material (including 12 patients with supratentorial tumors) this decrease in ICP usually became evident on the 2nd day of therapy and did not amount to more than one pressure class.

Barostabilization

The present report confirms the previous observation (5) that dexamethasone leads to a steepening of the pressure histogram with a narrowing of its base - Barostabilization. This corresponds to a decrease in intracranial pressure fluctuations, evident also in the absence of plateau waves (Figs. 3 and 4) and apparently independent of the net reduction of ICP alone, since other substances which lead to a more pronounced decrease in ICP than corticoids fail to induce Barostabilization (Fig. 5).

The pathophysiological importance of Barostabilization - no matter what its ultimate cause - consists in the fact that less fluctuation of ICP is obviously paralleled by less fluctuation of cerebral perfusion pressure and, consequently, a more homogeneous blood supply to the brain. The increased constancy of cerebral blood flow, in its turn, will exert a favorable effect on cerebral metabolism - mainly in diseased areas - contributing to improvement of the clinical condition of the patient. The observations on the effect of dexamethasone on rCBF (16, 34) are in agreement with this hypothesis. This is also why the effect of dexamethasone on the EEG "does not appear to be mediated by the effect of this drug on cerebral edema" (32). Further, the reduction in ICP fluctuations will decrease shearing forces and tissue pressure gradients within the cranium (2, 4, 4a). Barostabilization also takes place during the postoperative period following brain tumor extirpations and shunting procedures for disturbances of CSF circulation.

In conclusion, Barostabilization appears to be the final common pathway, for the effect of dexamethasone on the various individual mechanisms disturbed in the presence of intracranial hypertension.

Summary

Frequency analysis of ICP in eight patients with infratentorial intracranial tumors shows that dexamethasone (1) decreases the amount and total duration of plateau waves, (2) lowers intracranial pressure, and (3) markedly reduces fluctuations in ICP (independently of the occurrence of plateau waves and of the net decrease in ICP). The consequence of this latter effect, Barostabilization, is a more homogeneous cerebral perfussion pressure and an improvement of cerebral metabolism, possibly leading to an amelioration of the patient's clinical condition.

Key Words

Frequency analysis of ICP, Barostabilization, Dexamethasone, Brain tumors.

References

1. BECKS, J.W.F., DOORENBOS, H., and WALSTRA, G.J.M.: Clinical experiences with steroids in neurosurgical patients. In: Steroids and Brain Edema (H.J. REULEN, K. SCHÜRMANN, eds.), pp. 233-238. Berlin-Heidelberg-New York: Springer 1972.

2. BROCK, M., BECK, J., MARKAKIS, E., DIETZ, H.: Intracranial pressure gradients associated with experimental cerebral embolism. Stroke 3, 123-130 (1972).

3. BROCK, M., DIEFENTHÄLER, K., ZYWIETZ, C., PÖLL, W., MOCK, P., DIETZ, H.: Amplitude analysis of long-term intracranial pressure recordings. In: Advances in Neurosurgery 2 (W. KLUG, M. BROCK, M. KLINGER, O. SPOERRI, eds.), pp. 310-313. Berlin-Heidelberg-New York: Springer 1975.

4. BROCK, M., FURUSE, M., WEBER, R., HASUO, M., DIETZ, H.: Brain tissue pressure gradients. In: Intracranial Pressure II (N. LUNDBERG, U. PONTEN, M. BROCK, eds.), pp. 215-217. Berlin-Heidelberg-New York: Springer 1975.

4a. BROCK, M., HADJIDIMOS, A.A., DERUAZ, J.P., FISCHER, F., DIETZ, H., KOHLMEYER, K., PÖLL, W., SCHÜRMANN, K.: The effects of hyperventilation on regional cerebral blood flow. On the role of changes in intracranial pressure and tissue-perfusion pressure for shifts in rCBF distribution. In: Cerebral Vascular Diseases (J.F. TOOLE, J. MOOSSY, R. JANEWAY, eds.), pp. 114-123. New York and London: Grune & Stratton Inc. 1971.

5. BROCK, M., ZILLIG, C., WIEGAND, H., ZYWIETZ, C., MOCK, P., DIETZ, H.: The effect of dexamethasone on intracranial pressure in patients with supratentorial tumors, In: Brain Edema. Formation and Resolution. (H. PAPPIUS, W. FEINDEL, eds.). Berlin-Heidelberg-New York: Springer 1976 (in press).

6. BROCK, M., ZYWIETZ, C., MOCK, P., WIEGAND, H., ZILLIG, C., TAMBURUS, W.M.: Reliability and reproduceability of ICP frequency analysis. In: Intracranial Pressure III (J.W.F. BEKS, A. BOSCH, M. BROCK, eds.), pp. 288-294. Berlin-Heidelberg-New York: Springer 1976.

7. CABRINI, G.P., GIOVANELLI, M., INFUSO, L.: Influenza del desametazone sulla pressione liquorale ventricolare in casi si ipertensione endocrania. Minverva Neurochir. 11, 94-102 (1967).

8. CASTEL, J.P., COHADON, F.: Méthode d'analyse modale automatique des variations de la pression intra-cranienne chez l'homme. Neuro-Chirurgie 21, 205-212 (1975).

9. CRONQVIST, S., LUNDBERG, N.: Regional cerebral blood flow in tumors with special regard to cases with intracranial hypertension. Scand. J. Clin. Lab. Invest. 22 (Suppl. 102) 15:A (1968).

10. FLETCHER, J.W., GEORGE, E.A., HENRY, R.E., DONATI, R.M.: Brain scans, dexamethasone therapy, and brain tumors. J.A.M.A. 232, 1261-1263 (1975).

11. GALICICH, J.H., FRENCH, L.A.: Use of Dexamethasone in the treatment of cerebral edema resulting from brain tumors and brain surgery. Am. Pract. Dig. Treat. 12, 169-174 (1961).

12. GALICICH, J.H., FRENCH, L.A., MELBY, J.C.: Use of dexamethasone in treatment of cerebral edema associated with brain tumors. Lancet 81, 46-53 (1961).

13. GARCIA-BENGOCHEA, F.: Cortisone and the cerebrospinal fluid of noncastrated cats. Am. Surg. 31, 123-125 (1965).

14. GARCIA-BENGOCHEA, F.: The effect of cortisone on cerebrospinal fluid production in castrated adult cats. Neurol. 16, 512-514 (1966).

15. GARDE, A.: Experiences with dexamethasone treatment of intracranial pressure caused by brain tumors. Acta Neurol Scand. 41 (Suppl. 13) 439-443 (1965).

16. HADJIDIMOS, A., STEINGASS, U., FISCHER, F., REULEN, H.J., SCHÜRMANN, K.: The effects of dexamethasone on rCBF and cerebral vasomotor response in brain tumors. Europ. Neurol. 10, 25-30 (1973).

17. HERRMANN, H.-D., NEUENFELDT, D., DITTMANN, J., PALLESKE, H.: The influence of dexamethasone on water content, electrolytes, blood-brain barrier and glucose metabolism in cold injury edema. In: Steroids and Brain Edema (H.J. REULEN, K. SCHÜRMANN, eds.), pp. 75-85. Berlin-Heidelberg-New York: Springer 1972.

18. HINDO, W.A., DETRANA, F.A., LEE, M.-S., HENDRICKSON, F.R.: Large dose increment irradiation in treatment of cerebral metastases. Cancer 26, 138-141 (1970).

19. HUTTEN, H., DIEFENTHÄLER, K., BROCK, M.: Ein neues Gerät für die kontinuierliche telemetrische Messung des intrakraniellen Drucks beim Menschen. Biomed. Techn. 16, 170-172 (1971).

20. KOBRINE, A.I., KEMPE, L.G.: Studies in head injury. Part II: Effect of dexamethasone on traumatic brain swelling. Surg. Neurol. 1, 38-42 (1973).

21. KULLBERG, G.: A method for statistical analysis of intracranial pressure recordings. In: Intracranial Pressure (M. BROCK, H. DIETZ, eds.), pp. 65-69. Berlin-Heidelberg-New York: Springer 1972.

22. KULLBERG, G.: Clinical studies on the effect of corticosteroids on the ventricular fluid pressure. In: Steroids and Brain Edema. (H. REULEN, K. SCHÜRMANN, eds.), pp. 253-258. Berlin-Heidelberg-New York: Springer 1972.

23. KULLBERG, G., WEST, K.A.: Influence of corticosteroids on the ventricular fluid pressure. Acta Neurol. Scand. 41 (Suppl. 13) 445-452 (1965).

24. LANGFITT, T.W., WEINSTEIN, J.D., KASSELL, M.F.: Cerebral vasomotor paralysis produced by intracranial hypertension. Neurology 15, 622-641 (1965).

25. LEECH, P.J., MILLER, J.D.: The effect of mannitol, steroids and hypocapnia on the intracranial volume/pressure response. An experimental and clinical study. In: Intracranial Pressure II (N. LUNDBERG, U. PONTEN, M. BROCK, eds.), pp. 361-364. Berlin-Heidelberg-New York: Springer 1975.

26. LONG, D.M., MAXWELL, R.E., FRENCH, L.A.: The effects of glucosteroids upon experimental brain edema. In: Steroids and Brain Edema (H.J. REULEN, K. SCHÜRMANN, eds.), pp. 65-75. Berlin-Heidelberg-New York: Springer 1972.

27. LUNDBERG, N.: Continuous recording and control of ventricular fluid pressure in neurosurgical practice. Acta Psychiat. Scand. (Suppl. 149) 36 (1960).

28. MARTY, R., CAIN, M.L.: Effects of corticosteroid (dexamethasone) administration on the brain scan. Radiol. 107, 117-121 (1973).

29. MAYMAN, C.I.: Inhibitory effect of dexamethasone on sodium-potassium activated adenosine triphosphatase of choroid plexus in cat and rabbit. Fed. Proc. 31, 591 (1972).

30. MILLER, J.D., LEECH, P.: Effects of mannitol and steroid therapy on intracranial volume-pressure relationships in patients. J. Neurosurg. 42, 274-281 (1975).

31. MITUS, A.: Dexamethasone. Its effectiveness in the treatment of the acute symptoms of meningeal luekemia. Amer. J. Dis. Child. 117, 307-312 (1969).

32. PAPPIUS, H.M.: Effects of steroids on cold injury edema. In: Steroids and Brain Edema (H.J. REULEN, K. SCHÜRMANN, eds.), pp. 57-63. Berlin-Heidelberg-New York: Springer 1972.

33. RANSOHOFF, J.: The effects of steroids on brain edema in man. In: Steroids and Brain Edema (H.J. REULEN, K. SCHÜRMANN, eds.), pp. 211-217. Berlin-Heidelberg-New York: Springer 1972.

34. REULEN, H.J., HADJIDIMOS, A., SCHÜRMANN, K.: The effect of dexamethasone on water and electrolyte content and on rCBF in perifocal brain edema in man. In: Steroids and Brain Edema (H.J. REULEN, K. SCHÜRMANN, eds.), pp. 239-252. Berlin-Heidelberg-New York: Springer 1972.

35. RISBERG, J., LUNDBERG, N., INGVAR, D.H.: Regional cerebral blood volume during acute transient rises of the intracranial pressure (plateau waves). J. Neurosurg. 31, 303-310 (1969).

36. RUDERMANN, N.B., HALL, T.C.: Use of glucocorticoids in the palliative treatment of metastatic brain tumors. Cancer 18, 298-306 (1965).

37. SATO, O.: The effect of dexamethasone on cerebrospinal fluid production rate in the dog. Brain and Nerve 19, 485-492 (1967).

38. SATO, O., HARA, M., ASAI, T., TSUGANE, R., KAGEYAMA, N.: The effect of dexamethasone phosphate on the production rate of cerebrospinal fluid in the spinal subarachnoid space of dogs. J. Neurosurg. 39, 480-484 (1973).

39. WEINSTEIN, J.D., TOY, F.J., JAFFE, M.E., GOLDBERG, H.I.: The effect of dexamethasone on brain edema in patients with metastatic brain tumors. Neurology 23, 121-129 (1973).

40. WEISS, M.H., NULSEN, F.E.: The effect of glucocorticoids on CSF flow in dogs. J. Neurosurg. 32, 452-458 (1970).

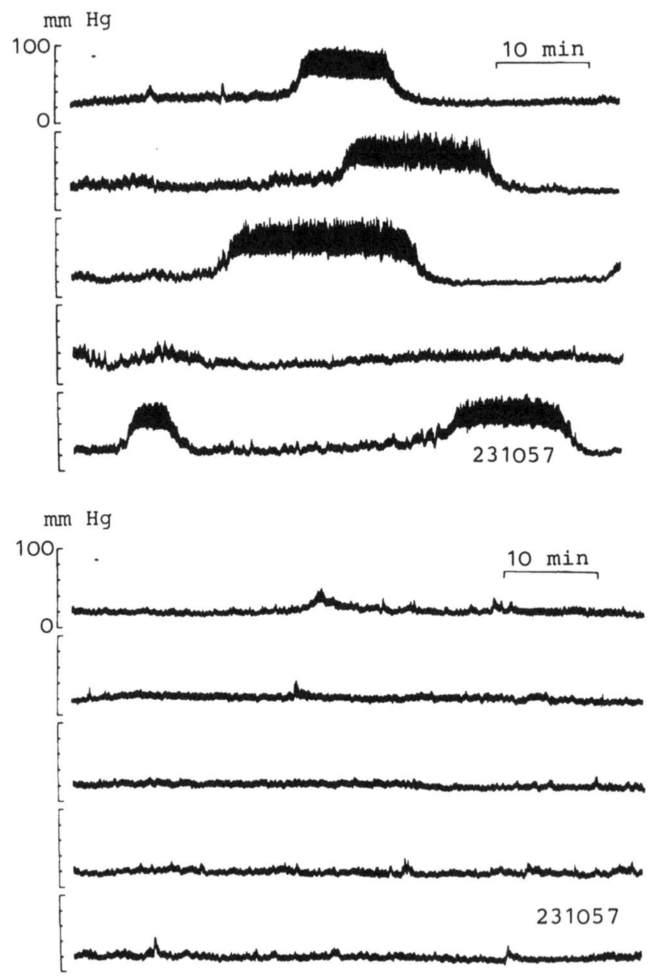

Fig. 1. Disappearance of plateau waves on the second day of dexamethasone therapy in a patient with a cystic cerebellar angioblastoma

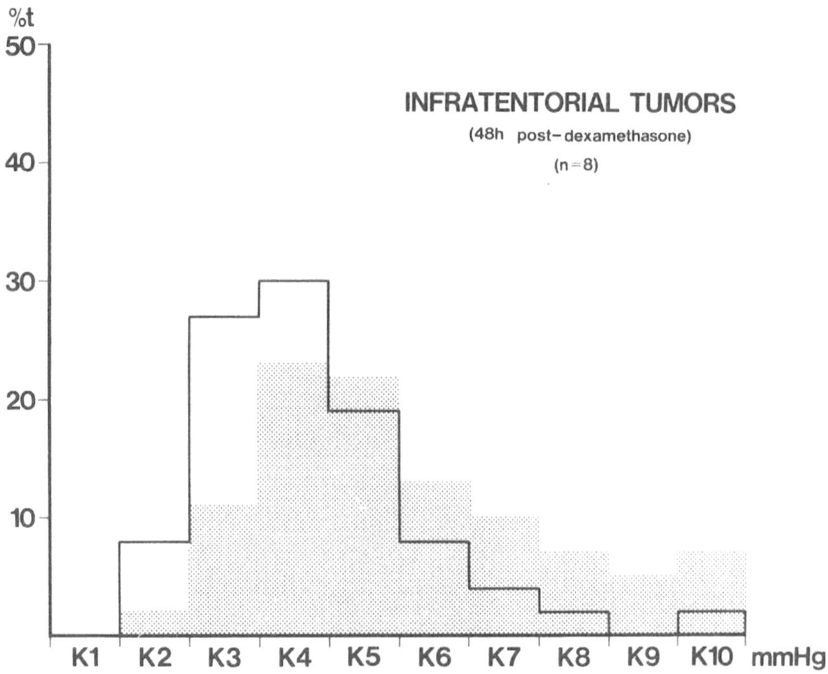

Fig. 2. Joint histograms of 8 patients with infratentorial tumors. Notice the significant shifting toward lower pressures (solid line histogram) on the second day of dexamethasone therapy as compared to the control histogram (hatched). Barostabilization is not evident from the joint histogram since the individual cases extend along the entire horizontal axis. The horizontal axis does not contain absolute pressure values as pressure-ranges varied from case to case

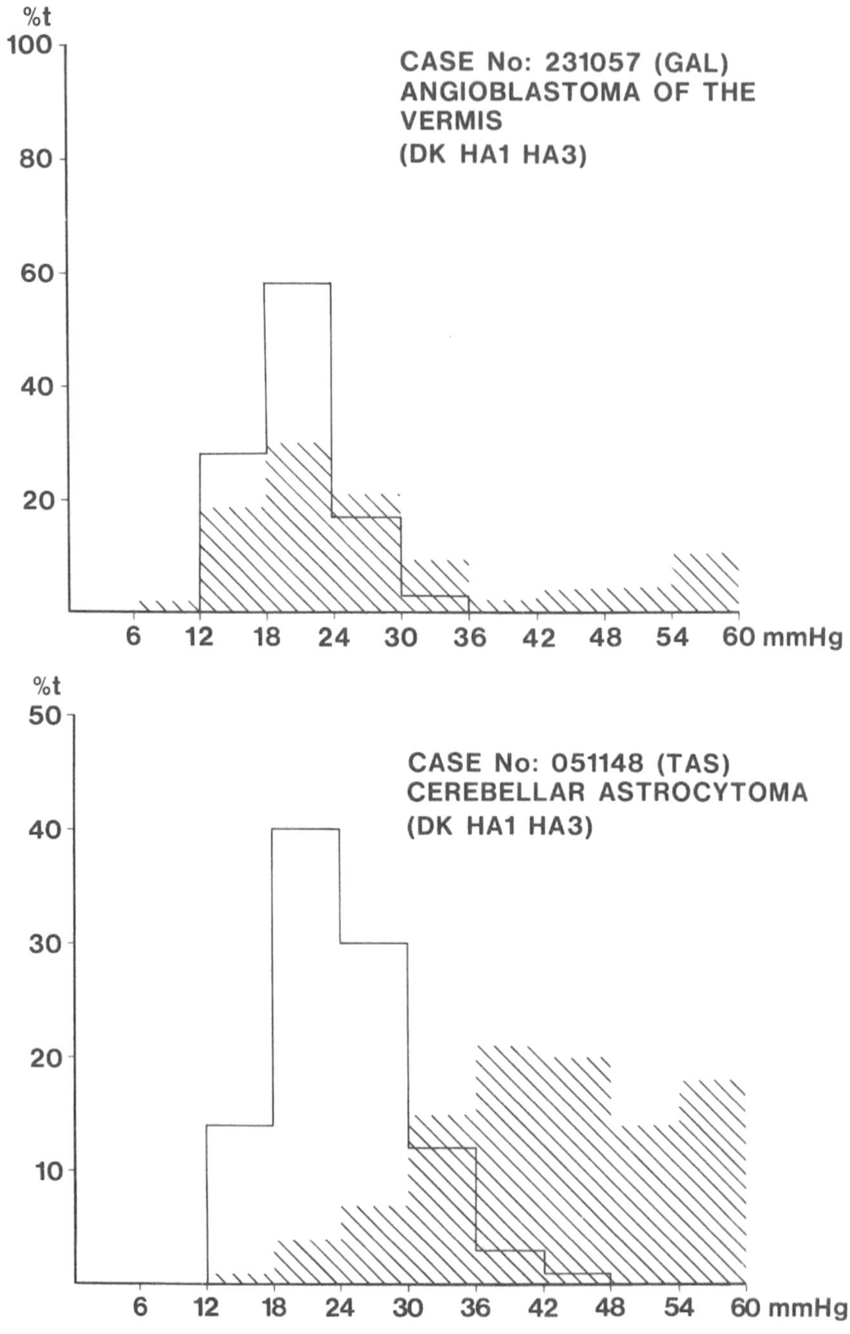

Fig. 3. Barostabilization is evident both in patients with (upper graph) and without (lower graph) plateau waves prior to therapy. The upper graph corresponds to the recording periods shown in figure 1, the lower graph corresponds to the recording periods showed in figure 4. Control histograms are hatched. Histograms following therapy are drawn with a solid line

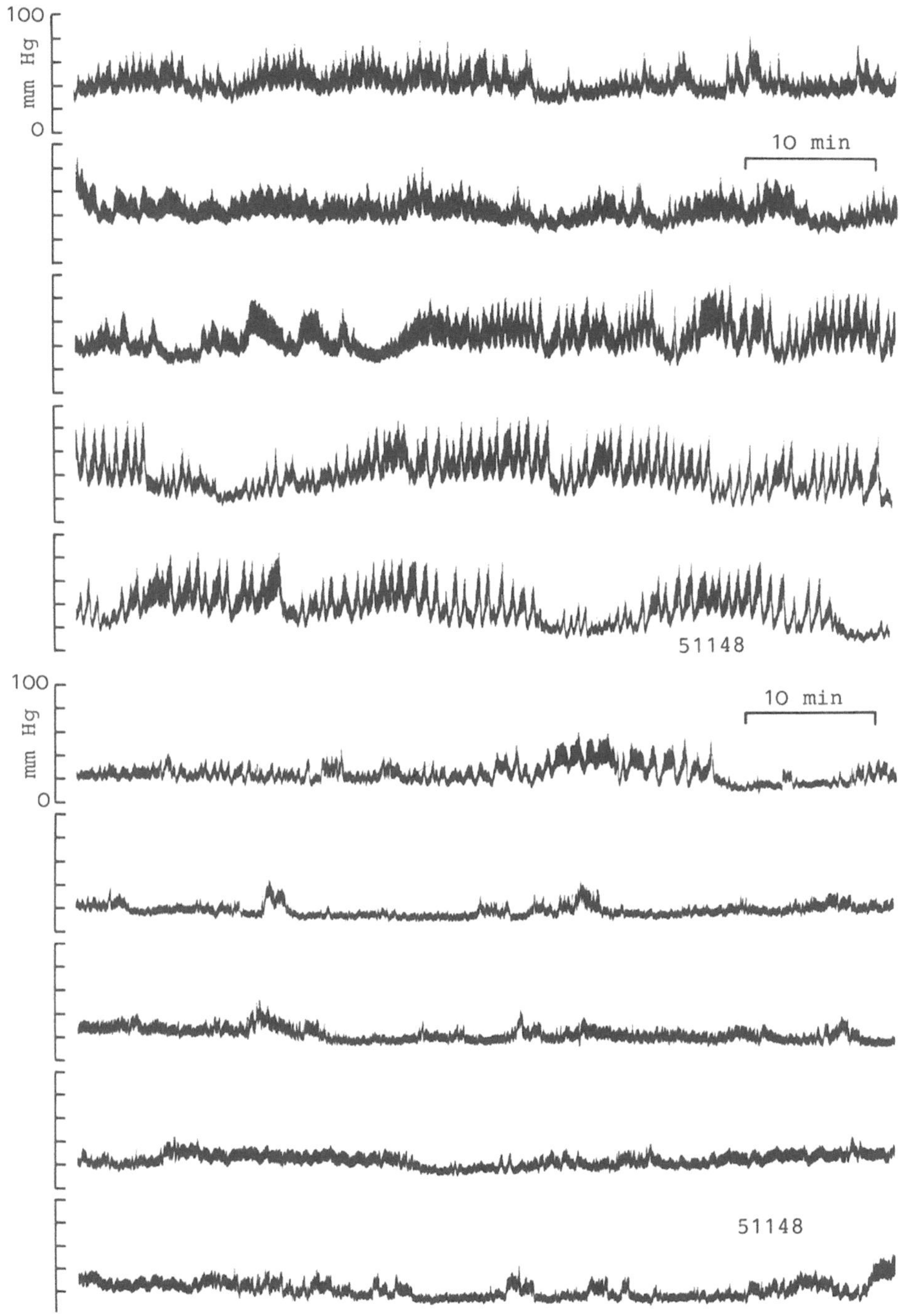

Fig. 4. Recording periods prior to (upper curve) and on the second day following decamethasone therapy (lower curve). Barostabilization is evident also the absence of plateau waves. (The corresponding histograms are shown in figure 3 lower part). In a patient with a cerebellar astrocytoma

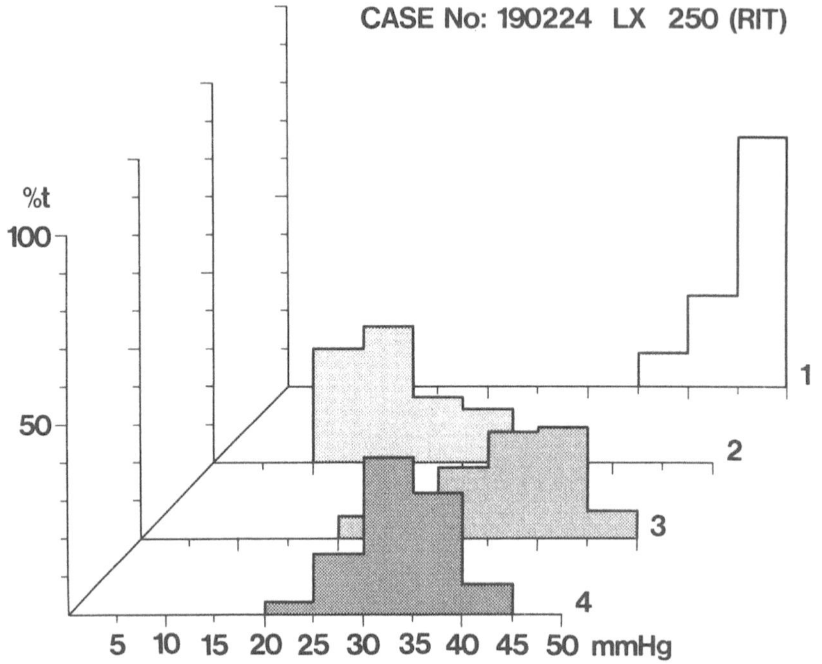

Fig. 5. Successive pressure histograms prior to (histogram 1), immediately (histogram 2), 4 hours (histogram 3) and 7 hours (histogram 4) following intravenous application of 250 mg of furosemide. Despite the marked decrease in ICP there is no Barostabilization

Summary

J. D. Miller and H. J. Reulen

The mechanisms of effect of therapeutic agents on ICP encompass their influence on arterial pressure and respiration, on the volume of intracranial constituents and on the lumped intracranial elastance which transduces changes in volume into given alterations in ICP.

SCHETTINI[1] indicated that halothane increased brain stiffness but Mc DOWALL questioned whether this property resided in brain tissue alone and suggested that what was being measured in this study was a parameter of intracapillary pressure. There was some agreement over the superiority of pancuronium over suxamethonium during induction of anesthesia in patients with a "tight brain" but questions arose concerning changes in arterial pressure, which may have contributed to the ICP changes seen by LEWELT and his colleagues (pp.215-218).

The apparent influence of THAM in restoring cerebral vascular reactivity and lowering ICP in post-compressive brain swelling (pp.219-223) was of considerable interest but it must be established whether it is a true effect or represents, in part, a tendency for the cerebrovascular system to regain tone in the time following the brain insult. This study could be pursued with profit to further compare the effects of sodium bicarbonate and THAM, but must include a control (non-treated) series.

KULLBERG (pp.224-230) was unable to demonstrate much effect on ICP of mannitol in comparatively low doses but GOBIET, BECKER, and McGRAW all had obtained more evident effects on ICP depending on higher doses, speed of administration and the initial ICP. The dangers of repeated mannitol infusions producing high serum osmolality (>330 mOsm/l) during treatment, leading to metabolic acidosis and renal failure, were emphasized by BECKER. He considered that if ICP could not be controlled at a pre-infusion serum osmolality of less than 310 mOsm/l the prognosis was bad.

TEASDALE commented on the assertion by GOBIET (pp.231-235) that high (>90 mg/day), but not normal (16 mg/day), dosage of dexamethasone reduced both ICP and mortality in serious head injuries. In an extensive combined stúdy of patients with severe head injuries, TEASDALE and JENNETT had seen no influence on mortality of steroids in the customary dosage (16 mg/day). REULEN confirmed that in a double-blind study carried out in Mainz high dosage of dexamethasone reduced mortality as compared with the usual steroid regime.

BROCK (pp.236-246) found that steroids produced a reduction in modal ICP and narrowing of the ICP range not only in patients with supratentorial tumors (presumably accompanied by edema) but also in patients with infratentorial tumors (accompanied by hydrocephalus). In discussion this was felt to be consistent with the effect of steroids on brain elastance with a reduced fluctuation of ICP as the P.V. curve flattens out under the steroid influence. As BROCK pointed out, however, an additional influence on CSF production/absorption might also be invoked to explain this effect in the latter group of patients.

[1] Manuscript not delivered for publication.

In summary, the papers and discussion in this session well exemplify the opening statement. The student of ICP must consider not only the changes in pressure produced by therapy but also the reasons for these changes, as techniques to evaluate such mechanisms in depth are now available.

Session H

Patient Management

Chairman: H. Troupp
Co-chairman: D. G. McDowall

The Significance of ICP-Monitoring in the Post-Operative Period

J. W. F. Beks, H. L. Journée, S. Albarda, and H. Flanderijn

Introduction

Monitoring intracranial pressure gives much important information concerning pathophysiology in patients in the post-operative period. From this monitoring we can learn how the intracranial situation in this period develops and it allows us in a number of cases to predict and to prevent complications.

Material and Methods

In this study we have monitored intracranial pressure in 86 patients. For this monitoring we used an epidural pressure-transducer which was developed by Philips in close cooperation with us. The transducer wad fixed in one of the burr holes of the craniotomy and connected with a polygraph and trend recorder. The 86 patients underwent operations for different neurosurgical lesions (18 patients with an aneurysm, 18 pituitary tumors, 50 supratentorial tumors). All operations were performed under steroid cover.

The operations on the 36 patients who underwent surgery for a pituitary tumor or an aneurysm were carried out under hypothermia and 100 cc of CSF was drained during the operation via a spinal catheter. The surgical treatment of the pituitary tumors was performed with operation by the frontal route.

Results

In this series we have seen no complications attributed to the implantation of the transducer. The mean epidural pressure at the start of the monitoring was in the patients with an aneurysm (group 1) 0.44 mm Hg (SD mean 2.7 mm Hg); in patients with a pituitary tumor (group 2) 2.9 mm Hg (SD mean 2.0 mm Hg) and in the patients with supratentorial tumors (group 3) 4.5 mm Hg (SD mean 1.2 mm Hg) (Table 1). In group 1 the average pressure was reached after about 16 h, in group 2 after 18 h and in group 3 after 24 h.

Table 1. Course of epidural pressure

	Aneurysms	Pituitary tumors	Brain tumors
Starting pressure	-0.44 mm Hg SD_{mean} 2.7 mm Hg	2.9 mm Hg SD_{mean} 2.0 mm Hg	4.5 mm Hg SD_{mean} 1.2 mm Hg
Time average pressure was reached	16 hrs	18 hrs	24 h
$\Delta P/_{\Delta T}$	16.5 mm Hg/$_{24\ h}$	16 mm Hg/$_{24\ h}$	9 mm Hg/$_{24\ h}$

In order to quantify the increase of pressure in the beginning of the curve, we calculated the quotient $\Delta P/\Delta T$, in which ΔP is the difference between the pressure at the moment when the curve reached the plateau and the initial pressure. ΔT is the time interval between those pressure values. These quotients were for group 1: 16.5 mm Hg/24 h, for group 2: 16 mm Hg/24 h, and for group 3: 9 mm Hg/24 h. According to LUNDBERG et al. (1965) 35 mm Hg was regarded as a critical level.

In group 1 we never saw an increase of the epidural pressure above 35 mm Hg (Fig. 1). In group 2 this happened 4 times (36 mm Hg, 39 mm Hg, 46 mm Hg and 50 mm Hg) (Fig. 2). In group 3 in 8 patients this level was reached or exceeded (40, 35, 45, 42, 45, 39, 49, 35 mm Hg) (Fig. 3).

When the intracranial pressure exceeded 35 mm Hg, the patient received mannitol in a dose of 1.5 g/kg intravenously over a 10-min period.

The intracranial pressure promptly reduced and remained on an acceptable level.
In none of the cases there was evidence of a rebound effect on intracranial pressure.
In our series we did not see plateau waves.

Discussion

It must be concluded that the intracranial pressure in patients who underwent surgery under hypothermia and had 100 cc of CSF taken off during operation, sooner reach the mean level of ICP than the other patients, though the starting value was lower. This possibly could result from a greater rate of CSF formation when the intracranial pressure is decreased.

The rate of CSF formation and absorption in man and the relationship of these to CSF pressure under both normal and abnormal conditions is still the subject of considerable controversy.

Another factor that possibly could play a role is that extirpation of a tumor gives a decompression that doubtless will interfere with the post-operative pressure course. That in the group who had surgery in the sellar region (pituitary tumors) significantly more patients showed an intracranial hypertension can be due to the fact that there was a temporary disturbance in the regulation of the body fluids caused by a transient change in the relation between the hypothalamus and pituitary gland.

Summary

Extradural monitoring of intracranial pressure in the post-operative period is a safe and satisfactory procedure. The course of postoperative pressure was studied in 86 patients who underwent surgery for different intracranial processes.

In only 14 of these patients was an increase in intracranial pressure above 35 mm Hg seen and never one above 50 mm Hg. The increase of ICP was significantly higher in patients wha had surgical treatment of pituitary tumors. Patients who during operation had a drainage of CSF, reached the average pressure level before those who had none.

Reference

LUNDBERG, N., TROUPP, H., LORNI, H.: Continuous recording of the ventricular fluid pressure in patients with severe acute traumatic brain injury. J. Neurosurg. 25, 581-590 (1965).

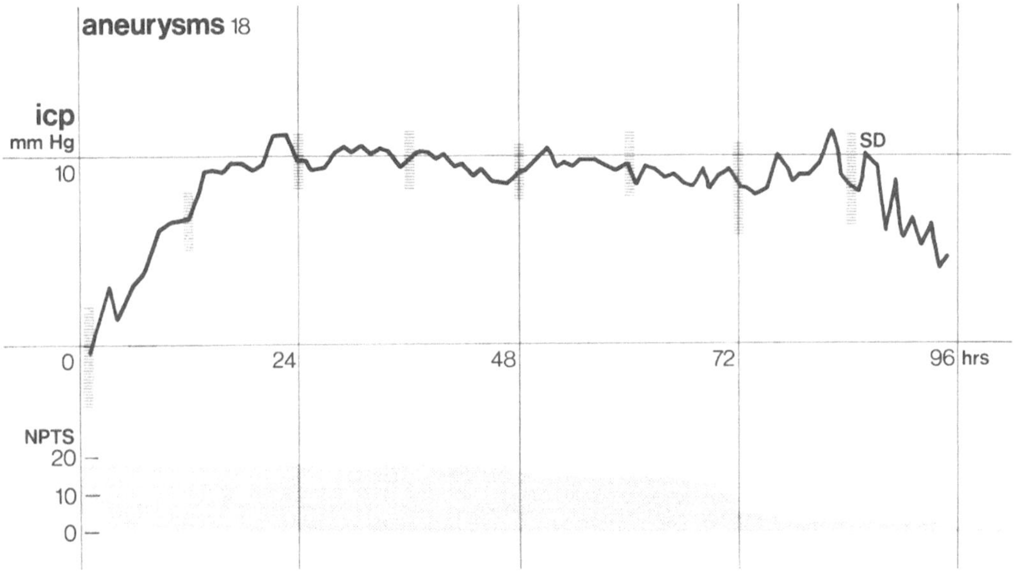

Fig. 1. Course of epidural pressure in patients who underwent surgery for an aneurysm

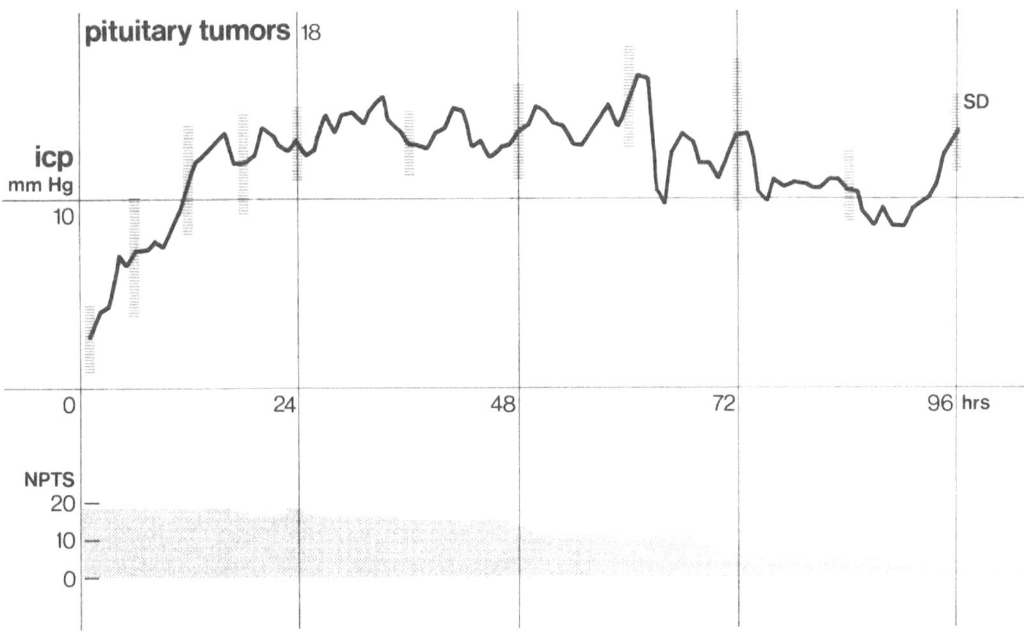

Fig. 2. Pressure recording in patients after surgery in pituitary region

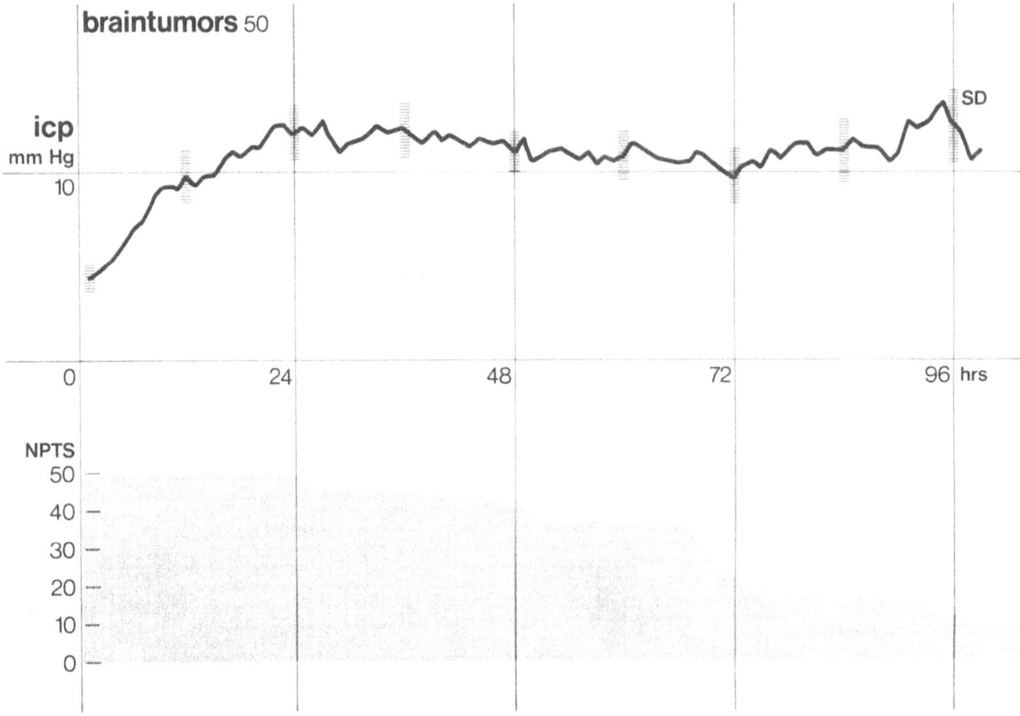

Fig. 3. Curve showing the epidural pressure course after surgery for brain tumors

The Clinical Value of Intracranial Pressure Monitoring

C.P. McGraw

Introduction

Intracranial pressure (ICP) monitoring has been accepted enthusiastically by some writers (2, 7), particularly since it has proven useful in patients with Reye's syndrome (1, 4).

At the First International Symposium on Intracranial Pressure, LANGFITT (5) summarized the results and concluded that the monitoring of ICP allows better therapeutic management of the individual patient.

Mortality at different levels of ICP has been investigated (3, 6, 8-10), but little has been done to correlate monitoring in the control of ICP with eventual mortality. In this study, an attempt was made to answer the question of whether ICP monitoring and subsequent maintenance of ICP within a normal range has improved the care of patients with clinical signs of elevated ICP.

Methods

Patients were selected from those with signs of increased ICP admitted to the North Carolina Baptist Hospital Neurosurgical, Pediatric, and Neurological Services over a 3-year period. The selection of patients for this group was made by an individual who was not in charge of the care of patients. Selection for inclusion was made on the basis of whether this individual believed that the patients might benefit from ICP monitoring. Usually, this was done on the basis of whether the patient has shown signs of elevated ICP, was expected to show increasing ICP, or did not have purposeful responses to pain without there being some operative approach to the problem.

Once the selection was made, the physician in charge of the patient was given the option to monitor the patients. The answer to this option was not always positive and there were, therefore, during this period, 100 monitored patients and 42 nonmonitored patients. It is of interest that in the first 18 months, only 20 patients were monitored, whereas in the last 18 months, 80 patients were monitored.

In the monitored group, the monitoring was continued for as long as it was considered useful to the patient. The deaths and survivals[1] were recorded and the overall mortality of the two groups compared.

---

[1]Deaths were those occurring during hospitalization and caused by the intracerebral condition (trauma, stroke, etc.); a patient was considered a survivor if he was discharged or transferred from the hospital.

Results

For the 3-year period, the mortality of the monitored and nonmonitored groups was not significantly different (Fig. 1). However, over the last 18 months, the mortality was significantly different ($P<0.02$), the nonmonitored group having a mortality of 87.5%, the monitored group a mortality of 52.5% (Fig. 2).

Discussion

An obvious weakness in this study is the many variables involved. There were a number of diagnoses, including severe head injury, stroke, intracerebral hemorrhaging, Reye's syndrome, meningitis, and postoperative brain tumor. The only common characteristic of these patients was the clinical indication of elevated ICP.

The assignment of patients to either of the two groups (monitored and nonmonitored) was affected by the familiarity of those caring for the patients with the value of the monitoring. With greater familiarity, a larger number of cases were monitored.

Summary

Continuous ICP monitoring was found to improve the care of patients with clinical signs of increased ICP. There was a decrease in mortality, and it was thought that this was brought about by improvements in monitoring techniques, more rapid initiation of monitoring, and more rapid response to data supplied by such monitoring to maintain ICP at normal levels.

References

1. BERMAN, W., PIZZI, F., SCHUT, L., RAPHAELY, R., HOLTZAPPLE, P.: The effects of exchange transfusion on intracranial pressure in patients with Reye syndrome. J. Pediat. 87, 887-891 (1975).
2. BROCK, M., DIETZ, H.: Intracranial Pressure: Experimental and Clinical Aspects. Berlin-Heidelberg-New York: Springer 1972.
3. JENNETT, B., JOHNSON, I.H.: The uses of intracranial pressure monitoring in clinical management. In: Intracranial Pressure (M. BROCK, H. DIETZ, eds.), pp. 353-356. Berlin-Heidelberg-New York: Springer 1972.
4. KINDT, G.W., WALDMAN, J., KOHL, S., BAUBLIS, J., TUCHER, R.P.: Intracranial pressure in Reye syndrome. Monitoring and control. J. Am. Med. Assoc. 231, 822-825 (1975).
5. LANGFITT, T.W.: Summary of First International Symposium on Intracranial Pressure, Hannover, Germany, July 27-29, 1972. J. Neurosurg. 38, 541-544 (1973).
6. LANGFITT, T.W., BEKS, J.W.F.: Comments to Session 7. In: Intracranial Pressure (M. BROCK, H. DIETZ, eds.), pp. 261-262. Berlin-Heidelberg-New York: Springer 1972.
7. LUNDBERG, N., PONTEN, U., BROCK, M.: Intracranial Pressure II. Berlin-Heidelberg-New York: Springer 1975.
8. NUMOTO, M., DONAGHY, R.M.P.: Effect of local pressure on cortical electrical activity and cortical vessels in the dog. J. Neurosurg. 33, 381-387 (1970).
9. TROUPP, H.: Ventricular fluid pressure recording after severe brain injuries. Europ. Neurol. 11, 227-235 (1974).

10. VAPALAHTI, M.: Intracranial pressure, acid-base status of blood and cerebrospinal fluid and pulmonary function in the prognosis of severe brain injury. From the Neurosurgical Department, University Central Hospital, Helsinki, Finland (1970).

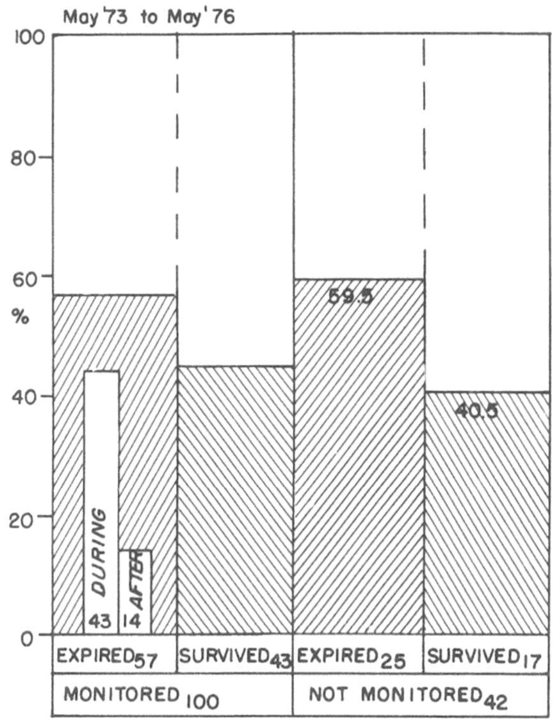

Fig. 1. Mortality and survival of monitored and nonmonitored patients over three-year period

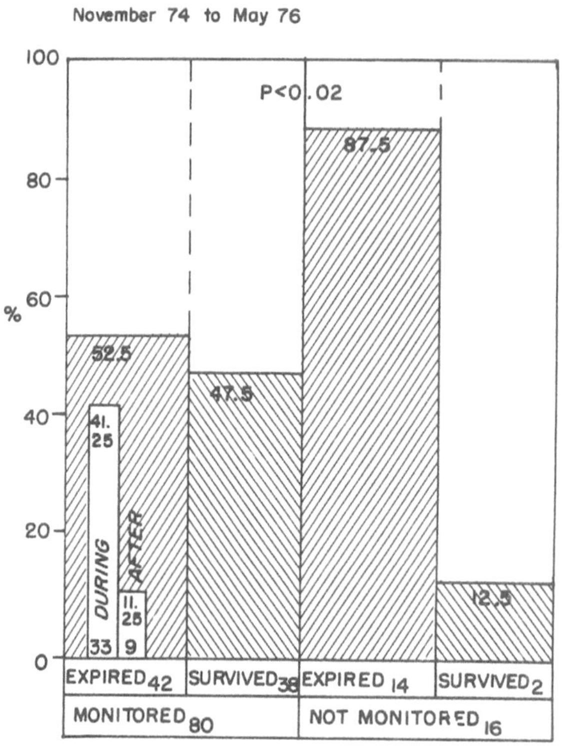

Fig. 2. Mortality and survival of monitored and nonmonitored patients over last 18-month period

The Effects of Head Position and Jugular Vein Compression (JVC) on Intracranial Pressure (ICP). A Clinical Study

A. Hulme and R. Cooper

It has been shown that large increases of ICP can be caused by flexion of the head in patients with posterior fossa tumors (6). Such increases might be harmful in some patients.
The present investigation was undertaken to study the magnitude and possible significance of changes of ICP associated with variations in head position and to compare these with changes caused by JVC.

Material and Methods

Studies were performed in 18 patients whose ICP was recorded continuously in the course of investigations for a variety of clinical conditions. The group consisted of 6 males and 12 females ranging in age from 17 to 60 years. They included two cases of posterior fossa and one of third ventricle tumor, three patients with partial occlusion of intracranial venous sinuses, three with "benign" intracranial hypertension, six cases of adult hydrocephalus and one each of aqueduct atresia, congenital occlusion of the foramen of Magendie and vascular hypertension with papilloedema.

In most cases ICP was recorded simultaneously by two methods.

The ventricular fluid pressure was measured by a catheter in the anterior horn of the lateral ventricle connected to an extracranial pressure transducer[1] set at the level of the foramen of Monro. Subdural pressure was recorded by a miniature transducer[2] in the subdural space.

The output from each was sampled and stored on a cassette magnetic tape at one per second intervals. The data were then transferred to the digital magnetic tape of a Link 8 computer for analysis. The average of the values from ventricular and subdural recordings was used in the calculations.

Each patient was studied lying quietly in bed. Recordings were first obtained with the head in the neutral position. Then a series of maneuvers was performed, each being maintained for 1-2 min, with intervals of similar length. The head was fully rotated to the right, to the left, and then flexed with the head and neck fully supported. Next JVC on the right, left and bilaterally was performed.

The mean pressure during the 5-s period immediately preceding any particular maneuver was compared with that recorded over the same period at the maximum level reached.

---

[1] Medical Transducer type 4-88. S.E. Laboratories (EMI) Ltd. North Feltham Trading Estate. Feltham, Middlesex. TW14 OTD.
[2] Implantable Pressure Transducer 3EA/b (ICT). Gaeltec Ltd. Stein Waternish, Isle of Skye, Scotland. IV51 9QA.

Results

The data are presented in Figure 1. With initial pressures below 10 mm Hg the responses to all maneuvers tended to be small and roughly similar, with the exception of bilateral JVC which caused somewhat larger increases. In a few instances of unilateral JVC a small reduction of pressure was recorded.

When the initial pressure exceeded 10 mm Hg, the magnitude of the increase varied widely among different patients and among various manipulations in the same individual. The maximum increase was associated with head flexion in 6 subjects, with bilateral JVC in 7, and with rotation to the right in 4. Rotation to the right caused a larger increase than rotation to the left in 14 patients and in no subject did leftward rotation produce the maximum increase.

Peak levels exceeding 50 mm Hg were recorded in 7 patients when the head was flexed or rotated to the right.

Typically the rise in ICP, which sometimes took the form of a plateau and in other instances of a peak, coincided precisely with the start and end of manipulation (Fig. 2).

In some patients however strikingly different responses were obtained.

A 43-year-old man had a large cholesteatoma in the posterior cranial fossa. Turning his head to the right caused a rapid and very large increase of ICP which persisted for 3 min after the head was returned to the neutral position before subsiding to the resting level (Fig. 3). This phenomenon was not produced by other manipulations, nor did it recur when rotation to the right was repeated. Intraventricular injection of 4 ml of CSF caused a similar rise which was reversed by voluntary hyperventilation.

A 48-year-old woman with clinical signs of raised ICP was shown on angiography to have a slow circulation rate and poor filling of the venous sinuses. A large plateau-like wave was initiated by rotating the head to the right but not by other manipulations (Fig. 4). The mean arterial BP remained at about 80 mm Hg indicating a reduction of cerebral perfusion pressure (CPP) to about 30 mm Hg at the height of the pressure increase.

In a patient with a congenital occlusion of the foramen of Magendie a very large increase of ICP was caused by head flexion. This persisted when the head was returned to the neutral position and she became extremely drowsy. Release of CSF led to prompt reduction of ICP and recovery of consciousness.

Discussion

The abrupt pressure changes observed in these experiments are best explained by interference with outflow of blood from the cranial cavity due to mechanical compression or distortion of veins in the neck or at the base of the skull, allowing an increment of arterial pressure to be transmitted downstream to the thin-walled cerebral veins and thus to the intracranial contents.

Although normally the dural venous sinuses and jugular veins are the major drainage route, other venous channels such as the pterygoid and orbital plexuses and emissary veins draining into the vertebral venous plexuses are also capable of conveying considerable volumes of blood (1). These channels are often enlarged in states of intracranial hypertension, especially if associated with some degree of venous sinus occlusion, and may be carrying a major proportion of the venous outflow. It could be anticipated that the rise of ICP would be greatly accentuated if they were temporarily occluded.

This hypothesis is supported by data from this study. In three of the patients who showed the largest pressure increases, angiography demonstrated impaired flow through the main venous sinuses. Two others, both with posterior fossa tumors, showed similar rises and a large increase followed flexion of the head in the patient with occlusion of the foramen of Magendie. Although no direct evidence of sinus occlusion was available in these three patients it has been demonstrated (3) that the lateral sinuses may be compromised in patients with posterior fossa space-occupying lesions. In a study in patients with severe head injuries OSTERHOLM found angiographic evidence of partial collapse of the lateral sinuses and enlargement of collateral channels with reversion to a normal pattern of venous drainage after relief of intracranial hypertension (7). The fact that alteration of head position caused a greater pressure increase than bilateral JVC in some of our subjects is interpreted as indicating significant dependence on collateral venous drainage and indicates the vulnerability of these channels to mechanical compression.

The pattern of pressure rise in several patients closely resembled the plateau waves described by LUNDBERG (5). We postulate that the reduction of CPP following an aute increase of ICP due to change of head position could result in the accumulation of acid metabolites in the brain thus tending to perpetuate cerebral vasodilatation, so that ICP remains high even after the postural stress is removed. The serious clinical significance of these phenomena is well established (2, 4) and underlines the importance of avoiding excessive rotation or flexion of the head in such subjects.

We are unable to offer any explanation for the interesting observation that turning the head to the right caused a larger increase of ICP than the reverse movement in most of the patients in this investigation.

Summary

Changes of ICP during head movement and JVC were recorded in 18 patients. Typically an abrupt rise and fall of ICP occurred with each maneuver. In some subjects with high ICP and especially those with evidence of venous sinus occlusion increases resembling plateau waves were evoked. It is suggested that these were initiated by temporary occlusion of collateral venous channels and that the sequential effects on CPP could cause clinical deterioration.

References

1. BATSON, O.V.: Anatomical problems concerned in the study of Cerebral Blood Flow. Fed. Proc. 3, 139-144 (1944).

2. COOPER, R., HULME, A.: Intracranial pressure and related phenomena during sleep. J. Neurol. Neurosurg. and Psych. 29, 564-570 (1966).

3. KINAL, M.E.: Infratentorial tumors and the dural venous sinuses. J. Neurosurg. 25, 395-401 (1966).

4. LANGFITT, T.W.: Pathophysiology of increased ICP. In: Intracranial Pressure (M. BROCK, H. DIETZ, eds.). Berlin-Heidelberg-New York: Springer 1972.

5. LUNDBERG, N.: Continuous recording and control of ventricular fluid pressure in neurosurgical practice. Acta Psych. et Neurol. Scan. Suppl. 149 (1960).

6. NORNES, H., MAGNAES, B.: Supratentorial epidural pressure recording during posterior fossa surgery. J. Neurosurg. 35, 541-549 (1971).

7. OSTERHOLM, J.L.: Reaction of the cerebral venous sinus system to acute intracranial hypertension. J. Neurosurg. 32, 654-659 (1970).

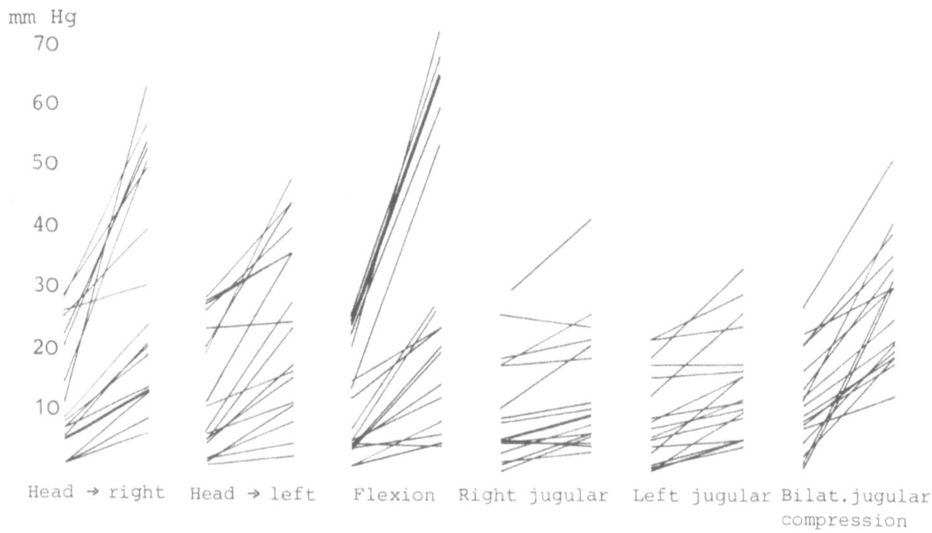

Fig. 1. Increase of resting to peak pressure during head manipulation and JVC in 18 patients. With initial pressure below 10 mm Hg, the effects are roughly comparable in all cases although bilateral JVC causes somewhat larger increases. With higher resting pressure the effects of rightward rotation and flexion are particularly striking

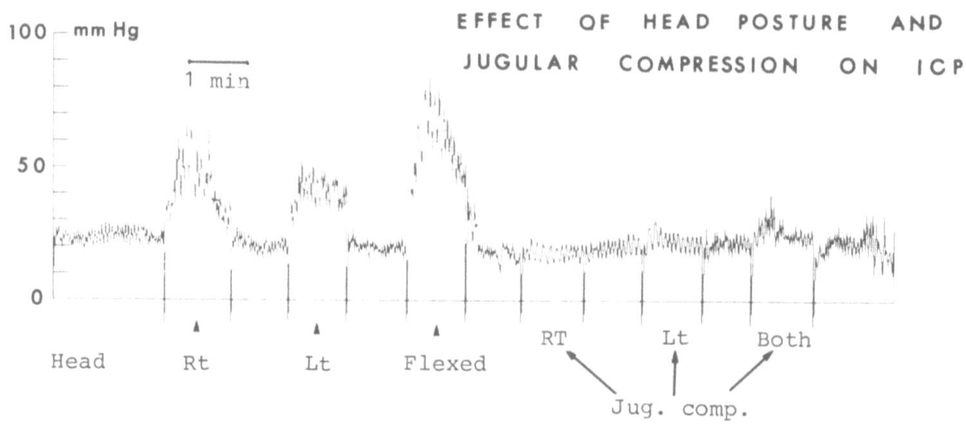

Fig. 2. Typical response. Peak type rise with right rotation and flexion; plateau with left rotation. In contrast the response to JVC was very small in this case

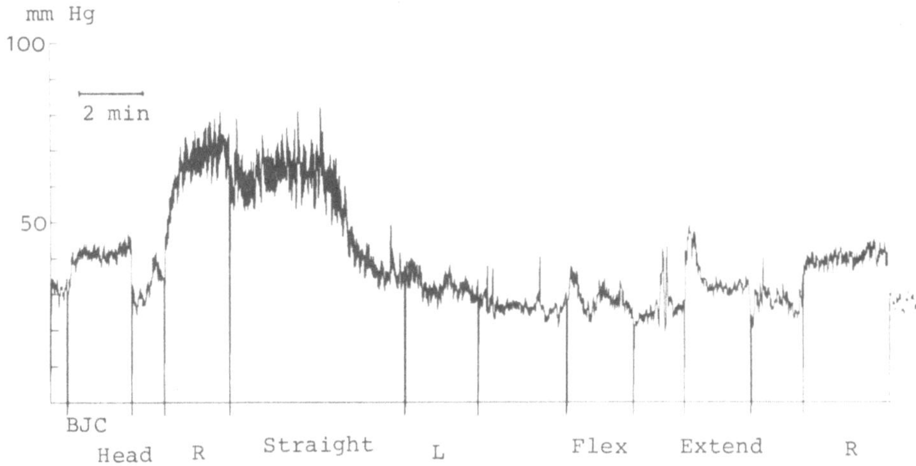

Fig. 3. Large sustained increase of ICP initiated by turning head to right in a patient with posterior fossa tumor. Note resemblance to spontaneous plateau wave

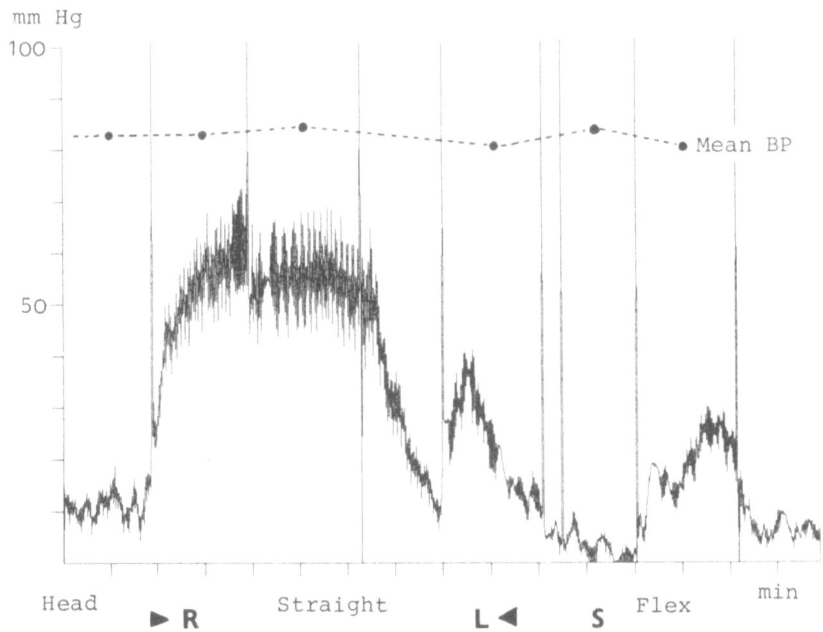

Fig. 4. Plateau wave provoked by head turning to right in patient with partial venous sinus occlusion. Rise with bilateral JVC was much smaller. Note reduction in CPP during period of high ICP

Sagittal Sinus Pressure and CSF Dynamics During Intracranial Hypertension in Man

E. Lamas, R. Diez Lobato, and J. Esparza

Introduction

Sagittal sinus hypertension (SSH), which can be primarily caused by different conditions (2), can also be found secondarily during intracranial hypertension (ICH) (3-5, 7). The CSF reabsorption rate, which is pressure-dependent, and the cerebral hemodynamics may be influenced by the response of the sagittal sinus pressure (SSP) to ICH. In this report we provide further evidence that ICH may induce severe SSH in man.

Materials and Methods

The clinical material presented, consists of six patients all with raised SSP due to chronic ICH (Table 1). All cases but one needed diagnostic ventriculography. Informed consent was obtained from the family or the patient to perform under local anesthesia right lateral and medial coronal burr holes with the purpose of simultaneously recording both intracranial pressure (ICP) and SSP. ICP recording was done through a

Table 1. Final diagnosis and mean arterial, intracranial and sagittal sinus pressures are shown. Grade of hydrocephalus and the ICP-SSP gradient variation are also shown

Cases ICH Clinical Evolution	Age years	Hydrocephalus	MAP mm Hg	Mean ICP mm Hg	Mean SSP mm Hg	VPR 1 cc mm Hg	ICP-SSP gradient variation	
1. Frontal astrocytoma 4 months	42	---	120	46	45	17.8 ±3.5	-4	+2
2. Aqueductal stenosis 7 months	68	+++	138	20	13	2.5 ±0.3	+2	+13
3. Subependymal astrocytoma 6 months	40	++-	108	36	28	14.0 ±2.9	0	+8
4. Recurring fibromyxoma 1 year	10	---	90	40	38	16.5 ±3.0	-3	+5
5. Colloid cyst 2 years	38	++-	106	33	30	13.1 ±2.1	0	+5
6. Posterior fossa cysticercosis 1 year	55	+++	120	38	31	15.1 ±1.8	+1	+10

polyethylene catheter introduced in the right frontal ventricular horn. SSP was recorded by means of 1 mm ID heparinized microcatheter placed in the middle third of the SS; the microcatheter position was verified by sinography in every case. A Philips electromanometer (Statham transducer) and an additional water manometer were used in the first four cases; in the remaining two, catheters were connected to transducers (Siemens polygraph). The patients were in the supine position during the recordings and the midaxillary line was taken as the zero point reference level for measurements. Mean arterial and central venous pressures were determined throughout the experiments. Arterial blood gas determinations were done in every case and in the last three cases blood gases were also measured in SS blood samples. ICP and SSP were continuous and simultaneously recorded for an hour; basal spontaneous oscillations of both pressures and their interrelation during ventricular drainage, rapid intraventricular injections and Queckenstedt maneuver, were observed. A constant-infusion ventricular test was performed in cases 2 and 5. ICP monitoring was maintained for an additional 24 h in every patient. Sedation was not needed and care was taken to maintain patients under normal respiratory conditions during the recordings.

Results

Central venous pressure in the supine position was normal in all cases, ranging between 4 and 10 mm Hg. There were no significant arterial pressure variations during the recordings and the arterial blood gases were within normal limits in all cases.

Intraventricular Pressure vs. ICP

In basal conditions all patients had variable degrees of ICH and all but case 5 showed true A waves being the "plateau waves" of only 23-24 mm Hg amplitude in case 2. Ventricular pressure response (VPR) to rapid intraventricular injection of 1 cc saline solution (6) was repeatedly high in all cases but case 2.

Sagittal Sinus Pressure

Under basal conditions variable degrees of SSH were found in every patient, SSP being highest in cases 1 and 4. All ICP variations, A waves included, were reflected on SSP recordings. The responses of SSP to a 1 cc intraventricular injection correlated with the VPR, but were very much attenuated, the relation being:
Mean VPR = Mean SSP response X 10.5.

ICP and SSP Interrelation

SSP almost constantly remained under ICP levels and faithfully followed ICP spontaneous oscillations in all patients (Fig. 2). In cases 1 and 4 this gradient was constantly minimum at different levels of ICP, being even inverted during brief periods of time. In cases 2, 3, 5 and 6 this gradient increased as ICP increased because SSP elevation was lower than ICP elevation. Case 1 histograms of SSP and ICP superimposed on a common diagram are shown in Figure 1. The linear correlation between ICP and SSP in a particular case and their relation in all the six cases are shown in Figures 3 A and B. Arterial and respiratory pressure fluctuations were always present on both ICP and SSP recordings, the relation between pulse amplitudes being variable. Bilateral jugular vein compression induced a similar pressure increase in both ventricular and SS compartments, SSP rise slightly preceding the ICP rise

(Fig. 2). Variable amounts of CSF ventricular drainage induced a similar fall in ICP and SSP. Ventricular constant infusion of 0.76 ml/min of artificial CSF in cases 2 and 5 raised ICP to 50 mm Hg in 12 min and 3.5 min respectively, the test being discontinued at this point. Opening pressures were 11 and 21 mm Hg, respectively. Recordings and ventricular injections or withdrawals of fluid did not cause any neurological or systemic alteration.

Discussion

The normal pressure values for the cerebral subarachnoid space and the SS have been established at 147 and 90 mm H_2O respectively by SHULMAN et al. in dogs (7). CSF drainage through the arachnoid villi starts when the CSF pressure reaches the so-called critical opening pressure, and the rate of drainage increases linearly with the ICP increase if SSP remains unchanged (1). In normal conditions SSP is mainly dependent on arterial pressure and its constancy during ICH has been theoretically presupposed in some experiments on CSF dynamics, but there are many clinical and experimental observations indicating that the dural sinuses are not always resistant to mechanical stress (3-5, 7), their anatomy being distorted with variable degrees of hemodynamic dysfunction. SSH will compromise CSF reabsorption, at least theoretically, in a degree dependent on the ICP-SSP gradient diminution. That means, as has been demonstrated in baboons (3), that when ICH induces SSH, the main vascular resistance in the cerebral venous outflow tract shifts from the lacuna lateralis to the sinus; as a consequence the "venting" action of the sinus, which represents a low pressure runoff for the cortical venous system, is compromised (7). When dural sinuses are subjected to hypertension brain venous drainage seeks out available and functional channels of collateral circulation that would be more or less efficient in discharging venous stasis; the difference in this capacity could explain in part the variability of both SSP and the intracranial dynamics observed in patients suffering from similar pathological conditions. In patients with SSH secondary to ICH, the buffering capacity of the cranial compartment to depress volumetric additions will be reduced in respect to other patients with similar ICP rates, but with a normal SSP. In the first situation there could be an impairment of the spatial compensatory volumetric reduction afforded by the transiently increased CSF drainage and the reciprocal change in the total volume of the intracranial venous bed. All patients but case 2 had a very high intracranial elastance ($\Delta P/\Delta V$) and in our experience the A-waves duration is longer when the ICP-SSP gradient is critically reduced or inverted. Moreover triggering A waves by certain maneuvers such as neck rotation or flexion is also facilitated in patients with SSH.

Summary

Chronic ICH in man may induce anatomical and hemodynamic alterations in the dural sinuses. Abnormally raised SSP is going to disturb both CSF reabsorption and the normal adjustments of the cerebrovascular resistance in the venous outflow tract; as a result craniospinal compliance will be further reduced in patients with sustained SSH.

References

1. CUTLER, R.W.P., PAGE, L., GALICICH, J., WATTERS, G.V.: Formation and absorption of cerebrospinal fluid in man. Brain 91, 707-720 (1968).

2. HAAR, F.L., MILLER, C.A.: Hydrocephalus resulting from a superior vena cava thrombosis in an infant. J. Neurosurg. 42, 597-601 (1975).

3. JOHNSTON, I.H., ROWAN, J.O.: Raised intracranial pressure and cerebral blood flow. 3. Venous outflow tract pressures and vascular resistances in experimental intracranial hypertension. J. Neurol. Neurosurg. Psychiatry 37, 392-402 (1974).

4. LANGFITT, T.W., WEINSTEIN, J.D., KASSELL, N.F., et al.: Compression of cerebral vessels by intracranial hypertension, I. Dural sinus pressures. Acta Neurochirurgica 15, 212-222 (1966).

5. MARTINS, A.N., KOBRINE, A.I., LARSEN, D.F.: Pressure in the sagittal sinus during intracranial hypertension in man. J. Neurosurg. 40, 603-608 (1974).

6. MILLER, J.D., GARIBI, J., PICKARD, J.: Induced changes of cerebrospinal fluid volume. Arch. Neurol. 28, 265-269 (1973).

7. SHULMAN, K., YARNELL, P., RANSOHOFF, J.: Dural sinus pressure in normal and hydrocephalic dogs. Arch. Neurol. 10, 575-580 (1964).

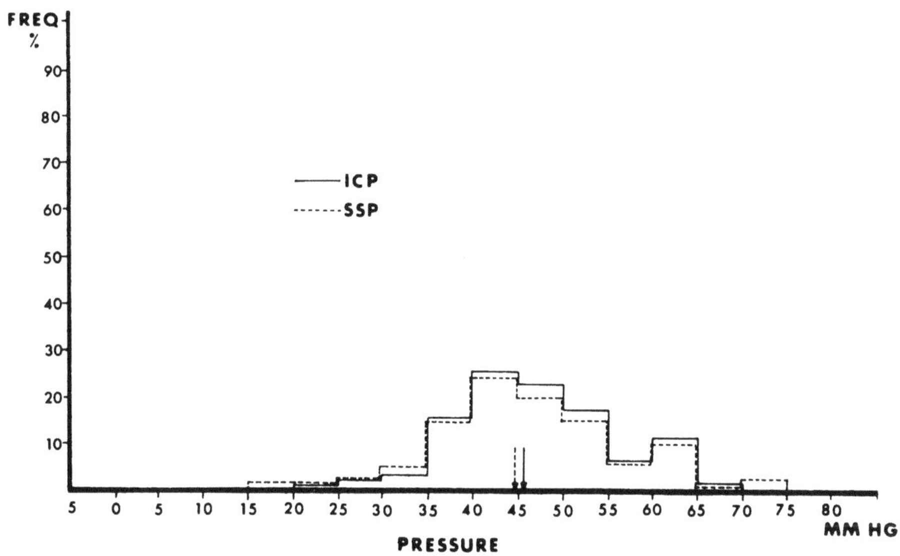

Fig. 1. ICP and SSP frequency histograms obtained from 1 h of simultaneous recordings in case 1

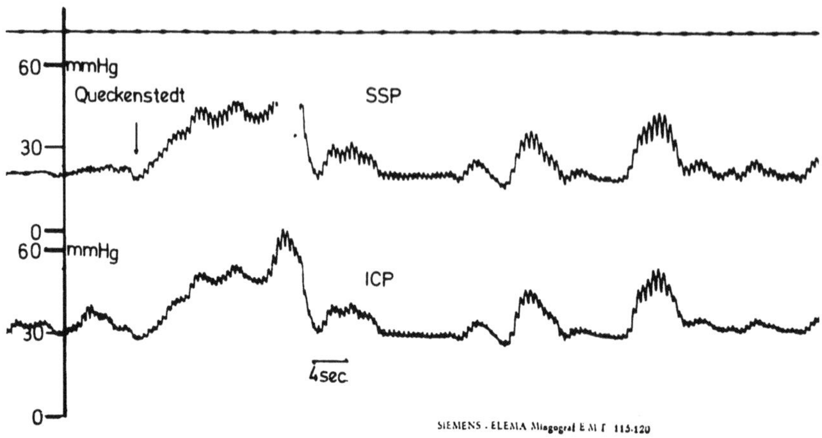

Fig. 2. Simultaneous ICP and SSP recording in case 6. Repercussion of Queckenstedt maneuver on ventricular and sagittal sinus compartments can be seen

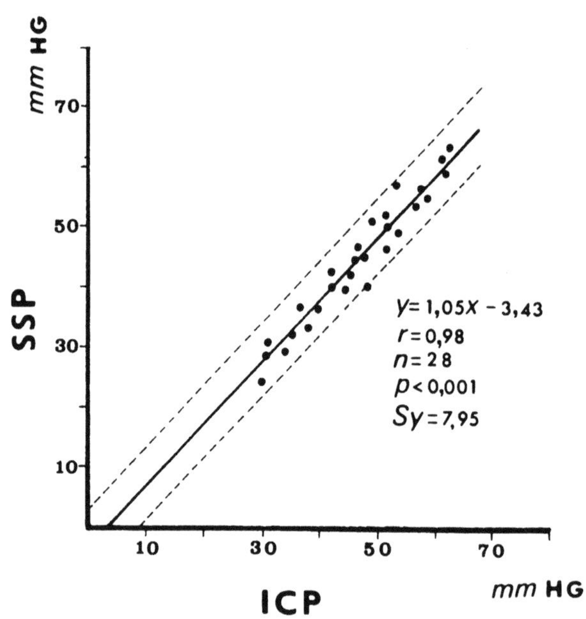

Fig. 3a. Graph showing linearity of relationship of ICP and SSP in case 1

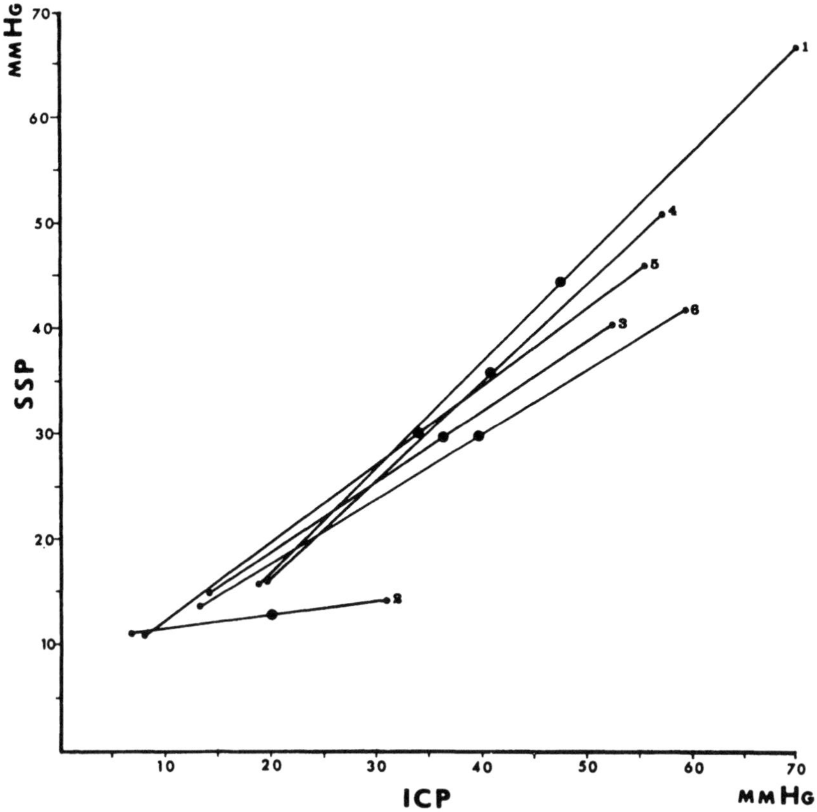

Fig.3b. Graphic representation of ICP and SSP correlation in total group of the patients. Black dots correspond to mean ICP and SSP in every case

The Cushing Response

R. Lorenz

Introduction

It is now over 100 years since the interrelationships between increased intracranial pressure and blood pressure were first investigated. Many details have been analyzed and explained but the so-called Cushing phenomenon still remains a problem.

During the last two symposia many authors reported on cardiovascular phenomena in connection with increased intracranial pressure. Cardiovascular disturbances were found in 27 patients who exhibited plateau waves: pulse rate decreased during the plateau wave changing towards tachycardia at the end of the wave (9). Other investigators stated that plateau waves are independent of blood pressure (3). From experimental studies it was concluded that cerebral ischemia, acute cerebral hypoxia, and increased intracranial pressure are related to the same type of blood pressure reactions (6). NORNES (7) distinguished four phases of the plateau wave and pointed out, as did LUNDBERG (5), that the unstable state in phase 4 of the plateau wave is due to the CUSHING response.

The present report deals with clinical observations on changes in vegetative parameters in cases of increased intracranial pressure, especially plateau waves.

Material and Methods

Sixty-five recordings in 35 patients were performed. Intraventricular pressure (IVP) was recorded through a catheter placed via a frontal burr hole; arterial pressure (ABP) was recorded directly or indirectly from the brachial artery; heart rate (HR) was recorded from the ECG and respiratory rate (RR) was recorded by the thermistor method. Fifteen patients had infratentorial space-occupying lesions, 4 had aqueduct stenosis, 4 communicating hydrocephalus, 7 obstructive hydrocephalus with tumor of the third ventricle region and 7 further patients had other supratentorial pathology.

Results

In four cases a steady increase of intracranial pressure from 0 mm Hg till 50 mm Hg was observed without any recognizable changes in vegetative parameters (Fig. 1). Only in few cases was a stable course (following de ROUGEMONT [9]) of intraventricular pressure noted. In the majority of patients the pressure curve was modulated and revealed small ondulations identical with the B and C waves described by LUNDBERG (6). In one patient pressure recording performed after Dimer X ventriculography showed an increased modulation of the pressure curve and the pulse rate without changes of the basic level of IVP. Another patient with thrombosis of the internal cerebral veins and thalamic hemorrhagic infarction had originally normal intraventricular pressure and arterial hypertension. Shortly before cerebral death IVP started to rise continuously. Further increase of the systolic ABP occurred when IVP reached the value of 50 mm Hg. This was followed by an abrupt fall of intraventricular pressure (the catheter being still patent), whereas the decrease of the arterial pressure and respiratory paralysis occurred with latency (11) (Fig. 2). The total of 137 A-waves (plateau waves) corresponding to the definition of LUNDBERG and to that summarized by LANGFITT were recorded in seven patients. The duration and the form of the plateau waves varied considerably (Fig. 3). In certain cases it was difficult to decide whether the wave should be classified as an atypical plateau wave or as some other irregular form of pressure increase. In some patients the plateau waves appeared in the form of oscillations reflecting the transition from suppressed to unsuppressed form. The behavior of the vegetative parameters during the plateau waves was not uniform - both increases and decreases of ABP, HR and RR were observed. Sometimes none of the parameters changed; on other occasions different combinations in the alteration of these parameters were seen. The latter included, as seen in Figure 4: parallel increase of ABP, HR and RR, increase of ABP and HR with constant RR, increase of ABP with unchanged HR and RR, parallel increase of ABP and HR with decrease of RR, increase of ABP followed by increase of RR and decrease of HR, increase of HR and RR with fall of ABP, decrease of RR with no change in ABP and HR and finally no change in all the three parameters during the occurrence of the plateau wave. Without considering all the possible combinations the analysis of 137 plateau waves (in eight cases no continuous recording of ABP was available and in one case the respiratory rate was not registered) is shown in Table 1. Only in a few cases was uniform distribution of alterations recognizable. The trend of change in individual patients was also different. For example, patient 3 mainly had constant blood pressure during plateau waves, decrease of HR and increase of RR; patient 2 had a preponderant increase of ABP with constant RR and HR during the plateau wave. The summary of the results shows that changes of ABP and HR are distributed almost similarly in contrast to changes of RR.

Discussion

LUNDBERG (5), LANGFITT (3), and NORNES (7) tried to describe the form and duration of the plateau wave or A-wave. Our experience is similar to theirs and corresponds with the opinion of TROUPP and de ROUGEMONT (10) that the plateau wave has a certain shape but that its characteristics are still not fully defined. Further analysis of the form and duration and possible subdivision seems to be desirable not only for pure morphological reasons but also for the analysis of accompanying phenomena and their causes. Considering the variability of changes of vegetative parameters, their decrease, increase or constancy with various combinations, the classification of the A-wave according to its importance for clinical practice becomes questionable. The analysis of vegetative changes reveals that even considerable increase of intracranial pressure is accompanied by changes of vegetative parameters which do not correspond to the so-called Cushing phenomenon. The increase of ABP may not only be lacking, but even a decrease of ABP can occur. The same is true for changes of HR and RR. Most probably the Cushing response constitutes only one of the possible phenomena.

Our previous studies on cardiovascular changes in patients with increased intracranial pressure (4) showed that the decrease of HR occurs as a particular form of reaction in patients with hypothalamic and bulbar lesions whereas the most common phenomenon is tachycardia with exaggerated additional heartbeat accelerations, particularly in patients with mesencephalic syndrome. Clinical analysis showed further that the ABP is influenced to a much lesser degree. Depending upon

Table 1. Number of plateau waves and type of alteration of vegetative parameters (↓ decreased, = constant, ↑ increased, Ø no registration)

Patient No.	Age (years)	No. of plateau waves	Arterial blood pressure (ABP)				Heart rate (HR)				Respiratory rate (RR)			
			↓	=	↑	Ø	↓	=	↑	Ø	↓	=	↑	Ø
071137051	39	11		5	5	1		9	2			10	1	
131120631	55	28	1	9	17	1	2	15	11		3	21	4	
171067622	7	27	5	12	6	4	13	9	5		6	10	11	1
150759282	15	9		8	1			8	1		1	6	1	
171165002	10	6	1	3	2			4	2		4	2		
200261281	14	15		5	10			1	14			2	13	
020559662	17	11		4	6	1			11		11			
211021722	54	15		5	10			4	11			7	8	
131264252	11	15		14		1		15				15		
Summary		137	7	65	57	8	15	65	57	0	25	73	38	1

the stage of herniation and topographic relation of the lesion to the brain stem, absolute increase of ABP and the increase of ondulations becomes larger. After different stimuli transient rises of ABP were observed as documented by interval registration in 149 patients and continuous registration in 100 patients. Moreover we were able to demonstrate that considerable variations of systolic and diastolic BP combined with marked increase of HR occur in patients prior to the development of decerebration if their basic ABP was already high. Few patients with normal original ABP values exhibited a gradual increase of the systolic ABP as the only vegetative sign before the development of decerebration. Patients with bulbar herniation showed either considerable dispersion of HR, systolic and diastolic ABP values occurring in addition to the already existing arterial hypertension, or marked variability of ABP values with irregular changes of HR and gradual decrease of RR.

The findings correlate well with data obtained from animal experiments, even if one bears in mind all the reservations bound to be raised against such an analogy. Own experiments in cats with an epidural balloon placed in different regions, with repeated compressive brain lesions and with induced intracerebral bleeding (each experimental series of 12 animals) demonstrated considerable variation of the cardiovascular reaction to the compressive lesion. The Cushing response (1) with the classical triad of ABP increase, bradycardia, and disturbances of respiration was not seen in these subacute experiments. Only in half the animals could a slight ABP increase and decrease of RR be seen.

In conclusion, CUSHING's (1) report of a raised ABP, slowing of heartbeat and respiratory disorders due to *extreme* values of intracranial pressure is often misinterpreted, and CUSHING's (2) important observation of sudden increase of heart rate in the clinical course of space-occupying lesions is undervalued.

Summary

By means of 65 recordings in 35 patients and analysis of 137 plateau waves and their relationship to ABP, HR and RR, the problem of the so-called Cushing response is discussed. Difficulties occur through the lack of clear definition of A-waves in respect to the number of combinations of responses of ABP, HR and RR that are possible during the phase of pressure increase.

Previous clinical investigations on the behavior of ABP and HR in patients with space-occupying intracranial lesions as well as animal experimental studies in raised intracranial pressure were confirmed. The Cushing phenomenon, understood as an increase of ABP and/or decrease of HR in response to increased intracranial pressure, should be considered as a particular form of reaction.

References

1. CUSHING, H.: Concerning a definite regulatory mechanism of the vasomotor centre which controls blood pressure during cerebral compression. Johns Hopkins Hospital Bulletin no. 126, 290-292 (1901).

2. CUSHING, H.: The blood pressure relations of acute cerebral compression, illustrated by cases of intracranial hemorrhage. A sequel to the mütter lecture for 1901. The American Journal of the Medical Sciences 125, 1017-1044 (1903).

3. LANGFITT, T.W.: Pathophysiology of increased ICP. In: Intracranial Pressure (M. BROCK, H. DIETZ, eds.), pp. 361-364. Berlin-Heidelberg-New York: Springer 1972.

4. LORENZ, R.: Wirkungen intrakranieller raumfordernder Prozesse auf den Verlauf von Blutdruck und Pulsfrequenz. Ein klinischer Beitrag zur Frage der Dysregulation vegetativer Funktionen durch zentrale Läsionen. Acta Neurochirurgica, Suppl. 20. Wien-New York: Springer 1973.

5. LUNDBERG, N.: Continuous recording and control of ventricular fluid pressure in neurosurgical practice. Acta Psychiat. Scand. 36, Suppl. 149 (1960).

6. McGILLICUDDY, J.E., KINDT, G.W., MILLER, C.A., RAISIS, J.E.: The interrelations between increased intracranial pressure, cerebral ischemia, cerebral hypoxia, and cerebral hypocapnia on the Cushing response. In: Intracranial Pressure II (N. LUNDBERG, U. PONTEN, M. BROCK, eds.), pp. 303-306. Berlin-Heidelberg-New York: Springer 1975.

7. NORNES, H., MAGNAES, B., AASLID, R.: Observations in intracranial pressure plateau waves. In: Intracranial Pressure II (N. LUNDBERG, U. PONTEN, M. BROCK, eds.), pp. 421-426. Berlin-Heidelberg-New York: Springer 1975.

8. de ROUGEMONT, J., BARGE, M., BENABID, A.L.: Correlative study of intracranial and systemic arterial pressures in neurosurgical patients. In: Intracranial Pressure (M. BROCK, H. DIETZ, eds.), pp. 232-238. Berlin-Heidelberg-New York: Springer 1972.

9. TINDALL, G.T., McGRAW, C.P., VANDERVEER, R.W., IWATA, K.: Cardiorespiratory changes associated with plateau waves in patients with head injury. In: Intracranial Pressure (M. BROCK, H. DIETZ, eds.), pp. 227-231. Berlin-Heidelberg-New York: Springer 1972.

10. TROUPP, H., de ROUGEMONT, J.: Pathophysiology of rapid variations of ICP. Chairmen's comments. In: Intracranial Pressure II (N. LUNDBERG, U. PONTEN, M. BROCK, eds.), pp. 419-420. Berlin-Heidelberg-New York: Springer 1975.

11. ZIERSKI, J.: Intracranial pressure recording in clinical practice. In preparation.

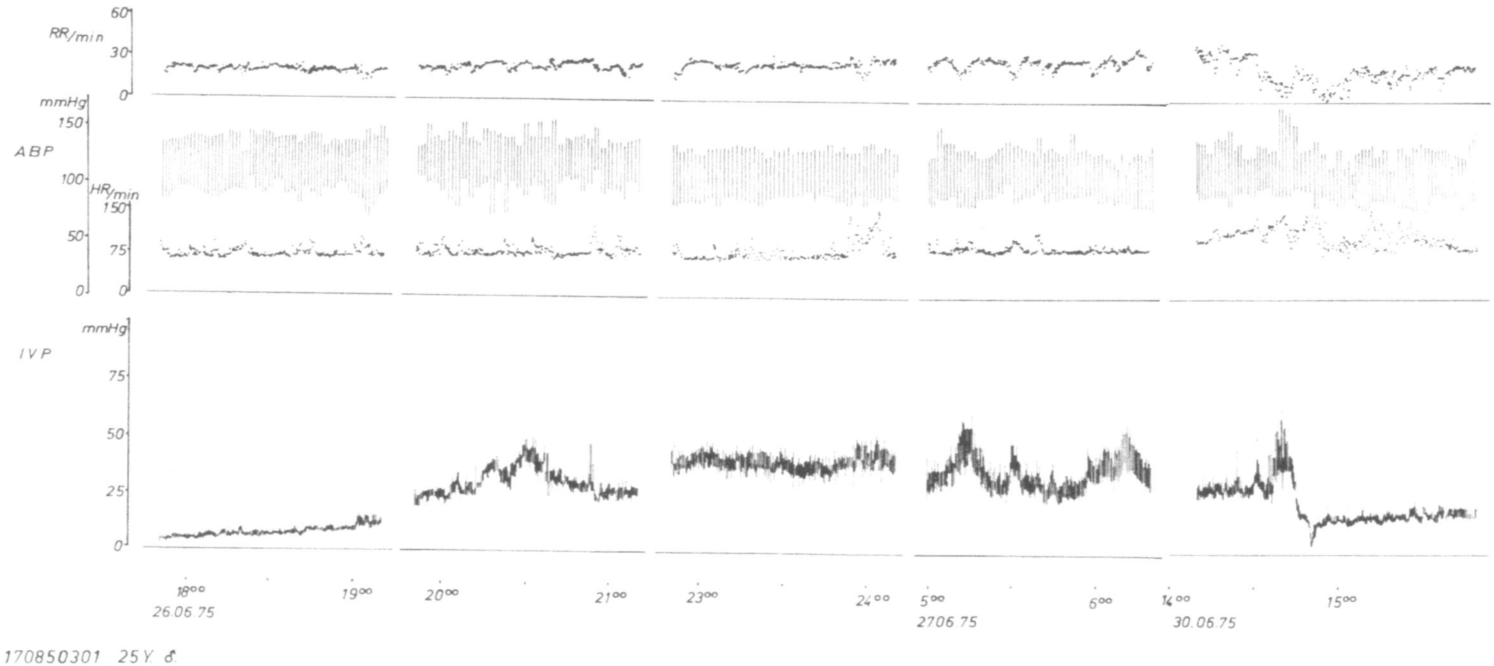

Fig. 1. Steady increase of intraventricular pressure without any recognizable changes of vegetative parameters

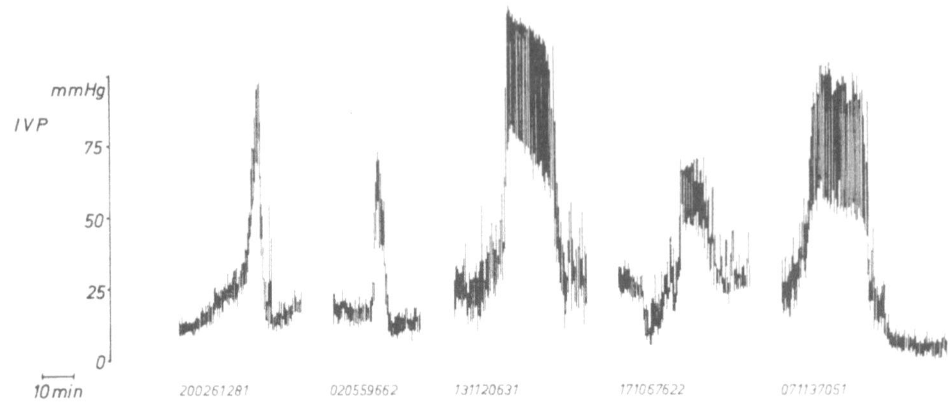

Fig. 2. Various types of A-waves

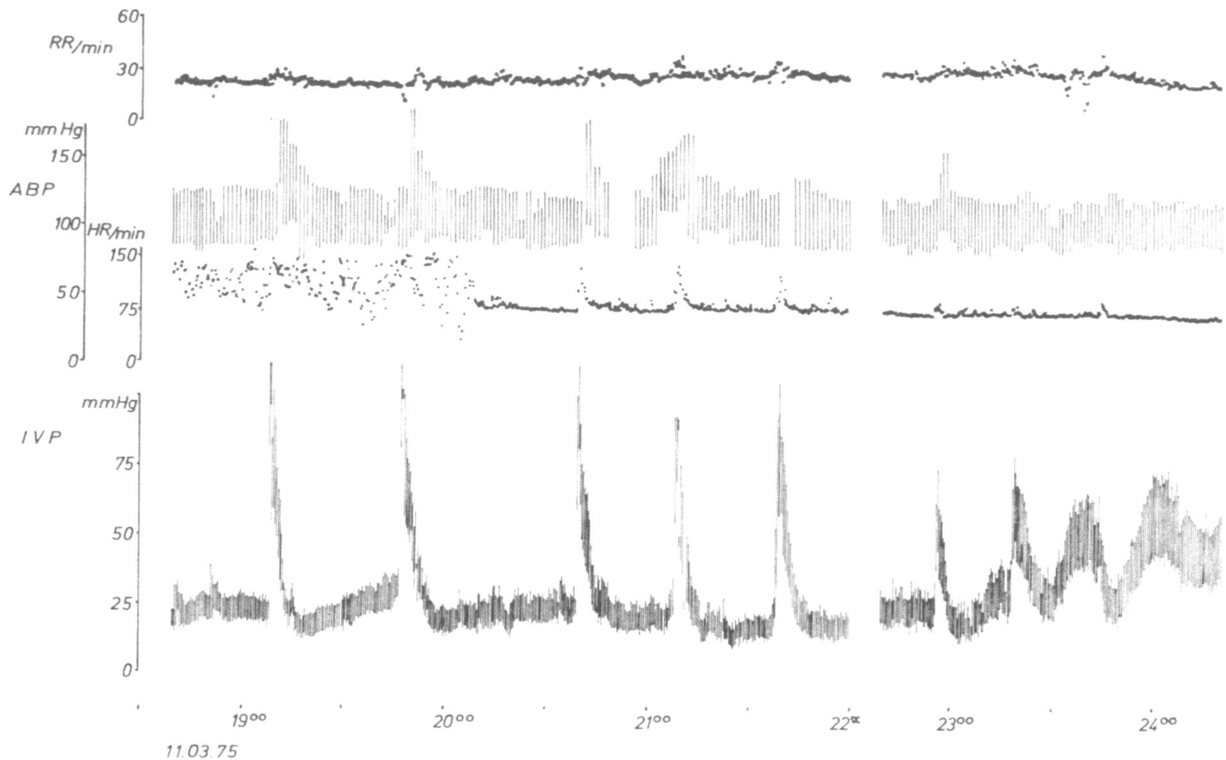

Fig. 3. Transition of vegetative reactions despite of persistence of pressure waves

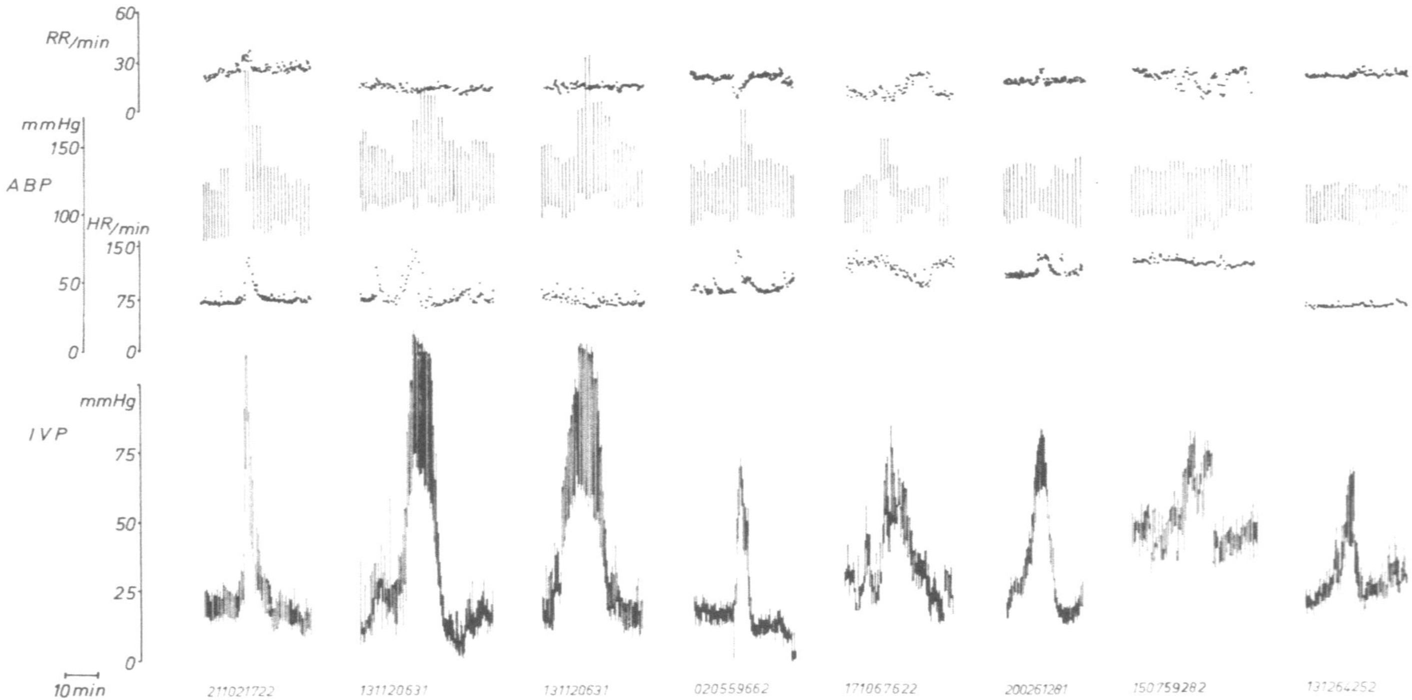

Fig. 4. Various reactions of vegetative parameters during A-waves

Summary

H. Troupp and D.G. McDowall

Direct measurement of intracranial pressure (ICP) has contributed immensely to our knowledge of the pathophysiology of various clinical neurosurgical conditions; it has also served to remove some unwarranted opinions and conclusions, for example, to correct the belief that blood pressure and pulse rate changes in neurosurgical patients are early indicators of rising ICP (see particularly the paper by LORENZ). But what has direct pressure measurement contributed to the management of the individual patient, to balance against the invasiveness of the technique? ICP monitoring is not in use in every neurosurgical department in the way that, say, angiography and air studies are and that, presumably, computerized axial tomography soon will be. Moreover, after the pioneering clinical work by JANNY and LUNDBERG, it took a long time for interest to become more widespread. What is the reason for this? An unconscious awareness that in many instances the actual level of the pressure is not so important, but the way it can be controlled? In his summing-up at the end of the symposium, BRYAN JENNETT asked the pertinent question that: "When high intracranial pressure occurs, does it always matter?". In Certain conditions the ICP usually remains within reasonable limits and a lot of monitoring is required before the occasional rise is seen, as, for example, in the post-operative period - as discussed by BEKS et al. When the diagnostic return is so low, is it justifiable to routinely leave a catheter in the ventricle, knowing that the reported incidence of infection is 0.5-3%? In the study of BEKS and colleagues, an epidural transducer was used, and it would seem clear that in such situations the epidural technique has a major advantage over the ventricular catheter method. The situation is very different where frequent abnormalities are revealed by ICP monitoring, or where therapy is partially controlled by this measurement, for then, in our view, the infection hazard can be justifiably accepted.

With the advent of computerized axial tomography it seems doubtful whether ICP recordings can be taken as an index of brain edema; it seems likely that very soon there can be no serious paper on clinical edema of the brain without access to computerized axial tomography.

The paper by HULME and COOPER was an eloquent reminder of the critical conditions under which we sometimes handle our patients, as NORNES pointed out in his comments; the positioning of the patient is extremely important, and KJALLQUIST showed a recording of a patient who developed a dangerous rise in ICP when his head was turned for shaving immediately before the operation. PRICE reminds us that, with a transducer mounted on the head, turning the patient's head could mean a difference of some 7 mm Hg, so not all changes should be interpreted as being due to obstruction of venous outflow. WILLIAMS pointed out that, when the patient's head is raised, downward movement of the brain might lead to blockage at the level of the foramen of Magendie, and that such blockage would tend to cut off the spinal compartment, making its capacitance unavailable to the rest of the cerebrospinal fluid circulation.

McGRAW's results in head-injured patients, showing a fall in mortality with increasing employment of ICP monitoring, were critically discussed. SYMON suggested that perhaps after McGRAW's colleagues had accepted the method, the pendulum had swung the other way, so that only those patients considered absolutely hopeless after a severe brain injury were left without a pressure recorder.

The paper by LOBATO et al. added to HULME and COOPER's findings of considerable variation from one patient to another. LOBATO et al. found a higher incidence of patients with parallel changes in ventricular and sagittal sinus pressures than reported in 1974 by MARTINS et al. (J. Neurosurg. 40, 603-608, 1974). This again brings up the usual question: How to select those patients who will benefit from ICP monitoring, for instance, in the diagnosis of post-operative pressure problems, as discussed by BEKS et al.? One cannot but speculate whether, for instance, patients whose ventricular and sagittal sinus pressures alter in parallel may be more prone to the dangerous effects of sudden rises in ICP?

LORENZ' impressive review, in which multi-channel circulatory and respiratory measurements were compared with ICP changes showed clearly that the so-called CUSHING response is but one of several possible responses; furthermore, compared to the acute experiments seen in the laboratory, clinical conditions are almost invariably more chronic. In the Discussion, ROWAN reported that he and TEASDALE had measured brain stem blood flow by the hydrogen clearance method in baboons and found no instance in which there was a drop in brain stem flow before the blood pressure started to rise; consequently, the so-called CUSHING response is *not* a response to brain stem ischemia. McDOWALL pointed out that sinus arrhythmia might have correlated better with changes in ICP in LORENZ' patients; it appeared that this sign had not been looked for.

Looking back a couple of weeks after the event, we see clearly that, although ICP monitoring has been extremely important to our understanding of what goes on within the skull, it has still not been accepted in many neurosurgical clinics as a routine monitoring technique, though its place, its limitations, and its hazards are becoming clearer.

Session I

Data Handling

Chairman: R. Cooper
Co-chairman: J. de Rougemont

Computer Analysis of Intracranial Pressure Measurements: Clinical Value and Nursing Response

J.M. Turner, D.G. McDowall, R.M. Gibson, and H. Khalili[1]

Introduction

Many workers (1, 2) have performed detailed analysis of intracranial pressure measurements in an attempt to obtain more information about the intracranial contents. In this paper we wish to present two aspects of our recent work. Firstly we have extended the use of computer analysis of ICP to the nursing staff in our wards, because we believe that such techniques greatly improve the understanding of the problems of the seriously ill neurosurgical patient by nurses, and secondly we have noted a potential use of simple analysis of ICP as an aid for the prediction of a rise in ICP.

Previous workers (2, 3) have made use of the frequency distribution of ICP displayed as a histogram and it was considered that this would be the most generally useful form of display. It therefore appeared to be important to assess the degree to which members of the nursing staff could understand the concept of a normal distribution curve.

Method

(a) The System

Intracranial pressure is measured from one lateral ventricle by standard, externally mounted pressure transducers, and the analogue trace is displayed on a chart recorder to ensure that there is no damping apparent. The electrical signal is passed through an analogue to-digital converter to a data logger which samples at preset time intervals. The numerical value for ICP is then stored on magnetic tape. For analysis the tape is transferred to a replay unit and the various statistical parameters and histogram are produced by the programmable calculator which controls the system. The statistical parameters are calculated from the original values for ICP, 500 consecutive measurements being used for the calculations and for the accompanying histogram, which is produced with 2 mm Hg class intervals. As the normal time interval between measurements is set to be 4 s, a histogram is compiled over approximately 33 min. Display of the histogram, and of the calculated results is either on a visual display unit, or for hard copy, a plotter can be used. Subsequent development has made possible a similar analysis on line.

[1]The authors wish to thank the members of the nursing staff of Wards 26 and 21 at the Leeds General Infirmary for their interest and support. Also Mr Michael Standen for technical assistance and Mrs Elaine Bent for secretarial help.

(b) Nursing Response

In view of the possibility that a slowly rising ICP could be demonstrated early by development of a skew distribution it was decided to assess the nursing staff response by the use of histograms exhibiting known degrees of skewness.
Therefore, 22 histograms were produced on a standard format and with an equal variance. For each histogram the moment coefficient of skewness was calculated by:

$$b_1 = \frac{m_3}{m_2^{1.5}}.$$

14 of the 22 histograms had a value for the skew coefficient which revealed a significant degree of skewness at the 5% level and 8 showed no significant degree of skewness.

The value of a normal distribution curve was explained to the nurses, particular emphasis being placed on the bell-shape of a normal distribution curve, and its symmetry, Each nurse was then asked to grade each histogram, shown in random order, as either "a normal distribution" or "a non-normal distribution". Of the 20 nurses involved in the test, 7 were trained staff on the neurosurgical ward or intensive care unit and 12 were nurses in training, and on the neurosurgical ward.

Results

(a) Nursing Response

Results of the testing are shown in Table 1. The figures in parentheses show for each category of staff the number of occasions that the appropriate grading should have been made, and the other numbers show the number of occasions a particular distribution actually was categorized.

Overall examination of Table 1 therefore shows a tendency for the eye to categorize a histogram as being that for skew distribution before the value of the skew coefficient reaches statistical significance - a tendency therefore to produce false positive results, and therefore for the system to fail safe. Examination of the individual records of the test show that a skew distribution was only categorized as "normal" by our nurses on three occasions (out of a total of 440) and these affected two histograms with a skew coefficient of -0.19 and 0.23 respectively (n = 1.000). So on 3 out of 440 occasions the system would have 'failed dangerous.'

Another interesting feature is that both trained and training staff were able to appreciate the display of histograms and that staff in training were as reliable as trained staff in their recognition of abnormal patterns so that as a monitoring aid the display of a frequency distribution would appear to be of particular value, as it does not necessarily appear to depend on skills acquired in training.

Table 1

		Category of staff	
		Trained	Training
Description of histogram	Normal	52 (64)	85 (96)
	Skew	124 (112)	179 (168)

(b) Prediction of Pressure Rise

Four out of 13 successive patients in whom ICP was measured developed an elevated ICP. Examination of each patient's record shows an appearance similar to that reproduced as Figures 1 and 2. In Figure 1 the mean ICP is normal and the distribution of the measurements is narrow. Figure 2 represents the next period of observation and shows that only a few measurements of ICP are above normal values, but that the distribution has greatly widened, as is reflected in the increase in variance.

Each histogram is composed of 500 observations taken at 4-s intervals, and the histogram with the widened distribution was followed in all four cases by the development of high ICP.

Discussion

A frequency distribution of ICP will include variations in ICP due to all sources, whether due to the cardiac impulse or to variations as a result of the respiratory cycle, or due to random variation, which is often increased in advanced neurosurgical disease. It is possible that such an increased variation existed before the pressure rise in our patients and this is reflected in Figure 3 which represents for three of the four patients who developed elevated ICP the relationship between pulse pressure and ICP at various periods of time before the development of high ICP. In each case the last point is that which applies to the period before the frank pressure rise and reflects, we believe, a period where there is an increased pulse pressure, which may in part account for the increased variation in the histograms.

Summary

The use of a histogram of the frequency distribution of pressure provides a display that nurses very easily appreciate. Such a display may lead to early recognition of ICP changes and possibly the prediction of an impending pressure rise if associated with simple statistical analysis.

References

1. AUGUSTYNIAK, B., DYTKO, P., DZIDUSZKO, J., KORSAK-SLIWKA, J., KUNICKI, A., SLIWKA, S., SZEWCZYKOWSKI, J.: Determination of critical ICP level in neurosurgical patients: A statistical approach. In: Intracranial Pressure II (N. LUNDBERG, U. PONTEN, M. BROCK, eds.), pp. 392-393. Berlin-Heidelberg-New York: Springer 1975.

2. JANNY, P., JOUAN, J.P., JAONNY, L., GOURGAND, M., GUEIT, U.M.: A statistical approach to long term monitoring of intracranial pressure. In: Intracranial Pressure (M. BROCK, H. DIETZ, eds.), pp. 59-64. Berlin-Heidelberg-New York: Springer 1972.

3. KULLBERG, G.: A method for statistical analysis of intracranial pressure recordings. In: Intracranial Pressure (M. BROCK, H. DIETZ, eds.), pp. 65-69. Berlin-Heidelberg-New York: Springer 1972.

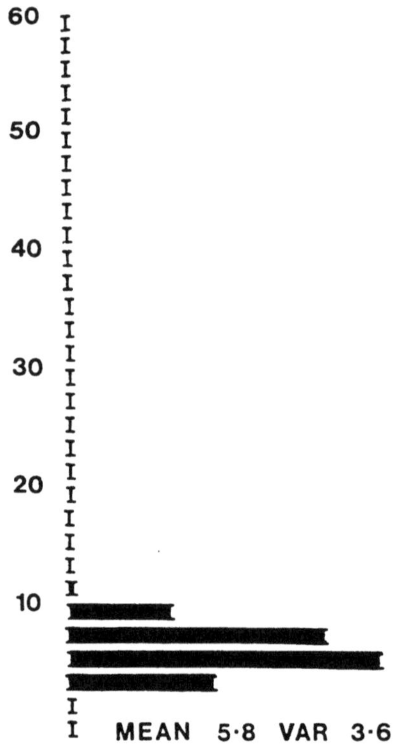

Fig. 1. Frequency distribution of ICP in a head injured patient, compiled from 500 consecutive readings, taken at 4-second intervals. Class interval is 2 mm Hg

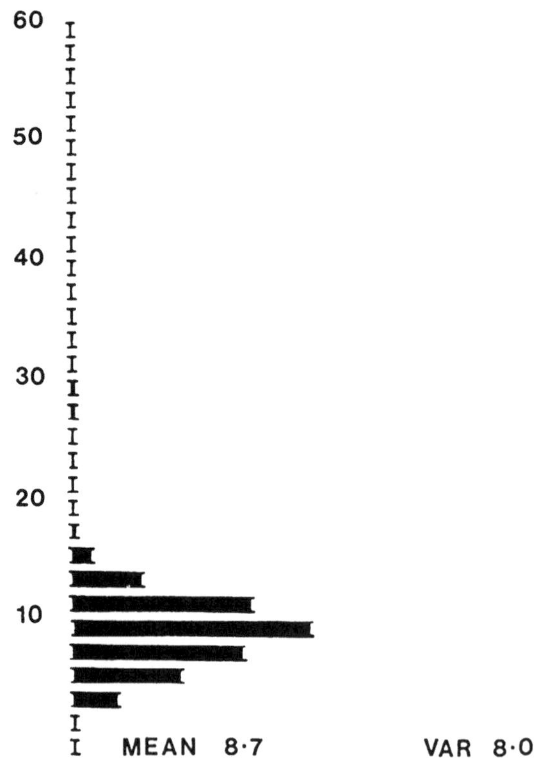

Fig. 2. Frequency distribution of ICP in a head injured patient, compiled from 500 consecutive readings, taken at 4-second intervals. Class interval is 2 mm Hg. This histogram immediately follows that of Figure 1

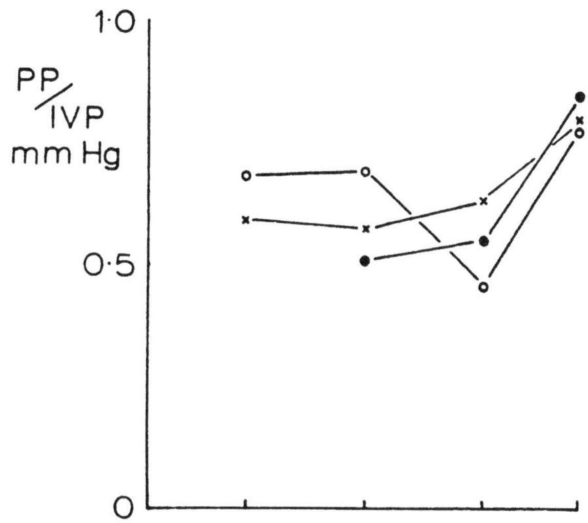

Fig. 3. Plot showing the relationship between intracranial pulse pressure and ICP in three patients who subsequently developed high ICP. In each patient the right hand point represents the relationship immediately before rise in ICP

Reliability and Reproduceability of ICP Frequency Analysis[1]

M. Brock, C. Zywietz, P. Mock, H. Wiegand, C. Zillig, and W. M. Tamburus[2]

Following the publications of KULLBERG and WEST (13), CABRINI et al. (6) and of JANNY et al. (12), several authors (1-5, 7, 9-11, 14, 16, 17) have employed some kind of computerized data sampling and statistical analysis as a complement to conventional ICP recording. However, little attention has been paid to the reliability and reproduceability of this method. Since ICP may undergo periodic variations of different origin and duration, several questions of practical importance arise:

1. Are ICP-histograms of 1-, 2-, 3-, and 6-h periods representative for the 24-h pressure histogram?
2. What are the spontaneous variations between histograms obtained from the same patient on 2 successive days?

Material and Methods

The above questions were studied in two groups of patients.

Group 1 consists of nine patients (Table 1) submitted to continuous monitoring of VFP (ventricular catheter connected to a Statham P23Db transducer at the level of the patient's forehead and to a conventional recorder).

In these patients a 24-h period of continuous frequency analysis was begun on the morning subsequent to the day of ventricular catheterization. The equipment used for this purpose has been previously described (2). The pressure range (15, 30 or 60 mm Hg) was subdivided into 10 equal pressure classes. The value of each class (% time) was recorded after 1 h, 2 h, 3 h, 6 h, and 24 h, and the corresponding histograms were calculated and printed (see below).

Group 2 consists of four patients (Table 2) from each of whom two 6-h histograms were obtained at similar times of day (either morning or afternoon) on 2 consecutive days following the day of ventricular catheterization. This group was originally constituted of six patients, two of whom had to be eliminated (a 7-year-old boy who was very restless during one of the periods of analysis, and a 17-year-old female submitted to frequency analysis at different times of day).

None of the patients of either group was under medication known to influence ICP directly.

The histograms as performed for the present study represent the relative frequency of pressure values recorded every second for a period T in a group m of patients.

---

[1]The equipment used for frequency analysis has been developed with the aid of the Deutsche Forschungsgemeinschaft.

[2]The authors are indebted to Miss. E. Riechers, Miss. I. Busche, Mrs. G. Wachholz and Mr. B. Aukskell for the valuable technical help.

Table 1

Patient No.	Sex	Age (years)	Diagnosis
100338	F	37	Craniopharyngioma
30831	F	44	Acoustic neurinoma
240468	M	7	Spongioblastoma 4th ventricle
90635	F	40	Craniopharyngioma
81246	M	34	Temporal glioma (unclassified)
40122	F	43	Glioma of the pons
80313	M	62	Frontal metastasis (Adenocarcinoma)
120833	F	40	Subdural hematoma
130139	F	36	Coma of unknown etiology (encephalitis)

Table 2

Patient No.	Sex	Age (years)	Diagnosis
70464	F	11	Medulloblastoma (4th ventricle)
20670	F	5	Tumor in 3rd ventricle (inoperable)
100338	F	37	Craniopharyngioma
90635	F	40	Craniopharyngioma

Since the relative frequencies in all pressure classes refer to the total duration of measurement T, taken at equidistant time intervals, their values also represent the percentage of time for each pressure class.

With the sampling rate S $\frac{1}{s}$ one obtains the pressure class frequency

$$t(n) = \frac{1}{m} \cdot \sum_{j=1}^{m} \frac{100}{TS} \sum_{j=1}^{T.S} \delta(K_{i,j} - Kn),$$

$n = 1, 2 \ldots 10.$

where δ means the Kronnecker symbol ($\delta(K_{i,j} - Kn) = 1$ if $K_{i,j} = Kn$). Kn are the pressure classes K1...K10 and $K_{i,j}$ is the normalized pressure (class) of the ith measurement of the j+n patient within the measurement period. Pressure normalization was done according to the amplitude range of the patient with P_o = 15, 30 or 60 mm Hg

$$K_{i,j} = \frac{Pi,J.}{P_o}$$

The product T.S gives the total number of measurements during the measurement period for each patient.

The value of t(n) may also be interpreted as amplitude density. A periodic pressure-time function results in a constant amplitude density when the measurement period T is large as compared with the period of the pressure frequency. All amplitudes occur with the same probability (flat distribution of t(n)), within their upper and lower peak amplitude. A constant pressure during the measurement period results in a Dirac-type function t(n).

The advantage of the histographic presentation is the high degree of data compression. Its disadvantage is the loss of information concerning the time-dependent behavior of intracranial pressure. The method is suitable when a more static level of ICP is of interest and a measurement duration of 1 h is long enough to filter out technical and biological "high frequency" noise (the technical noise lies normally above 1 Hz, biological "disturbances" like the heart-frequency-dependent blood pressure variations or respiratory influence may have a period length of 1...10 s).

For further insight into the dynamic nature of the ICP behavior, future investigations should include spectrum and interval analysis.

Results

Group 1

Provided the patient's condition remains stable, the 1-h histograms can be considered representative for the ICP distribution during longer periods or time (2 h, 3 h, and 6 h). This is illustrated by comparison of the corresponding joint histograms (Fig. 1). Although the agreement between the 1-h and the 24-h histograms can also be considered satisfactory, there is a tendency of lower pressure to increase (see discussion).

Group 2

Despite the small number of patients, this group confirms the tendency observed in group 1 at the end of the 24-h period of analysis, namely a progressive decrease of ICP during the first 2 days following the introduction of a ventricular catheter (Fig. 2). Such changes (of which no mention has been found in literature) are statistically significant ($\underline{P}<0.001$, Mann-Whitney test) although much less pronounced than those observed after 48-h under dexamethasone therapy (4, 5).

Comments

Since most authors employing ICP frequency analysis have used relatively long periods of time - mainly for fear that shorter periods might provide non-representative data - our observation that 1-h and 2-h histograms also reflect reliable information, is of direct practical relevance. It validates the use of brief sampling periods (1 h or 2 h) and permits saving equipment time, an important aspect of on-line computer processing. Obviously, one prerequisite is that the patient's clinical condition remains stable.

The reason for the shifting of lower pressure values in the course of a 24-h period of analysis (as compared to the histogram of the 1st hour) is not clear. It appears unlikely that statistical factors or circadian ICP variations (8, 11, 15) might account for such a shifting, since the trend toward lower pressure levels becomes even more pronounced during the 2nd day following ventricular catheterization (Fig. 2). Rather, we believe that the procedure of ventricular catheterization per se - and the removal of 1 or 2 ml of CSF for chemical studies at the moment of ventricular puncture - has a longer-lasting influence on CSF dynamics. This effect can scarcely be a direct consequence of the withdrawal of so small a volume of CSF. It is more probably due to a change in the dynamics (compliance or elastance) of the entire system. This phenomenon deserves further clarification and must be taken into account in studies on the pharmacotherapy of ICP.

We conclude, therefore, that frequency analysis for periods of 1 h or 2 h provides representative and significant information on the ICP distribution pattern. A progressive decrease in ICP during the first 48 h following ventricular catheterization must be taken into account when comparing histograms of the first 2 days immediately subsequent to ventricular puncture.

Summary

Studies with serial frequency analysis in two groups of neurosurgical patients have shown that ICP histograms obtained from periods of 1 h or 2 h significantly and reliably reflect the overall pressure distribution pattern of longer time intervals (up to 1 day) under conditions of clinical stability. This validates the use of shorter sampling periods. Our observations also suggest that ventricular catheterization per se leads to a decrease in ICP during the first 48 h, a fact which must be taken into account when performing long-term ICP studies.

Key Words

Intracranial pressure, Frequency analysis, Ventricular puncture.

References

1. BARNES, R.W., McGRAW, C.P.: A new on-line portable ICP data processor. In: Intracranial Pressure II (N. LUNDBERG, U. PONTEN, M. BROCK, eds.), pp. 389-390. Berlin-Heidelberg-New York: Springer 1975.
2. BROCK, M., DIEFENTHÄLER, K., ZYWIETZ, C., PÖLL, W., MOCK, P., DIETZ, H.: Amplitude analysis of long-term intracranial pressure recordings. In: Advances in Neurosurgery 2 (W. KLUG, M. BROCK, M. KLINGER, O. SPOERRI, eds.), pp. 310-313. Berlin-Heidelberg-New York: Springer 1975.
3. BROCK, M., DIEFENTHÄLER, K., ZYWIETZ, C., PÖLL, W., MOCK, P., DIETZ, H.: Amplitude analysis of intracranial pressure recordings. In: Intracranial Pressure II (N. LUNDBERG, U. PONTEN, M. BROCK, eds.), p. 391. Berlin-Heidelberg-New York: Springer 1975.
4. BROCK, M., WIEGAND, H., ZILLIG, C., ZYWIETZ, C., MOCK, P., DIETZ, H.: The effect of dexamethasone on ICP in cases of supratentorial tumors. In: Brain Edema (H.M. PAPPIUS, W., FEINDEL, eds.). Berlin-Heidelberg-New York: 1976 (in press).
5. BROCK, M., ZILLIG, C., WIEGAND, H., ZYWIETZ, C., MOCK, P.: The effects of dexamethasone on ICP in patients with tumors of the posterior fossa. In: Intracranial Pressure III (J.F.W. BEKS, D.A. BOSCH, M. BROCK, eds.), pp. 236-246. Berlin-Heidelberg-New York: Springer 1976.
6. CABRINI, G.P., GIOVANELLI, M., INFUSO, L.: Influenze del desametazone sulla pressione liquorale ventricolare in casi di ipertensione endocranica. Minerva Neurochir. 11, 94-102 (1967).
7. CASTEL, J.P., COHADON, F.: Méthode d'analyse modale automatique des variations de la pression intra-cranienne chez l'homme. Neuro-Chirurgie 21, 205-212 (1975).
8. COOPER, R., HULME, A.: Intracranial pressure and related phenomena during sleep. J. Neurol. Neurosurg. Psychiat. 29, 564-570 (1966).

9. CROCKARD, H.A., HANLON, K., GANZ, E., DUDA, E.E.: Intracranial pressure gradients in a patient with a thalamic tumor. Surg. Neurol. 5, 151-155 (1976).

10. GASPARETTO, B., SICCARDI, A., SIANI, C., ZATTONI, J.: Automatic analysis of some changes of intracranial pressure having clinical interest. Boll. Soc. Ital. Biol. Spar. 50, 382-385 (1974).

11. HEMMER, R., MOHADJER, M., SCHIEFER, K.: Untersuchungen zur cerebralen Dysregulation bei Tumoren der hinteren Schädelgrube mit Hydrocephalus occlusus. Neurochirurgie 17, 96-106 (1974).

12. JANNY, P., JOUAN, P., JANNY, L., GOURGAND, M., GUEIT, M.: A statistical approach to long-term monitoring of intracranial pressure. In: Intracranial Pressure (M. BROCK, H. DIETZ, eds.), pp. 59-64. Berlin-Heidelberg-New York: Springer 1972.

13. KULLBERG, G., WEST, K.A.: Influence of corticosteroids on the ventricular fluid pressure. Acta Neurol. Scand. 41 (Suppl. 13), 445-452 (1965).

14. KULLBERG, G.: A method for statistical analysis of intracranial pressure recordings. In: Intracranial Pressure (M. BROCK, H. DIETZ, eds.), pp. 65-69. Berlin-Heidelberg-New York: Springer 1972.

15. SYMON, L., DORSCH, N.W.C., STEPHENS, R.J.: Intracranial pressure monitoring in communicating hydrocephalus. Proc. Roy. Soc. Med. 65, 888-890 (1972).

16. SZEWCZYKOWSKI, J., DYTKO, P., KUNICKI, A., KORSAKSLIWKA, J., DZIDUSZKO, J., AUGUSTYNIAK, B.: Determination of critical ICP levels in neurosurgical patients: A statistical approach. In: Intracranial Pressure II (N. LUNDBERG, U. PONTEN, M. BROCK, eds.), pp. 392-393. Berlin-Heidelberg-New York: Springer 1975.

17. SZEWCZYKOWSKI, J., SLIWKA, S., KUNICKI, A., KORSAKSLIWKA, J., DZIDUSZKO, J., DYTKO, P., AUGUSTYNIAK, B.: Computer-assisted analysis of intraventricular pressure after mannitol administration. J. Neurosurg. 43, 136-141 (1975).

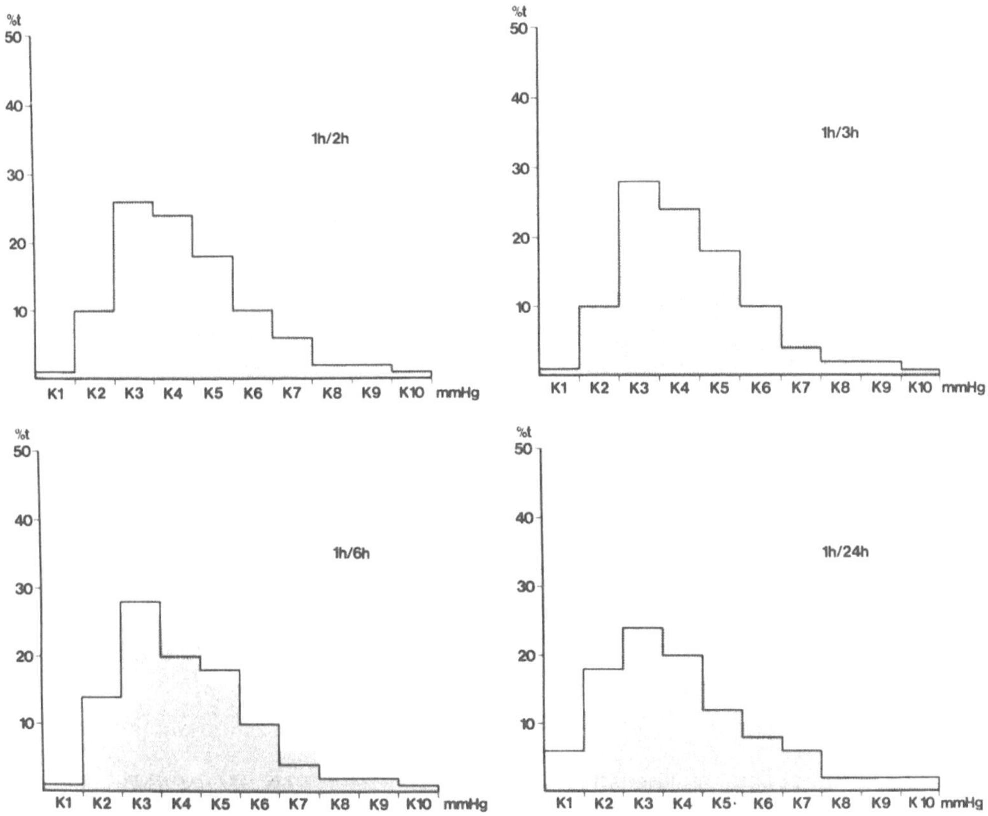

Fig. 1. Joint histograms of patients of group 1. Note good correlation between the 1-h histogram (*hatched*) and those obtained from sampling periods of 2 h, 3 h and 6 h (*solid lines*). The 24-h histogram shows a shifting toward the left (lower pressure classes). Vertical axis: percent of recording time. Horizontal axis: pressure classes

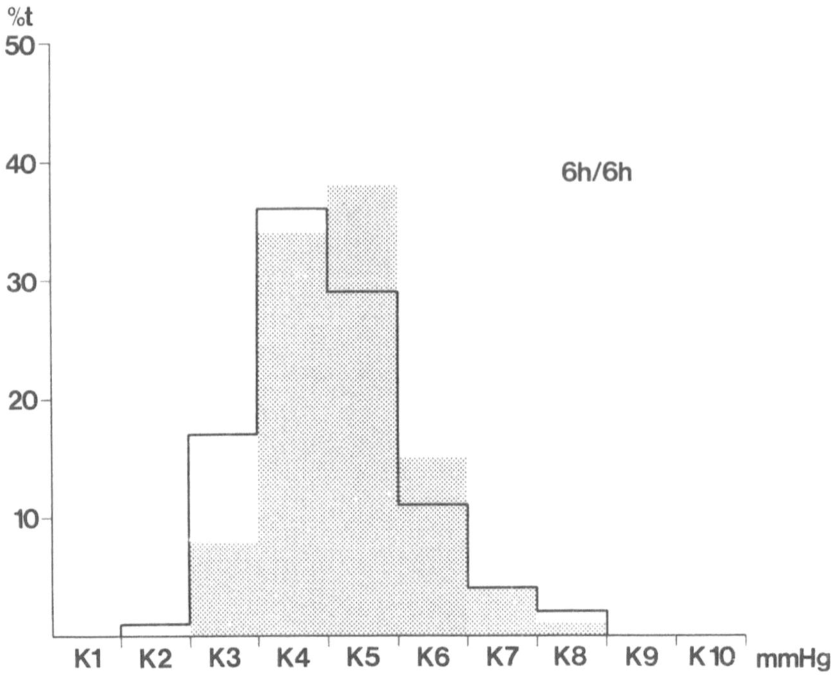

Fig. 2. Comparison of point histograoms of 6-h periods obtained 24 h (*hatched*) and 48 h (*solid line*) following ventricular catheterization. There is a shifting of the intracranial pressure pattern toward lower values. Vertical axis: percent of recording time. Horizontal axis: pressure classes

Computer-Assisted Determination of Optimum ICP Levels

J. Szewczykowski, J. Korsak-Sliwka, A. Kunicki, P. W. Dytko, S. Sliwka, and J. Dziduszko

Introduction

The condition known as "intracranial tightness" can constitute a grave risk to the patient. It is occasionally observed that patients with normal intracranial pressure (ICP) develop the condition of "tight brain" (7). The only dependable indicator of intracranial tightness is the behavior of intracranial elastance. The elastance of the intracranial system can be determined from the pressure volume (P-V) relationship (1, 3-6). However, the P-V method has limited application in neurosurgical practice.

In this work, elastance changes are determined from the relationship between the amplitude of pulse-related ICP oscillations and the basic ICP level (2, 8). This relationship, called the Amp-P curve (10), is shown in Figure 1.

By definition the elastance $E = dP/dV$; since P (pressure) is a nonlinear function of V (volume), E is a function of ICP. If the volume changes forced on the intracranial system are *sufficiently small and fast* then it can be assumed that

$$\Delta P = E/P/.\Delta V \qquad (1)$$

Hence, the same volume changes ΔV produced at different ICP levels will cause different ICP responses proportional to E (Fig. 2). Injections of additional volume increments ΔV in order to obtain the P-V curve, and hence the elastance-pressure (E-P) curve, may produce unexpected pressure rises endangering the patient. In our method of computerized elastance examination (CEE) we assumed that the physiological cerebral blood volume (CBV) changes generated by cardiac action are sufficiently small and fast to be used in the determination of intracranial elastance. The amplitude of pulse-related ICP oscillations is described by the equation:

$$Amp = E/P/.\Delta CBV_{pr} \qquad (2)$$

where ΔCBV_{pr} is the pulse-related CBV change.
Thus, in order to determine the E-P curve it is sufficient to obtain the Amp-P curve and to calculate ΔCBV_{pr}.

Material and Method

The CEE studies were performed on a group of 15 patients without intracranial pathology (a) and another group of 15 patients with raised ICP (b).

(a) In this group the measurements were made from the lumbar subarachnoid space. We elevated the ICP by giving a series of 2 ml injections of physiological saline in intervals of 1 min. The data coming in from the patients were processed in the real time by a minicomputer (9) according to the program represented by the flow-chart of Table 1. The

Table 1. Flow-chart of data acquisition and processing program

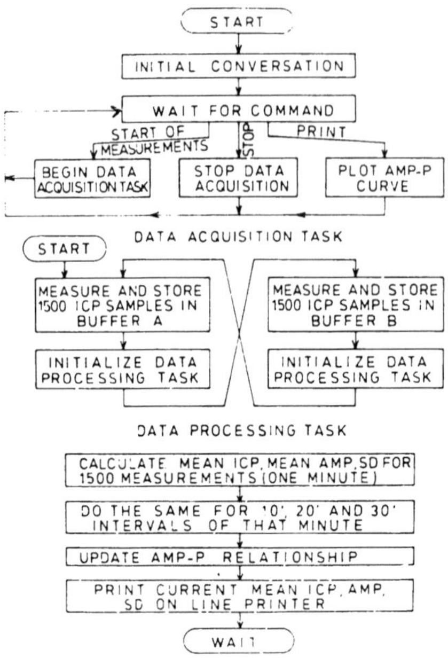

Amp-P curve was printed out and ΔCBV_{pr} was computed from the formula:

$$\Delta CBV_{pr} = A/P/ \cdot \frac{\Delta V}{\Delta P} \qquad (3)$$

where: ΔV is the volume of injected saline, ΔP the resulting pressure response, and A/P/ the amplitude of pulse-related oscillations at ICP level concerned.

Next, the E-P curve was computed from ΔCBV_{pr} and the Amp-P slope.

(b) In patients with intracranial pathology the ICP was measured from one lateral ventricle by the method of Lundberg. All the patients had ventricular CSF drainage. For the time of the CEE examination the drainage catheter was closed and the rising ICP was monitored by the computer system. In this way, without injecting saline, it was possible to monitor the ICP over a pressure range sufficient for the determination of the Amp-P curve. ICP rises above approximately 35 mm Hg were prevented by opening the catheter. The short duration of the examination as well as the continuous monitoring of the pressure permitted full control over the intracranial situation. Once the character of the Amp-P curve and the location of its transition zone were known, it was possible to determine ΔCBV_{pr} by giving a single injection of a suitable quantity of saline (normally 1 or 2 ml, depending on the Amp-P slope). The E-P curve was then computed, as in the physiological group.

The CEE method makes it possible to limit the number of intraventricular injections, which is of great importance in clinical practice. Table 2 shows a block diagram of the procedure.

Table 2. Block diagram of CEE procedure

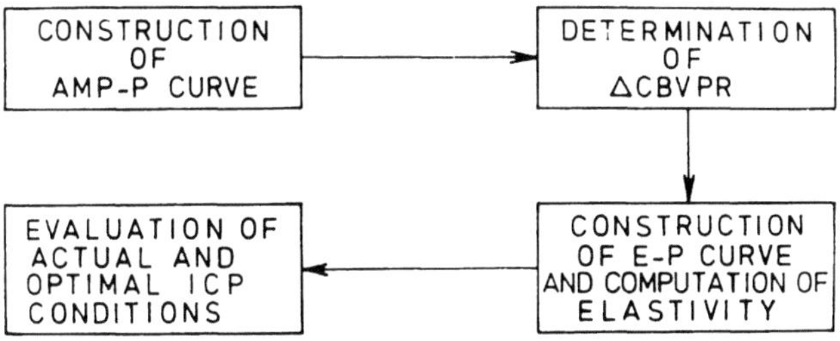

Results

The results obtained in 24 patients are given in Table 3. A typical E-P curve (case 22) is shown in Figure 3. Figure 4 shows three E-P curves obtained in 1 patient (case 25) before surgery, after administration of lasix, and after surgery.

Table 3. Summary of CEE results obtained in 24 neurosurgical patients

CASE Nº		ICP RANGE EXAMINED	OPENING PRESSURE	TRANSITION ZONE	SLOPE AMP-P	ΔCBV PR	ELASTIVITY	ELASTANCE AT OPENING PRESSURE	ELASTANCE AT TRANSITION ZONE
1	PHYSIOL	14-30	15-16	16-18	0.325	1.04	0.312	1.2	1.4
2	PHYSIOL	6-24	8-9	8-10	0.323	0.67	0.416	0.6	0.6
3	PATHOL	2-40	9-10	8-10	0.305	—	—	—	—
4	PATHOL	12-30	16-17	14-16	0.247	—	—	—	—
5	PATHOL	4-30	9-10	8-10	0.287	—	—	—	—
6	PHYSIOL	6-20	6-7	6-8	0.230	0.55	0.419	1.3	1.3
7	PATHOL	8-30	9-10	8-10	0.443	1.03	0.430	1.3	1.3
8	PATHOL	2-18	6-7	—	0.263	0.93	0.282	1.1	—
9	PHYSIOL	4-26	9-10	6-8	0.481	0.93	0.517	0.4	0.4
10	PATHOL	2-38	9-10	8-10	0.426	—	—	—	—
11	PATHOL	4-50	7-8	—	0.511	0.67	0.763	3.0	—
12	PHYSIOL	0-30	4-5	2-4	0.440	1.80	0.244	0.55	0.55
13	PHYSIOL	4-26	4-5	—	0.391	1.24	0.316	2.0	—
14	PHYSIOL	0-14	7-8	6-8	0.305	0.82	0.372	1.0	1.0
15	PHYSIOL	4-36	9-10	8-10	0.382	1.23	0.311	0.6	0.6
16	PATHOL	0-28	7-8	8-10	0.357	0.60	0.594	0.5	0.5
17	PHYSIOL	4-34	4-6	8-10	0.283	0.72	0.393	1.3	1.3
18	PHYSIOL	4-24	6-8	8-10	0.352	0.87	0.404	1.6	1.7
19	PHYSIOL	2-34	8-10	6-8	0.485	0.89	0.433	1.5	1.0
20	PATHOL	12-28	15-16	—	0.215	0.99	0.217	1.5	—
21	PATHOL	0-46	7-8	10-12	0.496	0.53	0.936	2.8	3.0
22	PATHOL	6-54	20-21	6-8	0.360	0.72	0.500	5.6	1.0
23	PHYSIOL	2-24	8-9	6-8	0.478	1.34	0.357	0.7	0.7
24	PATHOL	6-32	7-8	8-10	0.328	0.79	0.415	1.0	1.0

All pressures are given in mm Hg; elastances in mm Hg/ml; ΔCBV_{pr} in ml.

Discussion

Changes in the amplitude of pulse-related ICP oscillations at different ICP levels constitute a valuable diagnostic indicator; however, the Amp-P curve alone does not make it possible to compute the elastance and elastivity (E-P slope) of the intracranial system, without which the degree of intracranial tightness cannot be evaluated accurately. If, in addition to the Amp-P curve, ΔCBV_{pr} is known, then the behavior of elastance at different ICP levels, and hence the optimum ICP range for the patient concerned, can be determined. The CEE studies of the physiological group show that there is good agreement between the value of opening pressure and the value indicated by the transition zone of the Amp-P curve. Therefore, knowledge of the E-P slope and of the transition zone makes it possible to determine with good probability whether or not the patient's intracranial system is in a state of pathological tightness. This is of great importance in the proper administration of drugs and in determining the optimum CSF drainage level.

In the physiological group the mean E-P slope (i.e. elastivity) was 0.386, SD 0.062. Case 22 presents a good illustration of the use of the CEE method. The patient, aged 23, was hospitalized because of headaches which started 2 months after head trauma caused by a ball. There were no distinct neurological symptoms except for a slightly narrower left pupil and a sensory deficit in the region of the first and second branches of the fifth cranial nerve. The CEE examination showed a high elastivity of 0.500 and an opening pressure of 20 mm Hg, the transition zone being at approximately 7 mm Hg. Elastance at opening pressure was 5.6 mm Hg/ml. The CEE results pointed to a considerable tightness of the intracranial system and indicated that its compensating ability was severely impaired. Angiography indicated a possible hematoma over the left hemisphere. At surgery an extensive subdural hematoma (150 ml in volume) was removed. Post-operatively the CEE examination showed an elastivity of 0.100.

The expansion of brain edema is also reflected in the CEE method, which in this case constitutes a valuable aid in determining the extent and intensity of anti-edema treatment. Figure 4 shows three E-P curves obtained in patient No. 27 with posterior fossa symptoms. The CEE examination before surgery showed a relatively high elastivity of 0.521. Lasix was administered in a dose of 40 mg and elastivity fell to 0.398. At surgery arachnoidal adhesions were separated and CSF circulation was restored; elastivity fell to 0.225. The low value of post-operative elastivity was suggestive of relative intracranial hypotension, though the patient's ICP was about 8 mm Hg. It was therefore decided to put the patient in the anti-hypotonic position, which resulted in the elimination of hypotonic headaches.

Summary

The CEE method provides information on the behavior of intracranial elastance in neurosurgical patients. Knowledge of such parameters of the E-P curve as transition zone, elastivity, and elastance at opening and transition pressures, makes it possible to determine the best ICP conditions for individual patients. Because of the elimination of serial injections the CEE method is particularly suitable for clinical use; however, a real-time computer system is needed.

References

1. COHADON, F., CASTEL, J.P., NOUILLANT, A., VANDENDRIESSCHE, M.: Volume pressure relationship in clinical and experimental conditions of raised ICP. In: Intracranial Pressure II (N. LUNDBERG, U. PONTEN, M. BROCK, eds.), pp. 107-112. Berlin-Heidelberg-New York: Springer 1975.
2. GILLAND, O., TOURTELLOTTE, W.W., O'TAUMA, L., HENDERSON, W.G.: Normal cerebrospinal fluid pressure. J. Neurosurg. 40, 587-593 (1974).
3. LANGFITT, T.W.: Increased intracranial pressure. Clin. Neurosurg. 16, 436-471 (1969).
4. LOEFGREN, J.: Mechanical basis of the CSF pressure-volume curve. In: Intracranial Pressure II (N. LUNDBERG, U. PONTEN, M. BROCK, eds.), pp. 79-81. Berlin-Heidelberg-New York: Springer 1975.
5. MARMAROU, A.: A theoretical and experimental evaluation of the cerebrospinal fluid system. Drexel University, PhD thesis, 1973.
6. MATAKAS, F., v. WAECHTER, R., KNUPLING, R., POTOLICCHIO, S.J.: Increase in cerebral perfusion pressure by arterial hypertension in brain swelling. A mathematical model of the volume-pressure relationship. J. Neurosurg. 42, 282-289 (1975).
7. MILLER, J.D., CARIBI, J.: Intracranial volume/pressure relationships during continuous monitoring of ventricular fluid pressure. In: Intracranial Pressure (M. BROCK, H. DIETZ, eds.), pp. 270-274. Berlin-Heidelberg-New York: Springer 1972.
8. RYDER, H.W., ESPEY, F.F., KIMBELL, F.D., PENKA, E.J., ROSENAUER, A., PODOLSKY, B., EVANS, J.P.: Modification of effect of cerebral blood flow on cerebrospinal fluid pressure by variations in craniospinal blood volume. Arch. Neurol. Psychiat. 68, 170-174 (1952).
9. SZEWCZYKOWSKI, J., KORSAK-SLIWKA, J., KUNICKI, A., SLIWKA, St., DYTKO, P.: A computerized neurosurgical intensive care system. Europ. J. Intensive Care Medicine 1, 189-192 (1975).
10. SZEWCZYKOWSKI, J., SLIWKA, St., KUNICKI, A., DYTKO, P., KORSAK-SLIWKA, J.: A fast method for estimating the elastance of the intracranial system. J. Neurosurg. submitted (1976).

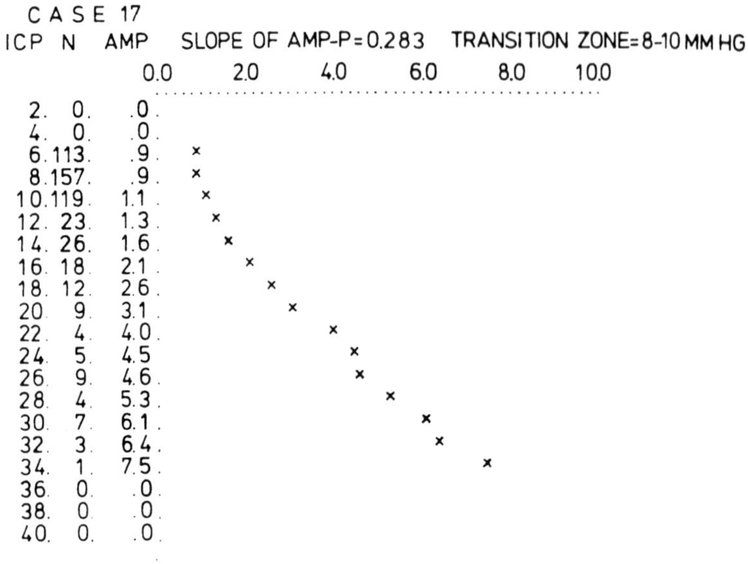

Fig. 1. Computer plot of typical Amp-P curve. Top row gives amplitude in mm Hg of pulse-related ICP oscillations, which corresponds to points on abscissa; middle row gives frequency of occurrence of particular ICP intervals; bottom row gives consecutive ICP levels in mm Hg for which amplitudes were calculated

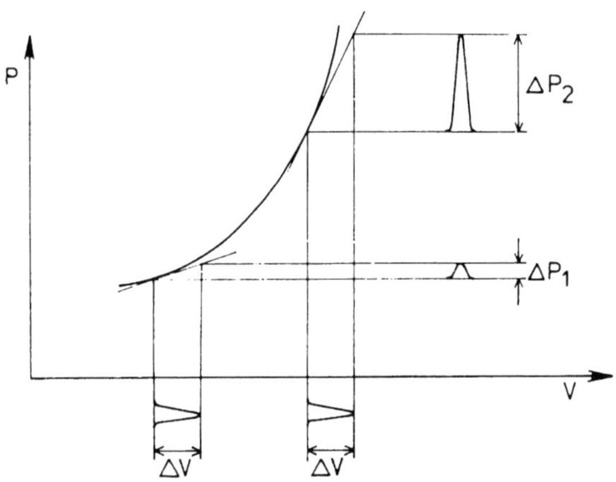

Fig. 2. Pressure responses ΔP_1 and ΔP_2 for same volume changes ΔV obtained at two different ICP levels

CASE 22

ICP N E ELASTIVITY=0.500 TRANSITION ZONE=6-8 MM HG

ICP	N	E
2.	0.	.0.
4.	0.	.0.
6.	26.	1.0.
8.	52.	1.0.
10.	5.	1.4.
12.	36.	1.9.
14.	9.	2.6.
16.	14.	3.3.
18.	29.	4.3.
20.	49.	5.1.
22.	24.	6.0.
24.	9.	7.2.
26.	6.	8.1.
28.	9.	9.9.
30.	1.	10.0.
32.	3.	11.4.
34.	4.	12.6.
36.	3.	14.7.
38.	1.	15.0.
40.	0.	.0.

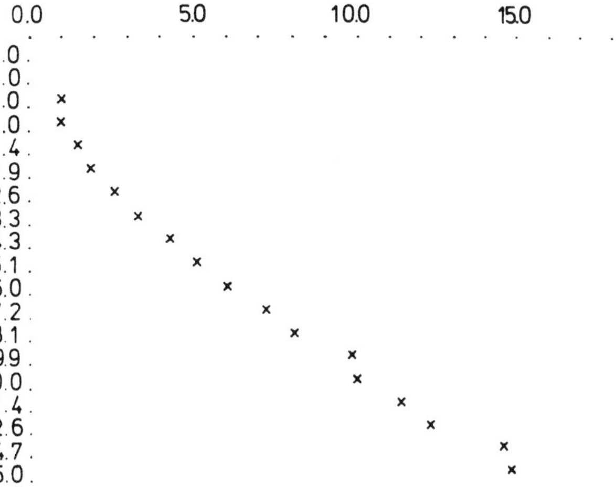

Fig. 3. Computer plot of pathological E-P curve. Top row gives respective values of elastance in mm Hg/ml corresponding to points on the abscissa; middle row gives frequency of occurrence of particular ICP intervals; bottom row gives consecutive ICP levels in mm Hg, for which elastances were calculated

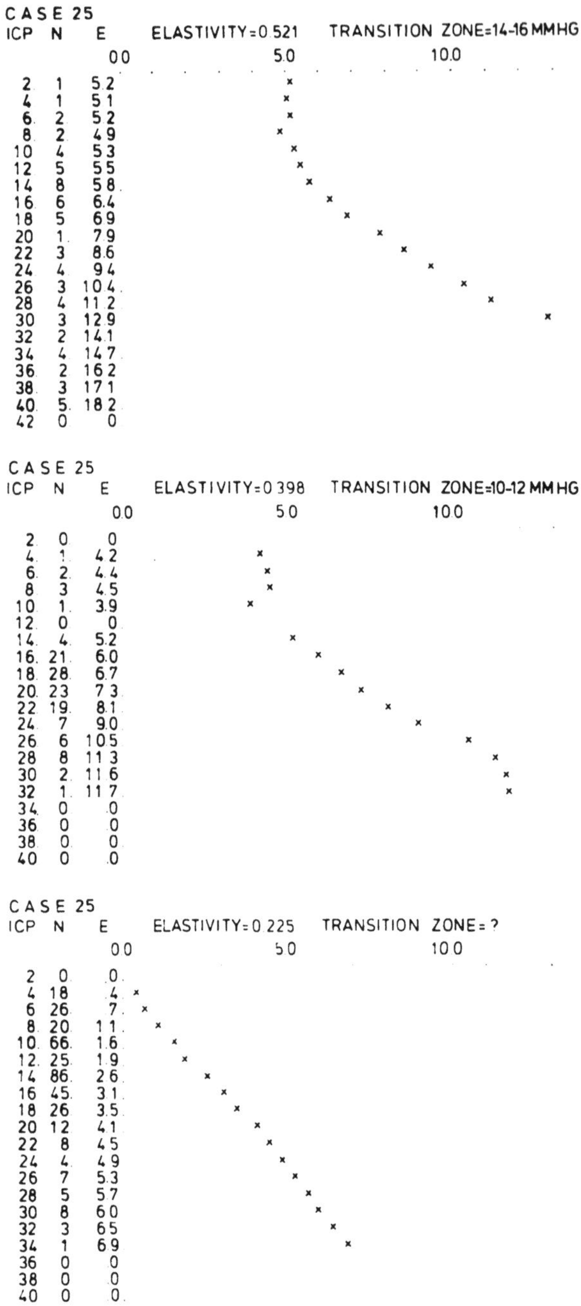

Fig. 4. Computer plots of three E-P curves obtained in one patient. From left to right: before surgery, after lasix, after surgery

The Pattern of Cerebral Pulse: Automatic Analysis

J. P. Castel and F. Cohadon

Introduction

The arterial origin of the intraventricular pulse wave is generally accepted (1, 2, 3, 7); like any systemic arterial signal the ICP signal is composed of a diastolic and a systolic component. This intraventricular systolic pulse (IVSP) may be considered a a rhythmic increment injected in the cranial cavity. The pressure response induced by this systolic increment of volume will reflect the overall elasticity of the intracranial contents, and so the ISVP may be used as a P/V response.

It has been shown that a linear relation does exist between the amplitude of the IVSP and the mean ICP level. Beyond this well-documented point our objectives are:

1. To study the morphological variations of the IVSP at different levels of mean ICP, when ICP is artificially or spontaneously raised.
2. To study the morphological variations of the IVSP at normal or normalized level of mean ICP in different physiopathological situations, i.e., situations where the overall elasticity of the intracranial contents is supposedly different.

Materials and Method

During routine IVP recordings, 44 patients were simultaneously recorded on magnetic tape.

These patients were classified within three groups:
Group I: "Normal patients" - 8 cases.
Group II: Active hydrocephalus - 24 cases.
Group III: Tumoral expansive process - 12 cases.

These three groups may be regarded as three physiopathological different situations where the total amount of the CSF volume is different within the cranial cavity, which total volume is constant according to the Monro-Kellie hypothesis. Thus three different situations of the elastic intracranial system may be studied.

In each case and at different levels of mean ICP (after substraction or infusion of CSF) one hundred IVSP were computed and added together in a multichannel analyser synchronized to the R peak of the ECG.

After this automatic analysis, each mean digital IVSP is normalized and its spectral pattern of frequency is set up using Fourier's harmonic analysis.

Results

1. Morphological Variations of the IVSP at Different Levels of Mean ICP

At a normal mean ICP level (Fig. 1), the normal IVSP is composed of a main initial peak PI followed by smaller peaks decreasing in amplitude: P2, P3, P4. The first peak PI is generally accepted to be directly generated by the arterial input within the cranial cavity; the other decreasing peaks are thought to result from a water-hammer phenomenon due to the venous side of the vascular bed (1, 2, 5, 7).

When ICP is artificially (CSF infusion) or pathologically (spontaneous variations) increased, the IVSP shows marked morphological changes (Fig. 2) not only on the amplitude of the first peak PI but also on the second peak P2 which seems now to bear the maximal amplitude of the signal. When ICP drops down by CSF substraction, the reverse phenomenon is seen.

The maximal amplitude of the IVSP bears a linear relationship to the mean ICP level (Table 1); but the mean amplitude of the signal represented by the first coefficient of the Fourier's harmonic analysis is found to reflect this relationship better than PI or P2 amplitude values.

However, spectral analysis fails to demonstrate any other reliable statistical correlation between the spectral pattern of the IVSP and the mean ICP level, although the morphological pattern of the IVSP appears to be really distorted according to the mean ICP level.

Table 1

	N	R coefficient	Student's test	P
Y max	65	0.5741	5.52130	0.001
1st coefficient $\hat{Y}$ (t)	65	0.5858	5.69070	<0.001

2. Morphological Variations of the IVSP within Three Physiopathological Situations at Normal ICP Value

Groups II and III of patients in which the total CSF volume is different, and thus the overall elasticity supposedly different, showed marked morphological differences of the IVSP (Fig. 3). In group II named "active hydrocephalus", the IVSP is characterized by a non-differentiated PI peak and a round-shaped second peak that seems to be P2 and P3 confused peaks. In group III ("expansive tumoral process") the IVSP is characterized by sharply individualized peaks.

To confirm these apparent morphological variations each IVSP numerically defined by the first ten coefficients of Fourier's series has been classified automatically using Fisher's discriminative method. Two-thirds of the total available samples of IVSP were used as a control group and the remaining third automatically classified. In reference to the clinically diagnosed pathological situation, these patients were classified without error using the automatic classification of their IVSP.

Discussion

As stated by DARDENNE, the intracranial CSF pulse is a complex function of arterial and venous hemodynamics (primary factors) and of intracranial conditions (secondary factors). In a hypothetical hemodynamically constant situation, the pattern of the intracranial CSF pulse will reflect the elastic response of the system related to: (1) the mean intracranial pressure level, and (2) the physiopathological situation.

These two conditions are indistinctly mixed and could not be distinguished with accuracy in the genesis of the CSF pulse pattern (2, 3, 4, 6). But as was noted using Fourier's harmonic analysis of the IVSP:

1. The mean amplitude of the signal bears a linear relationship with the mean ICP level.
2. Fourier's modulus reflects its relationship with the physiopathological situation.

We then supposed that, regardless of the primary generating factors (extracranial hemodynamics) that would change the CSF pulse pattern, the physiopathological situation, through variations of the elasticity within the system, has a distinct influence on the spectral pattern of the IVSP. Controlling the statistical difference between the three groups studied, we found that these primary generating factors, certainly different and complex in each patient, may be disregarded.

The IVSP is a rather complex P/V response, but it may be used clinically as an indirect approach to the ICP level and as a numerical pattern of the overall elasticity within the cranial cavity. To this purpose, Fourier's harmonic analysis of the IVSP appears to be a suitable computer analysis since the spectral pattern of IVSP brings quantitative information on these two main points: the mean ICP level and the pathological condition of the patient.

Summary

The intraventricular systolic pulse has been studied on ICP recordings from patients classified within three clinically and physiopathologically different groups. The IVSP is modified morphologically by the mean ICP level and by the elastic condition of the system resulting from the physiopathological situation. Fourier's harmonic analysis seems to be a suitable digital method for representation of these morphological variations, since it brings useful quantitative information regarding the mean ICP level and the elastic condition.

References

1. BERING, E.A., INGRAHAM, F.O.: The arterial pulsation of the CSF. Trans. Amer. Neurol. Ass. 78th Annual Meeting, pp. 49-54 (1953).

2. DARDENNE, G., DEREYMAEKER, A., LACHERON, J.M.: Cerebrospinal Fluid Pressure and Pulsatility. Europ. Neurol. 2, 193-216 (1969).

3. DEREYMAEKER, A., STEVENS, A., ROMBOUTS, J.J., LACHERON, J.M., PIERQUIN, A.: Study on the influence of the arterial pressure upon the morphology of cisternal CSF pulsations. Europ. Neurol. 5, 107-114 (1971).

4. DUNBAR, H.J., GUTHRIE, T., KARPELL, B.: A study of the CSF pulse wave. Arch. Neurol. 14, 624-630 (1966).

5. JANNY, P.: La pression intra-cranienne chez l'homme. Thesis Paris (1950).

6. SATO, K., YAHAGI, Y.: CSF pulse wave changes in cases with normal pressure hydrocephalus. In: Intracranial Pressure II (N. LUNDBERG, U. PONTEN, M. BROCK, eds.), pp. 133-136. Berlin-Heidelberg-New York: Springer 1975.

7. TINEL, J.: Etudes sur le pouls cérébral. Encéphale 22, 229-244 (1927)

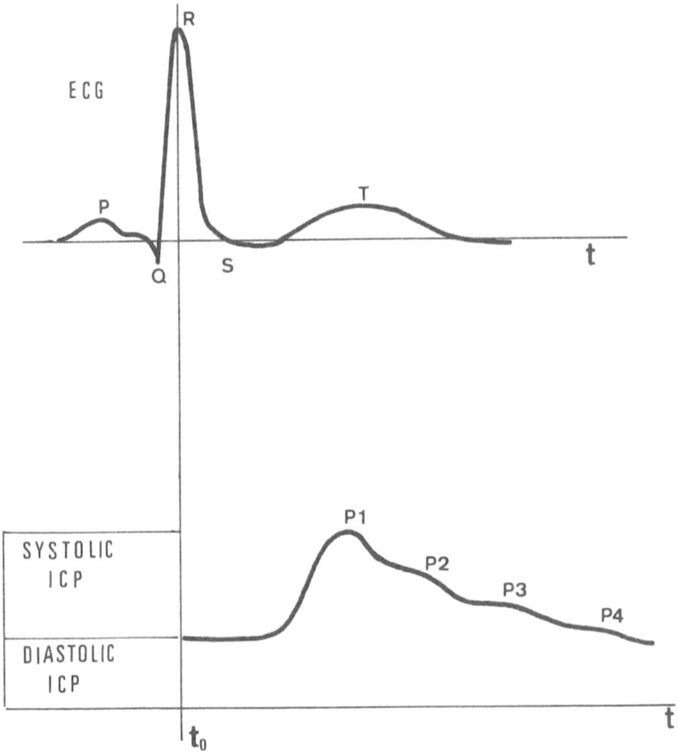

Fig. 1. Normal mean IVSP (*below*) from multichannel analysis synchronized on the R peak of ECG (*above*)

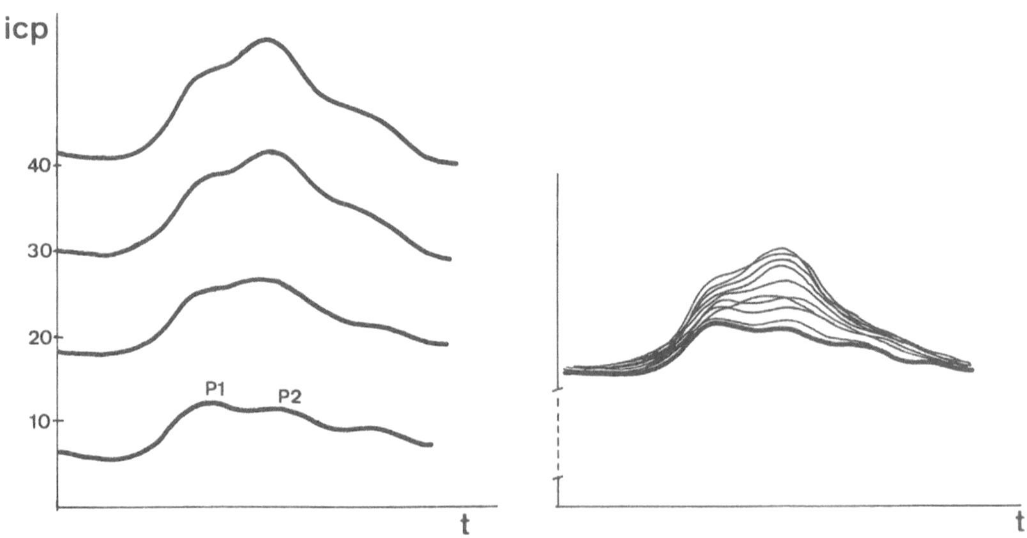

Fig. 2. (*Left*) Morphological variations of IVSP at different mean ICP levels. (*Right*) Superimposed mean IVSP showing maximal amplitude on peak P2

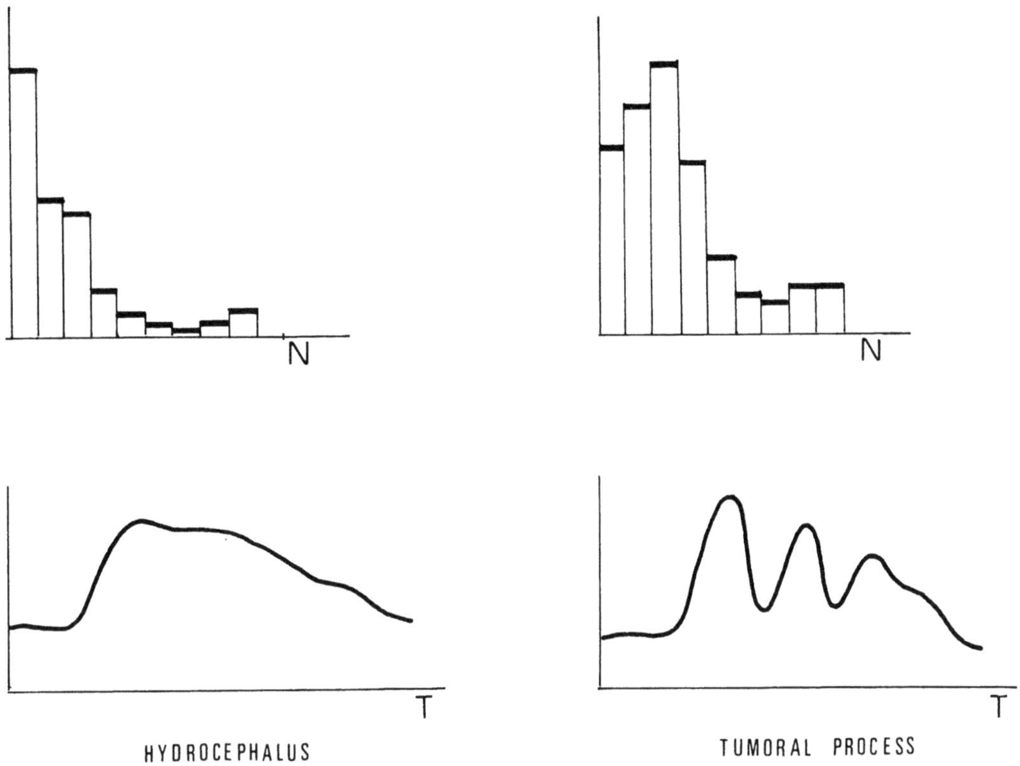

Fig. 3. (*Below*) Morphological variations of IVSP within different pathological conditions. (*Above*) Spectral pattern of IVSP

A New Method of Monitoring Intracranial Volume/Pressure Relationship

C.J.J. Avezaat, J.H.M. van Eijndhoven, D.A. de Jong, and
W.C.J. Moolenaar

Introduction

The volume/pressure test (VPT) has been reported to yield valuable clinical information additional to that obtained from routine ventricular fluid pressure (VFP) monitoring. It assesses the risks that patients with space-occupying lesions run from further increases in intracranial volume (2-5). In our experience, however, the clinical applicability of the VPT is limited for the following reasons. The volume/pressure response shows a wide variability in the individual patient. The VPT can only be used in pressure measurements with access to the CSF compartment and not, e.g., in epidural techniques. The test adds to the infection hazards. And finally, in patients with a high intracranial elastance the addition of extra volume may provoke secondary rises in pressure, sometimes even plateau waves.

Analogous to the volume/pressure response, the CSF pulse pressure can be regarded as the pressure response to the net increase in intracranial volume during each cardiac cycle. The purpose of this study was to investigate whether the relationship of CSF pulse pressure to CSF mean pressure could yield information on the volume/pressure relationship (VPR). If such were the case, we should be able to monitor continuously any change in the VPR.

Materials and Methods

An equation for the pulse pressure/pressure relationship (PPPR) was derived, departing from an exponential volume/pressure curve which can be described by the following equation:

$$P^* = A \exp(BV^*) \qquad (1)$$

where $P^* = P - P_0$ and $V^* = V - V_0$;
V_0 is the volume where $P = A + P_0$.

A and B are constants. The constant B characterizes the slope of the volume/pressure curve, a higher value for B meaning a more unfavourable VPR.

When V^* increases with a volume ΔV (injected volume during VPT or the volume change per cardiac cycle), P^* increases with a pressure response ΔP (volume/pressure response or CSF pulse pressure), thus

$$P^* + \Delta P = A \exp[B(V^* + \Delta V)] \text{ or} \qquad (2)$$
$$P^* + \Delta P = A \exp(BV^*) \cdot \exp(B\Delta V) \qquad (3)$$

From the equations (1) and (3) the equation for the PPPR can be derived:

$$\Delta P = P^*[\exp(B\Delta V) - 1] \qquad (4)$$

This relationship depends on two, still unknown, parameters: the coefficient for the volume/pressure curve B, and ΔV, defined as the net volume change per cardiac cycle.

If both B and ΔV remain constant, it follows from Equation (4) that there is a linear relationship between pulse pressure and pressure.

By carrying out a VPT with a known volume, 1 ml, B can be computed from Equation (4), which gives:

$$B = \ln \frac{P_2 - P_0}{P_1 - P_0} \qquad (5)$$

where P_1 = resting level of VFP, P_2 = resting level of VFP + volume/pressure response (ΔP).

P_0 = intersection point of Equation (4) with the pressure axis (Fig. 2).

Finally, ΔV can be calculated from the slope of the PPPR, which is known from the pressure recording (Fig. 2), using Equation (4).

In conclusion, it is evident from Equation (4) that if, during VFP monitoring, there is a change in the PPPR, this means a change either in the VPR (B) or in the volume change per cardiac cycle (ΔV). It takes a VPT to distinguish between these two possibilities.

To verify these theoretical considerations a clinical investigation was carried out in a group of 31 unselected neurosurgical patients in whom VFP was monitored for various reasons. The pressure recording was performed as described by LUNDBERG (1). The pressure signal together with the electrocardiogram (ECG) was recorded on tape (Philips Analog 7) and analyzed off-line by computer (DEC PDP 15) with a sampling frequency of 80 Hz. The mean VFP and the CSF pulse pressure were computed for each RR-interval of the ECG (Fig. 1). The pulse pressure was computed using the following equation:

$$\Delta P = \frac{1}{2}[2P_{max}(N) - P_{min}(N) - P_{min}(N+1)] \qquad (6)$$

This corrects the pulse pressure for trends in the pressure curve. The whole recording period was subdivided into periods of 4000 heartbeats, i.e. approximately 1 h. For the purpose of this study only the first hour of the recording period was taken into consideration. Figure 2 shows an example of a computer plot in a patient with a glioma. Both mean VFP and the pulse pressure are plotted against the time-course expressed in number of heartbeats. In a separate diagram the pulse pressures are plotted against the mean VFP and the regression line is drawn.

A number of VPT's was done in each patient. The volume/pressure response was defined as the immediate change in VFP following an addition of 1 ml in 1 second to the ventricular CSF volume. From the results of these series of VPT's the constant for the VPR, B, was computed for each patient using Equation (5). Next, the net volume change per cardiac cycle, ΔV, was calculated from the value for B and the slope of the regression line in the pulse pressure/pressure diagram using Equation (4).

The PPPR was compared with the VPR by plotting the slopes of the pulse pressure/pressure regression lines against the values for B, the constant of the volume/pressure curve.

Since the PPPR is dependent on both B and ΔV, it was investigated whether there was any correlation between B and ΔV.

Results and Discussion

In all 31 patients a linear relationship was found between the CSF pulse pressure and mean VFP (Fig. 2), the regression lines showing high correlation coefficients (mean r = 0.87; SD = 0.02).

A total of 14g VPT's were done in 31 patients, comparison of the volume/pressure responses with the resting levels of VFP showing a high correlation.

There was no significant correlation between the slope of the PPPR and the constant for VPR, B (Fig. 3). The reason is that the slope is also influenced by ΔV, the volume change per cardiac cycle. This would mean that on the basis of the PPPR no predictions can be made on the VPR without the aid of VPT's. Whether this also holds for the individual patient still remains to be seen, since the changes of ΔV in the individual patient are not known. In any case, in monitoring the individual patient the VPT can now be applied more rationally: the indication to perform a test would be a change in the slope of the PPPR. The number of tests can then be reduced, which at the same time diminishes the risks of infection.

A significant negative correlation was found between the coefficient for the VPR, B, and the volume change per cardiac cycle, ΔV (Fig. 4). Further knowledge of the correlation between B and ΔV might enable us in the individual patient to translate changes in the PPPR into changes in the VPR without the aid of VPT's. An example is given in Figure 5 which shows a distinct change of the PPPR during the formation of a plateau wave, strongly suggesting a change in VPR.

Summary

By means of computerized data analysis the pulse pressure/pressure relationship can be monitored continuously. A change in this relationship during patient monitoring means a change either in the volume/pressure relationship or in the net volume change per cardiac cycle. A volume/pressure test is required to differentiate between these two possibilities. This has the advantage that the volume/pressure test can be applied more rationally. Further knowledge of the relationship between the volume/pressure relationship and the volume change per cardiac cycle might make the volume/pressure test superfluous.

References

1. LUNDBERG, N.: Continuous recording and control of ventricular fluid pressure in neurosurgical practice. Acta Psychiat. Scand. (Suppl. 149) 36 (1960).
2. MILLER, J.D., GARIBI, J.: Intracranial volume-pressure relationships during continuous monitoring of ventricular fluid pressure. In: Intracranial Pressure (M. BROCK, H. DIETZ, eds.), pp. 270-274. Berlin-Heidelberg-New York: Springer 1972.
3. MILLER, J.D., GARIBI, J., PICKARD, J.D.: Induced changes of cerebrospinal fluid volume: Effects during continuous monitoring of ventricular fluid pressure. Arch. Neurol. 28, 265-269 (1973).
4. MILLER, J.D., PICKARD, J.D.: Intracranial volume/pressure studies in patients with head injury. Injury 5, 265-268 (1974).
5. MILLER, J.D., LEECH, P.J., PICKARD, J.D.: Volume-pressure response in various experimental and clinical conditions. In: Intracranial Pressure II (N. LUNDBERG, U. PONTEN, M. BROCK, eds.), pp. 97-100. Berlin-Heidelberg-New York: Springer 1975.

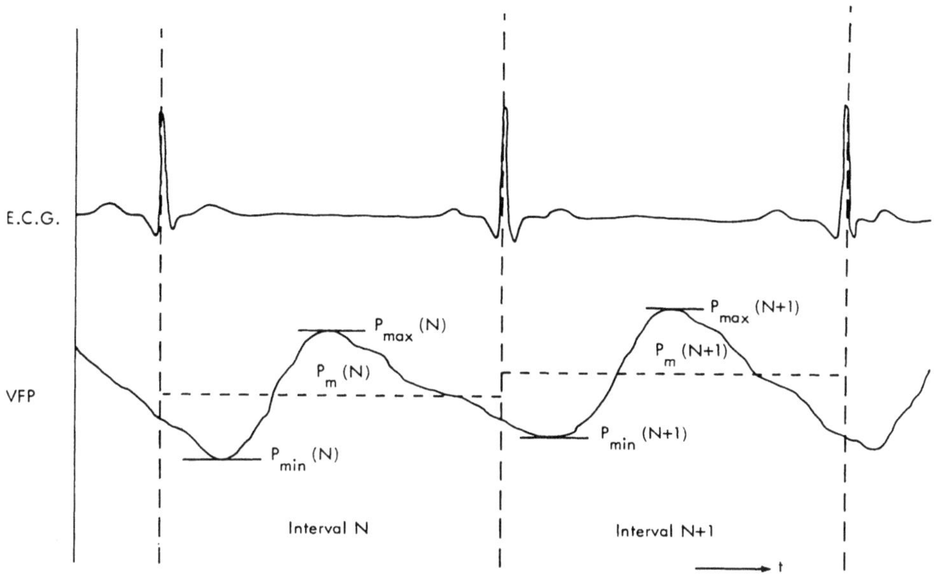

Fig. 1. Relationship between ventricular fluid pressure (VFP) and electrocardiogram (ECG)

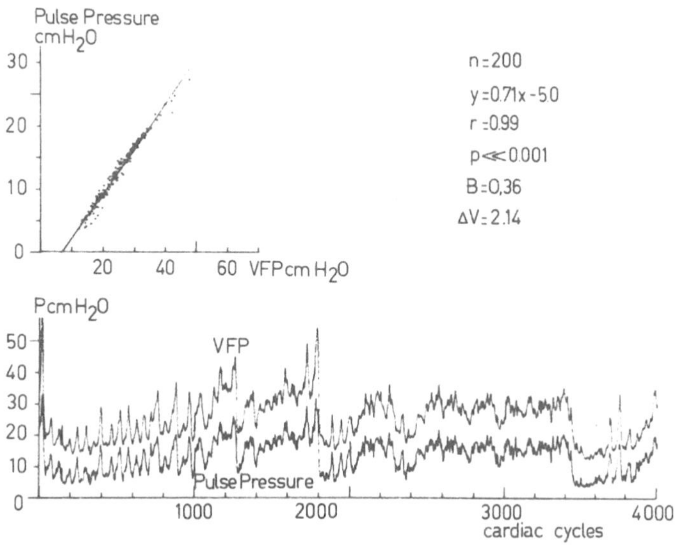

Fig. 2. Computer plot of a pressure recording during approximately 1 h (4000 cardiac cycles) in a patient with a glioma. Mean VFP and CSF pulse pressure plotted against time-course in number of heartbeats. Diagram at top shows a linear relationship between CSF pulse pressure (ordinate) and mean VFP (abscissa). Regression equation is given. B, the constant for the VPR, has been calculated from the VPT's in this patient. ΔV, the volume change per cardiac cycle, has been computed from the slope of the regression line. The equations are given in the text

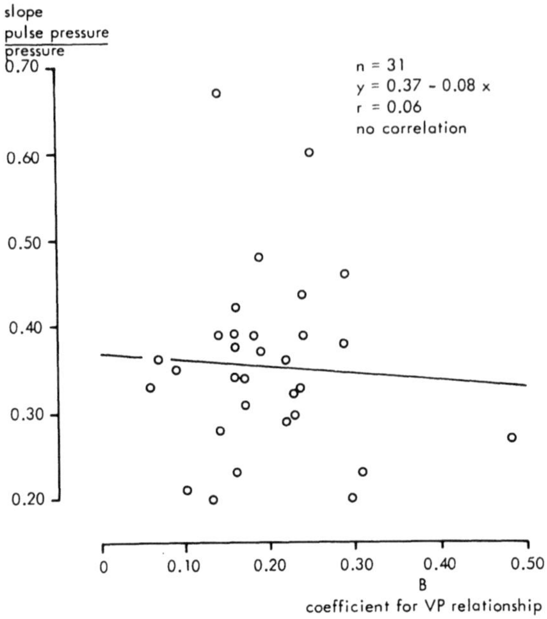

Fig. 3. The slope of the regression line of the pulse pressure/pressure relationship plotted against the coefficient for the volume/pressure relationship, B

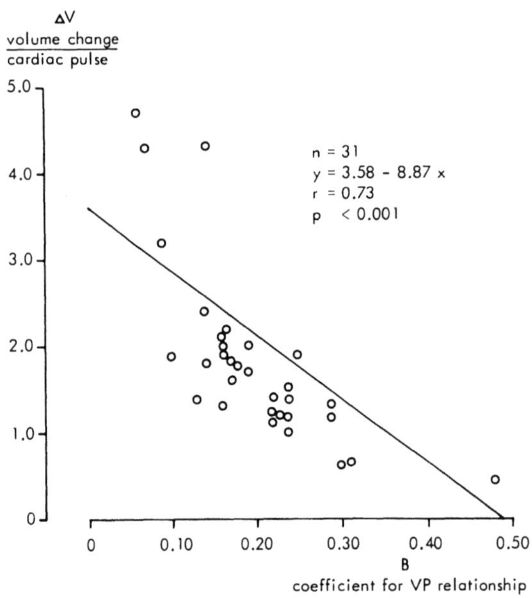

Fig. 4. Relationship between volume change per cardiac cycle, ΔV (ordinate) and coefficient for the volume/pressure relationship, B (abscissa). Regression line is shown

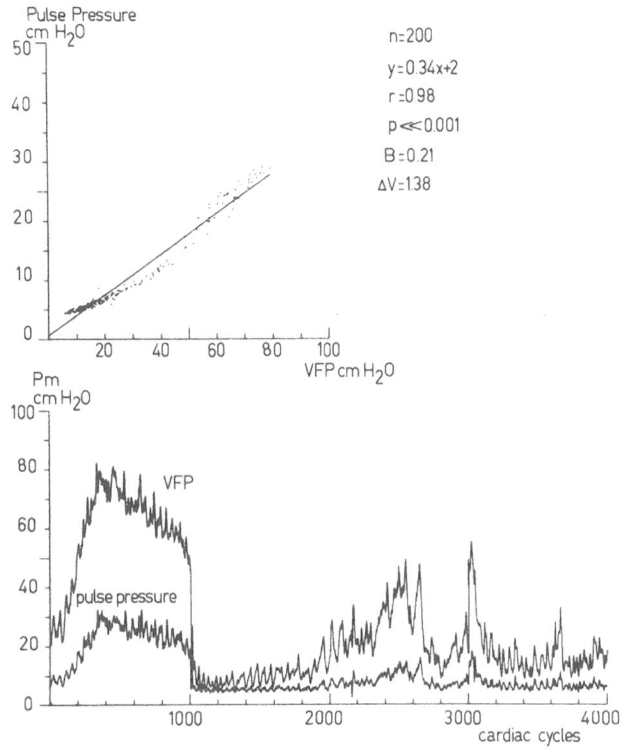

Fig. 5. Computer plot of a pressure recording during a plateau wave. Computer has drawn only one regression line, but there is a distinct change in the slope of the scatter diagram, suggesting a difference in volume/pressure relationship during plateau wave and during baseline VFP

A Dynamic Pressure Profile in the Management of Patients with Glioma

D.J. Price and S. Onabanjo

Introduction

We have attempted to extend the use of intracranial pressure (ICP) measurement to study the baseline pressure and the response to saline infusion in a group of 25 patients with supratentorial gliomas, with the hope that this additional information will improve the selection of patients for radiotherapy.

We are often faced with the ethical dilemma as to whether it is kind to the patient and his relatives to subject him to radiotherapy after glioma surgery. If we can improve our present methods of prediction based on clinical and pathological data, it may be possible to select only those patients who will, with certainty, have a reasonable quality of survival for at least 1 year.
The aim of the study is therefore to compare the traditional clinical methods of selection with the data provided by a 'profile' of ICP data.

Methods

We found it difficult to select the most useful method of measurement of the reserve of compensation. We overcame this by using every method we knew and applied them to every patient, hoping that at least one of these would prove to be useful.

Intermittent Bolus Method

The intermittent bolus method of measuring the *Volume Pressure Response* (2) seemed the simplest and quickest but, on repeating the test, the pressure rises varied and we suspect that this may be due to the uncertainty of each starting point of the *Pressure Volume Curve*. Unfortunately with very rapid infusions of saline, the pressure rise is not totally dependent on the natural compensatory mechanisms of the cerebrospinal fluid (CSF) and venous hydraulic systems, but also reflects the speed of CSF transmission through the ventricular system.

Continuous Infusion Methods

The gradient of the rise in mean ICP with continuous infusion of saline was measured and plotted on both linear and logarithmic graphs.

Unfortunately, these gradients varied from one infusion speed to another and all attempts to correlate this variation with the speed failed. The *Pressure Volume Index* as measured by the volume of fluid required to raise the ICP by a factor of 10 (1) was unsatisfactory as the standard deviations were too great for the mean to be acceptable. Equations combining the *Pressure Volume Index* with the data from sin-

Table 1. Comparison of methods of measurement of available intracranial compensation reserve

	'Compliance'		'Outflow resistance' by continuous infusion
	Intermittent bolus	Continuous infusion	
Measure			
Speed of CSF shifts	++	-	-
Speed of turning taps	+	-	-
Starting point on P-V curve	++	-	-
Infusion speed	-	++	-
Venous exit resistance	++	++	++
CSF outflow resistance	+	++	++

gle bolus responses to calculate the *Compliance* and *Outflow Resistance* merely served as combinations of the inaccuracy of the two methods with mathematically questionable logic (Table 1).

After many months of frustrated attempts to achieve a dynamic pressure profile of ICP data which truly represented the reserve of compensation available to the brain and which could be used as a diagnostical management tool in neurosurgical practice, we decided to re-examine the basic concepts of the hydraulic mechanisms within the cranio-spinal compartments.

Basic Concepts

We compared the ventricular cavity with a bath filled by a continuous flow of water from the choroid plexus 'tap'. The outflow resistance of the bath outlet represents the outlet foramina of the fourth ventricle leading to the spinal space with its compliant dural sac.

The level of bath water remains constant when both inflow and outflow are identical and will rise if the rate of inflow is increased. The level of water then gradually rises until a new state of equilibrium is achieved and again, the now increased rate of outflow due to the higher fluid pressure becomes equal to the new rate of inflow. An increase in outflow resistance due to obstruction at the outlet or inadequate drains would cause a similar rise in water level until sufficient pressure had been created to return the rate of outflow to normal when an equilibrium would again be established.

This crude analogy should not be taken too seriously, but if both the hydraulic systems within the cranium are now considered, Figure 1 may in some way represent the principles involved.

In the adult, the only compliant compartment is the spinal dural sac and this has to be filled from the ventricular outflow. It could therefore be assumed that a measure of '*Outflow Resistance*' would be more appropriate than any attempts to estimate the compliance of a virtually incompressible brain within a solid skull.

CSF *Outflow Resistance* is measured by plotting the mean steady-state pressures for each infusion rate against that rate. The gradient of this plot should represent the combined CSF *Outflow Resistance* and *Venous Exit Pressure*. This method has already been described by several workers and Figure 2 shows a typical linear plot. We contend that it provides a more significant estimate of the combined reserve capacity of ICP compensation within both CSF and venous capacitance hydraulic systems.

As a supratentorial tumor increases in size, this reserve of available compensation becomes less and is inversely related to the *Outflow Resistance*. After discarding *Compliance* and *Elastance*, the 'ICP Profile' has been restricted to mean ICP, *Mean Pulse Pressure* (PP), the gradient of the linear plot PP/ICP and *Outflow Resistance*. Figure 3 demonstrates the ranges of *Outflow Resistance* in various pathological conditions and shows some diagnostic discrimination (Fig. 3). The other components of the profile showed less discrimination.

The Patients

Twenty five patients with supratentorial gliomas were treated with as much surgery as thought applicable followed by a standardized steroid regime and radiotherapy. This selection for radiotherapy was purposefully wider than our normal practice. The ICP studies were carried out after surgery (Fig. 4).

Clinical Assessment

We attempted to rationalise the clinical aspects which would normally be taken into consideration in the decision as to whether radiotherapy should be given after surgery. The length of history, tumor pathology, surgical achievement and the degree of disability at the time of decision were thought to be the most relevant indicants. Severe disability or death within a year of surgery was considered as confirmation that radiotherapy should not have been given.

Prediction with Clinical Indicants

There was no clear correlation between surgical achievement and final outcome, but by selecting the three remaining indicants, the outcome of 22 out of 25 patients could be predicted correctly.

Prediction with Additional ICP Profile

The ICP rejection indicants on their own did not improve the accuracy of prediction but when taken into account with the clinical data, 100% prediction was achieved. Patients with large tumors and low outflow resistance died particularly rapidly as this indicated necrotic tumors with much tissue destruction (Table 2).

Summary

The measurement of *Outflow Resistance* appears to be the most repeatable and reliable test for estimating the available compensation reserve of the CSF and venous hydraulic compartments. Whenn applied to this small series of patients with supratentorial gliomas, it proved to have more predictive significance in evaluating final outcome than any other single parameter. The series of patients is too small to male a definite conclusion that this addition to the clinical indicants provides a worthwhile improvement in prediction.

Table 2

Clinical rejection indicants	Correct prediction		
1. History <30 days	22/25 (1–3)	22/25 (Clinical 1–3 + ICP 1–3)	25/25
2. Glioblastoma multiforme			
3. Moderate or severe diability			
ICP Profile Rejection Indicants			
1. Mean ICP >35 mm Hg	10/25 (1–3)	21/25 (ICP 1–5)	
2. Mean pulse pressure >15 mm Hg			
3. PP/ICP gradient >0.6			
4. Outflow resistance <30 mm Hg/ml/min	19/25 (4–5)		
5. Outflow resistance >70 mm Hg/ml/min			

References

1. MARMAROU, A., SHULMAN, K., LAMORGESE, J.: Compartmental analysis of compliance and outflow resistance of the cerebrospinal fluid system. J. Neurosurg. 43, 523-534 (1975).
2. MILLER, J.D., GARIBI, J.: Intracranial volume-pressure relationships during continuous monitoring of ventricular fluid pressure. In: Intracranial Pressure (M. BROCK, H. DIETZ, eds.), pp. 270-274. Berlin-Heidelberg-New York: Springer 1972.

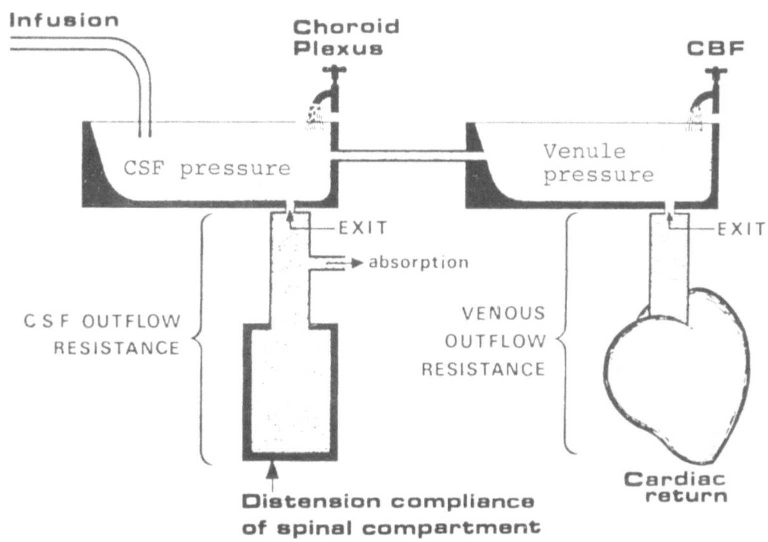

Fig. 1. Intracranial hydraulic mechanisms

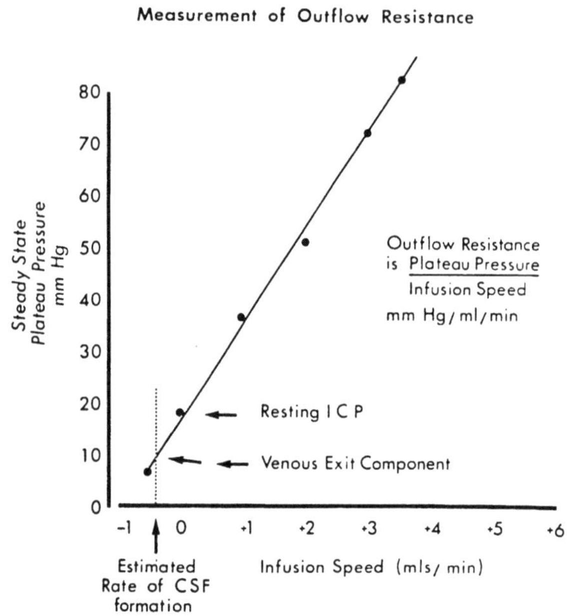

Fig. 2. Estimation of outflow resistance by continuous saline infusion

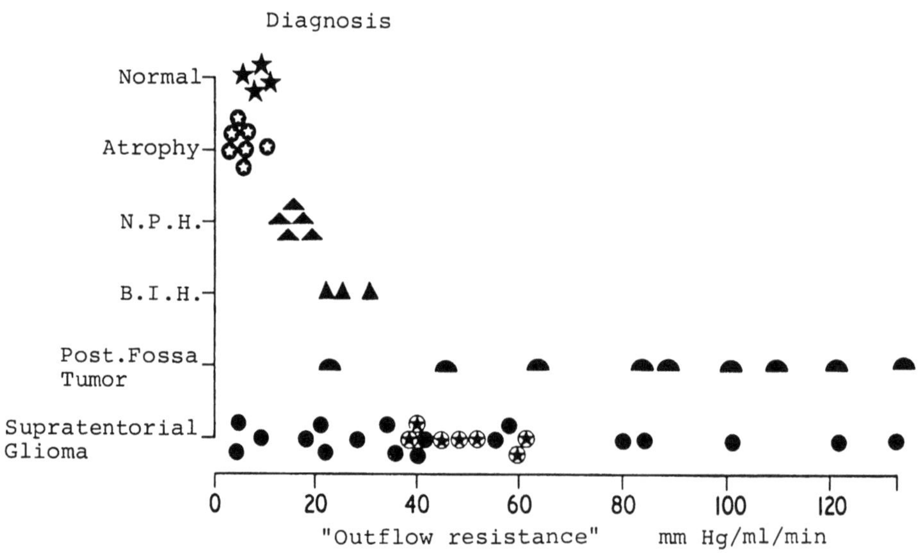

Fig. 3. Outflow resistance in various pathological conditions

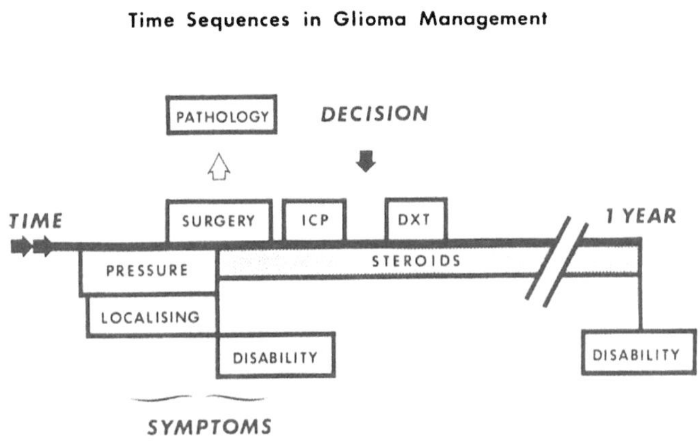

Fig. 4. Time sequences in glioma management

Summary

R. Cooper and J. de Rougemont

The underlying theme of all the papers in this session is that the data collected during ICP measurements contain more information than that expressed by the mean value and that the variability contains potentially valuable clinical information.

The source of variation in intracranial pressure recordings is due to arterial pulse, respiration, blood pressure changes, plateau waves and non-specific changes such as coughing and straining. Both the papers by TURNER et al. and WIEGAND et al. are concerned with the distribution of amplitude (expressed as a histogram) over a period of time. TURNER et al. compare successive histograms generated over periods of 30 min and in the initial stages of the work spent considerable effort in training and testing the ability of the nursing staff to detect changes in shape of the distribution. Of particular interest in their paper is the increase of variance which precedes a rise in ICP. If this is confirmed in more patients it will have prognostic value. WIEGAND et al. show that pressure histograms are similar from hour to hour but can vary from day to day. Both groups are concerned whether to include such changes of pressure as plateau waves in the analyzed data. The German group make a point of trying to record in "stable" conditions though there was discussion whether sich patients existed! In further discussion an interval class between 2 and 5 mms was thought to be satisfactory and the difference between clinical and statistical significance was emphasized with the clinicians, as usual, having to work with changes that statisticians consider inadequate.

The papers by SZEWCZYKOWSKI et al., AVEZAAT et al. and CASTEL and COHADON are concerned with analysis of the pulsatile component of the ICP. The first two groups measure the pulse amplitude and relate this to the changes of mean level of pressure. In the discussion the difficulties of converting changes of pressure to changes of volume and elastance and the relationships of these factors to the clinical state were repeatedly emphasized. A major problem in the interpretation of the ICP pulsatile component is the lack of knowledge of the pulse amplitude of blood pressure.

The paper by CASTEL and COHADON concentrates on the analysis of the shape of the pulse pressure wave and shows that Fourier analyses of the waveform are different in "normal" patients, patients with active hydrocephalus and expanding space-occupying lesions. In the discussion the limitations of frequency analysis when there was damping of the components by extracranial monitoring was stressed. Dr. WILLIAMS (Smethwick) emphasized that the analysis of the pulse waveform must take into account the behavior of the fluid within the spinal cavity which provides a resonant chamber resulting in frequency components of about 12 Hz.

The last paper by PRICE and ONABANJO is concerned with the change of intracranial conditions when some form of disturbance (by infusion) is imposed. The problems of standardisation of amount and rate or infusion are considerable.

The whole group of papers represent a significant advance in the analysis of the data obtained from pressure recordings and it is to be hoped that standardisation of procedures, acceptance by the nursing staff and correlation with clinical conditions will permit prediction of impending damaging intracranial events.

Session J

Pediatric Aspects

Chairman: N. Lundberg
Co-chairman: J. W. F. Beks

The Role of Intracranial Pressure Monitoring in a Pediatric Intensive Care Unit

D.A. Bruce, L. Schut, and L.A. Bruno

Introduction

The specific use of the technique of intracranial pressure (ICP) monitoring in children has received little attention in the literature. Diffuse brain swelling is a common finding in patients dying from head injury (3) frequently with minimal focal damage (1). A similar picture is seen in Reye's syndrome and other encephalitides and in anoxic encephalopathy. The time course of the brain swelling and its role in the patient's demise are not clear.

The greater the disturbance of brain function the more difficult it is to estimate the level of the ICP. Clinical signs: opisthotonos, decerebration, episodes of bradycardia, and intermittent pupillary dilatation may or may not be associated with an elevated ICP. If the initial estimation of ICP is difficult, equally so is the evaluation of the response to therapy. Finally, when the ICP is high and difficult to control, intensive therapy (i.e., paralysis with hyperventilation or barbiturates) can only be safely used if the ICP and cerebral perfusion pressure (CPP) is known.

Material

The records of 50 consecutive patients in whom the ICP was monitored were examined. The age range was 1-13 years with a mean age of 5.3 years and the interval, January 1975 to April 1976. Table 1 shows the pathological diagnoses and number of patients in each category. Thirty-nine patients had monitoring with a subarachnoid screw (2) and 13 with an intraventricular catheter. Two patients, 1 with encephalitis and 1 with pseudo-tumor cerebri, had monitoring with both methods. More than half of the patients in whom an intraventricular catheter was used had posterior fossa tumors. All but 3 had significant ventricular enlargement.

Table 1. Diagnosis in 50 cases of pediatric patients with ICP monitoring, January 1975 to March 1976

Disease	No.	Subarachnoid Bolt	Cannula
Reye's syndrome	13	13	0
Head injury	15	14	1
Tumors	8	1	7
Intracerebral hemorrhage	4	1	3
Encephalitis	4	4	1
Anoxic encephalopathy	3	3	0
Pseudo tumor	2	2	1
Meningitis	1	1	0
	50	39	13

Results

Table 1 shows that head injury and Reye's syndrome (fatty infiltration of the liver and kidneys plus encephalopathy) are the two most common conditions to be monitored. Monitoring is begun within the first 6-12 h of the insult in patients with head injury, anoxic encephalopathy, and intracranial hemorrhage. In patients with Reye's syndrome or encephalitis, monitoring is usually begun within 12 h of the onset of coma.

We have found the subarachnoid screw (2) a reliable means of monitoring pressure in children aged 1 and up for periods of time up to 3 weeks. Complications with the bolt were 7 superficial infections requiring topical therapy and 1 requiring excision and secondary closure of the wound. One of the 13 patients in whom a cannula was used developed ventriculitis and 2 had positive cultures from the catheter tip at the time of removal.

Table 2 shows the mean time course of monitoring, the interval from commencing monitoring to the increase in ICP and the duration of therapy required. In head injury and anoxia the rise in ICP was delayed to the 2nd or 3rd day and therapy was required for a mean of 6.5 and 8 days respectively.

Thirteen of the 15 head-injured patients had CT scans and in 7 (54%) a picture of diffuse swelling with obliteration of the ventricles and cisterns was seen. This picture is seen in 24% of all scans for head-injured children and in 56% of these the clinical history is of a mild injury followed by headache, vomitting, prostration, and progressive obtundation. A review of the CT scans in this group shows a decrease in brain density as the ventricles return to normal size and recovery ensues. This is against the presence of edema early. Local cerebral blood volume (LCBV) measurements show a marked increase in volume in the early stages and cerebral blood flow (CBF), a marked hyperemia. ICP is not elevated in this group initially. However, in 5 of the 7 patients with this picture the ICP rose significantly after 24 hours and required intensive therapy.

Although volume pressure responses (VPR) are impossible through the subarachnoid screw, we have been able to tentatively identify the head injury patient with low compliance. Figure 1 shows two ICP trac-

Table 2. Mean duration of recording: time to onset of elevated ICP, duration of elevated ICP, and % in each group with elevated ICP

Disease	Mean length of recording[a]	Onset of↑ICP[a]	Duration of↑ICP[a]	% with ↑ICP	Expired
Reye's syndrome	4 ±1.0	Immediate	2.7±1	77	6
Head injury	6.2±1.1	2	6.5±1.1	53	1
Intracranial hemorrhage	5.6±1.5	Immediate	3 ± .48	75	0
Encephalitis	2.2± .48	Hours	1	25	1
Encephalopathy	7 ±2.8	2	8	66	2

[a]In days.↑ ICP > 25 Torr. Mean values ± SEM.

In head injury, intracranial hemorrhage, and encephalopathy the monitoring was always instigated within 12 hours of ictal event. In Reye's syndrome and encephalitis the monitoring was instigated within hours of the onset of coma.

ings. The upper trace shows that with hourly chest therapy and suctioning ICP spikes occur that immediately fall to the baseline. When the compliance is low, small plateau waves are triggered by the suctioning process.

In these few patients there was a good correlation between an increased ICP and a poor neurological status at the end of 2 weeks. One of the 8 patients with increased ICP died from progressive pulmonary interstitial fibrosis. Three of the others were vegetative, 3 severely hemiplegic, and 1 aphasic at the time of transfer to a rehabilitation hospital. Five of the 6 patients without increase in ICP were intellectually and physically intact at the time of discharge. All of the 7 with increased ICP have shown improvement: 2 are now normal, 3 remain hemiparetic but are back in school, an 2 are only beginning to smile and move spontaneously.

The early aggressive treatment of elevated ICP in Reye's syndrome has enabled the pressure to be controlled in all but 2 of the 13 patients. Therapy is with decadron, hyperventilation, hypothermia, barbiturates, and exchange transfusion (4).

The use of ICP monitoring to control the early stages of intraventricular hemorrhage or intracerebral hemorrhage allow us (a) to save the patient's life by controlling the ICP and (b) to pick an opportune moment for the surgical intervention.

We cannot compare therapeutic modalities since only 1 of the 27 patients who required therapy for elevated ICP had a single modality. Eighteen patients had at least three separate therapeutic modalities. Mannitol had a shorter duration of effect than in adults (3 h) and with time became less effective. Frequently, after cooling or barbiturates mannitol would again be effective. Following anoxia and head injury, if the ICP was still high at 3-4 days and no mass lesion was present on the CT scan, LP's or small amounts of ventricular drainage were now an extremely effective way of controlling the ICP. The mortality rate was 24% (6 Reye's syndromes). The mortality rate for the 7 who received barbiturate therapy was 42.8%.

Discussion

The data shows that ICP monitoring has a significant role in the intensive care of the child in whom an elevated intracranial pressure is suspected. The procedure is safe and effective. In over 50% of patients monitored, therapy is required. In most cases, the ICP can be controlled. However, in Reye's syndrome, despite ICP control progressive brain stem dysfunction and death may occur.

The realization that in head-injured patients and post-anoxic encephalopathy the ICP problems occur late and last long is most important. This differs from the classical concepts and must be borne in mind if adequate therapy is to be given. In our unit as many patients required therapy for elevated ICP as required surgery and twice as many are monitored.

In conclusion, ICP monitoring gives information that is available by no other method. It may be life-saving by measuring the height of the ICP, dictating the need for therapy, recording the results of therapy and defining the duration of therapy in a variety of diseases of childhood.

Summary

A review of 50 consecutive patients with ICP monitoring is presented. The most frequent cause for ICP monitoring is head injury and Reye's syndrome. In patients with head injury, a diffuse cerebral hyperemia is frequently found that leads after 24 h to an elevated ICP. Treatment may need to be prolonged for 6-8 days. In 50% of all patients monitored, the ICP rises. The ICP can usually be controlled, although three or four modalities of therapy are frequently necessary. It is the authors' opinion that ICP monitoring is a necessary part of the intensive care of pediatric patients in whom an elevated ICP is suspected.

References

1. COURVILLE, C.B.: Contre coup injuries of the brain in infancy. Arch. Surg. 90, 157-165 (1965).
2. JAMES, H.E., BRUNO, L.A., SCHUT, L.: Intracranial subarachnoid pressure monitoring in children. Surg. Neurol. 3, 313-315 (1975).
3. LINDENBERG, R., FISHER, R.S., DURLACHER, S., LOVITT, W.V., Jr., FREYTAG, E.: The pathology of the brain in blunt head injuries of infants and children. Internat. Congr. Neuropath. Proc., Excerpta Medica (Amsterdam) Vol. 1, 477-49 (1955).
4. PIZZI, F.J., SCHUT, L., BERMAN, W., HOLTZAPPLE, W.: Intracranial pressure monitoring in Reye's syndrome. Child's Brain 2, 59-66 (1976).

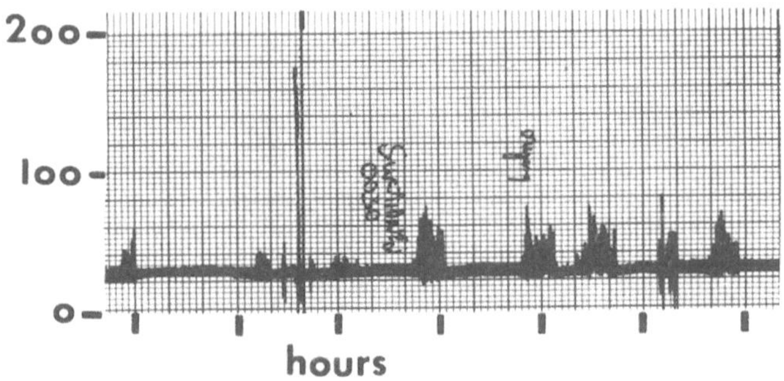

Fig. 1.
Two ICP recordings

(A) Spiking occurring with suctioning returning immediately to baseline

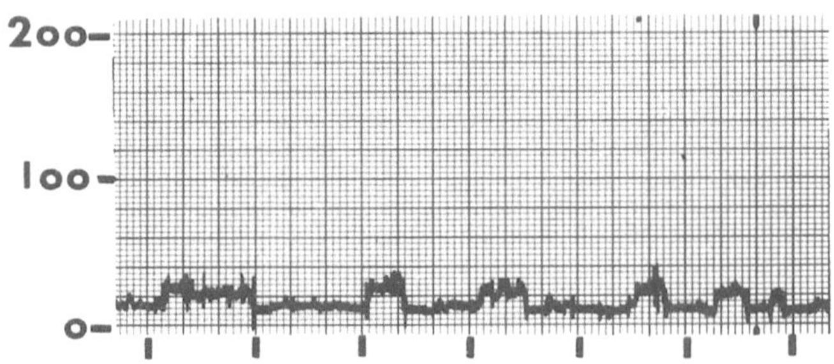

(B) Small plateau waves triggered by suctioning suggesting low compliance

Intracranial Pressure in Reye Syndrome

M.P. Horta and P.A. Mello

Introduction

Every year, during March and April, just after the rainy season, cases of Reye's syndrome are referred to the pediatric unit of the Hospital Distrital de Brasilia. The reversibility of this entity is well known (3, 6). Nevertheless, the brain edema and increased intracranial pressure (ICP) occurring with this disease have been reported to be life-threatening (1, 4).

We decided to study this model of pseudotumor cerebri under the following aspects: common values of ventricular fluid pressure (VFP), response to clinical treatment, indication for decompressive surgery, and prognosis as related to the values of the VFP.

Material and Methods

During the years 1974 and 1975 VFP was monitored (5) in 6 patients with Reye syndrome. All were in coma and the diagnosis was established according to clinical and laboratory data indicated by SAMAHA et al. (7) (Table 1). The main signs and symptoms were: vomiting (5 patients), hypertonia (6 patients), deep brisk reflexes (6 patients), decerebrate rigidity (3 patients), bilateral mydriasis (4 patients), sign of Babinski (4 patients) and lack of superficial reflexes (2 patients). All patients had metabolic acidosis, which was promptly corrected. No patient had papilledema. Four patients were submitted to bilateral decompressive craniotomy.

Results

Figure 1 shows the VFP values in all 6 patients. In each graph infusions of mannitol and/or time of surgery are indicated. In one patient surgery was performed before the beginning of VFP monitoring. In the first 4 patients VFP levels were elevated to maximal values of 50, 45, 40 and 125 mm Hg. In the second patient the pressure of 45 mm Hg was coincidental with decerebration. This picture reverted immediately, after the use of mannitol. The fourth patient died during a pressure wave of 125 mm Hg. Decrease in VFP preceded clinical improvement in the 3 patients that recovered without sequelae.

Comments

The main cause of death in Reye syndrome has been reported as being the increase in ICP (1) due to brain edema (2). Some of the results observed here appear to confirm this. However, the fact that ICP was 25 mmHg in the third patient when he died might suggest that increased ICP is not always the main cause of death in this syndrome. In patient No. 6 VFP was already zero at admittance. We believe this to indicate

Table 1. Reye syndrome. Laboratory data

	TGP	Glycemia	Protr. (%)	Protr. (SEG)	Na	K	Cl	A.R.	Amylase	Bilirrubin	HC
1. R.V.R. 444407	700	55	43	13/42	138	4	105.9	20	315	T=1.5 I=1.0 D=0.5	Htc=36% Hb=11.9g% WBC=13100/mm^3 (2-1-37-59-1)
2. S.P.L. 496713	850	76	23	23/12	148	4.9	111.1	22	154	T=0.7 I=0.2 D=0.5	Htc=45% Hb=13.2g% WBC=5400/mm^3 (2-1-30-65-2)
3. H.R.S. 496886	700	48	8	12/45	150	5.6	105.9	10	-	T=3.1 I=0.8 D=2.3	Htc=45% Hb=14.0g% WBC=5800/mm^3 (1-0-12-85-2)
4. G.C.R. 498858	800	60	6	12/52	150	4.9	105.9	16	320	T=3.6 I=1.3 D=2.3	Htc=39% Hb=12.0g% WBC=5400/mm^3 (2-0-66-32-0)
5. I.M.D.L. 504264	300	97	6	12/52	152	5.2	105.9	22	96	T=0.5 I=0.2 D=0.3	Htc=38% Hb=11.3g% WBC=4600/mm^3 (3-1-23-70-3)
6. C.L.C.S. 519012	650	43	5	12/52	152	3	117	14	-	T= 1 I=0.5 D=0.5	Htc=37% Hb=11.0g% WBC=4400/mm^3 (1-1-29-68-1)

cerebral death, since she had bilateral fixed pupils, and lack of superficial and deep reflexes despite spontaneous respiration.

In view of the reversible character of the disease, we had initially adopted the policy of performing bilateral decompressive craniotomy in all patients in coma at admission. This is what happened in cases 1, 2, 3 and 4 of this series. Our experience since then has led us to believe that ICP monitoring may serve as a valuable aid in posing the indication for this form of treatment. TROUPP and VAPALAHTI (8) related the levels of VFP to prognosis in severe brain injuries in children. According to these authors, we admit the value of 30 mm Hg as an indication for decompressive craniotomy, provided all clinical measures fail.

Summary

The authors have continuously recorded VFP in a group of 6 patients with Reye syndrome. Continuous monitoring of VFP has proven to be a valuable guide for the therapeutic management of such patients. The authors have also considered the effects of bilateral decompressive craniotomy and conservative treatment in such cases.

References

1. AOKI, Y., LOMBROSO, C.T.: Prognostic value of electroencephalography in Reye's syndrome. Neurology 23, 333 (1973).
2. CHANG, L.W., GILBERT, E.F., TANNER, W., MOFFAT, H.L.: Reye's syndrome: light and electron microscopic studies. Arch. Pathol. 96, 127 (1973).
3. HUTTENLOCHER, A.M., SCHWARTZ, A.D., KLATSKIN, G.: Reye's syndrome: ammonia intoxication as a possible factor in the encephalopathy. Pediatrics 43, 443 (1969).
4. KINDT, G.W., WALDMAN, J., KOHL, S., BAUBLIS, J., TUCKER, R.P.: Intracranial pressure in Reye's syndrome. JAMA 231, 822 (1975).
5. LUNDBERG, N.: Continuous recording and control of ventricular fluid pressure in neurosurgical practice. Acta Psychiatr. Neurol. Scand. 149 (Suppl.) 1 (1960).
6. PARTIN, J.C., SCHUBERT, W.K., PARTIN, J.S.: Mitochondrial ultrastructure in Reye's syndrome (encephalopathy and fatty degeneration of the viscera). N. Engl. J. Med. 285, 1339 (1971).
7. SAMAHA, F.J., GLAN, E., BERARDINELLI, J.L.: Reye's Syndrome: clinical diagnosis and treatment with peritoneal dialysis. Pediatrics 53, 336 (1974).
8. TROUPP, H., VAPALAHTI, M.: Ventricular fluid pressure in children with severe brain injuries. In: Advances in Neurosurgery 1 (K. SCHÜRMANN, M. BROCK, H.J. REULEN, D. VOTH, eds.), pp. 62-66. Berlin-Heidelberg-New York: Springer 1973.

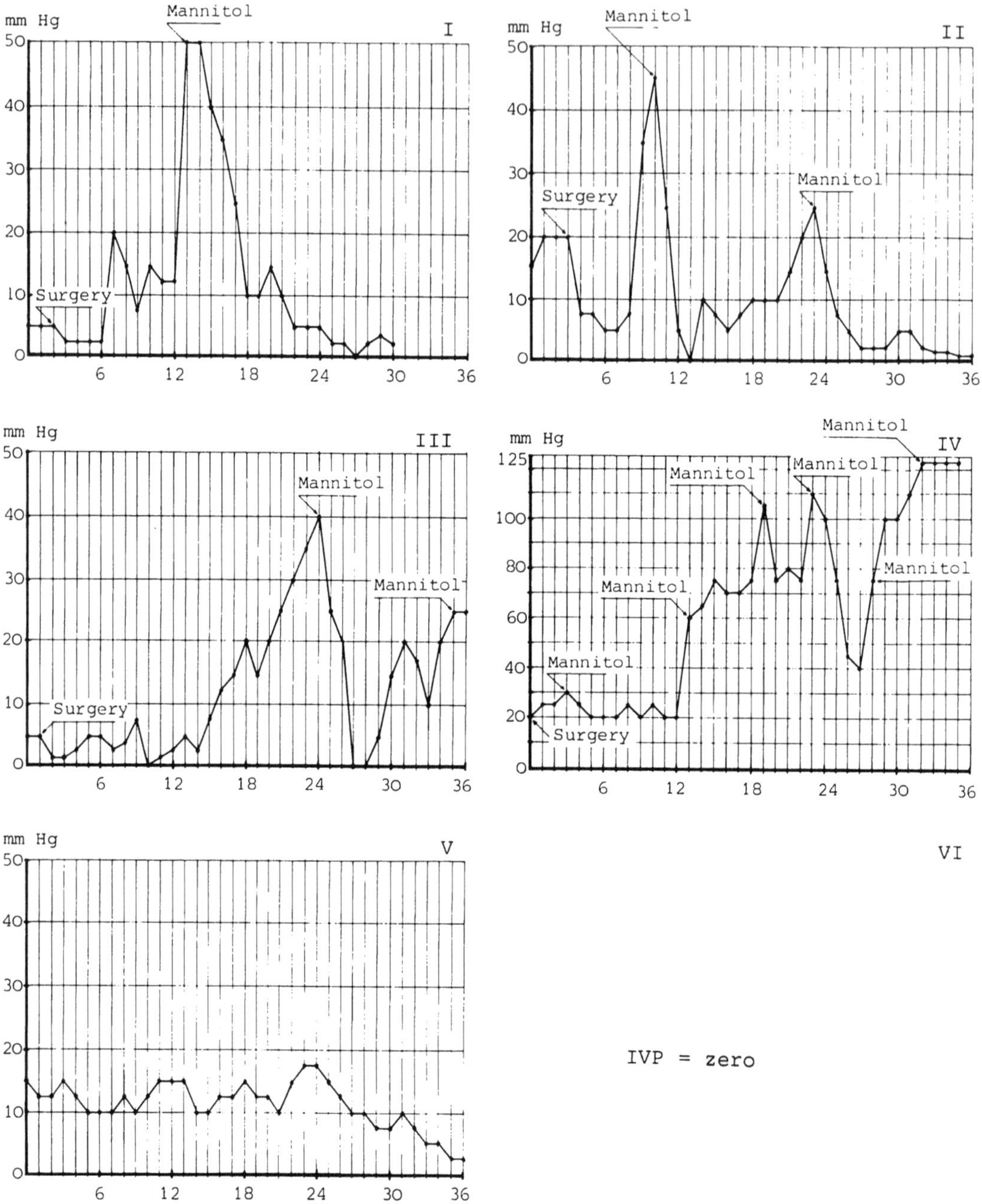

Fig. 1. Course of ICP during the first 36 h following admission in 6 patients studied

The Importance of Preventing Increased Intracranial Pressure in Patients with Cerebral Edema not Related to Trauma

G.W. Kindt, W.F. Chandler, and H.H. Gosch

Introduction

The presence of elevated intracranial pressure (ICP) in patients with cerebral edema secondary to non-taumatic, non-neoplastic encephalopathies has been well documented, usually via lumbar puncture. Few reports exist however of continuous ICP monitoring of patients with non-traumatic cerebral edema (5, 6, 11). We are reporting our experience in monitoring and controlling ICP in 15 such patients.

Materials and Methods

The ICP was monitored by simple subdural pressure monitoring system reported previously (4). All 15 patients were comatose with non-focal neurologic examinations. They were on respirators with close monitoring of arterial blood gases, central venous pressure, and arterial blood pressure. The patients were monitored from 2 to 14 days, and there were no monitor failures or infections.

The 15 patients included 11 children, aged 3-14, with the diagnosis of Reye's syndrome. All of the children had grade III to IV EEGs by the classification of AOKI and LOMBROSO (1). Two underwent peritoneal dialysis and none had exchange transfusions. A 5-year-old boy was monitored with a severe encephalopathy secondary to mushroom poisoning. A 16-year-old boy, who had undergone a meso-caval shunt at age 3 for portal vein stenosis, was monitored when he developed hepatic coma secondary to a massive gastrointestinal hemorrhage. Two additional patients, age 20 and 24, had the diagnosis of viral encephalitis, one having elevated titers for herpes simplex.

All 15 patients were treated with dexamethasone, 12-16 mg i.m. All patients were hyperventilated such that the pCO_2 was between 20 and 25 mm Hg, and additional hyperventilation was done during pressure spikes. All of the patients received either i.v. mannitol or urea, up to 1 g per kg, to control sudden rises in intracranial pressure. Hypothermia, to 31°C, was carried out in six patients, and two patients received i.v. barbiturates, both long and short acting.

Results

The 11 children with Reye's syndrome all showed elevated ICP, usually greater than 40 mm Hg, and with waves up to 90 mm Hg. Eight of these 11 survived and are neurologically normal. Three children died, and necropsies done in two showed marked cerebral edema. No correlation could be made between survival and the degree of EEG abnormality, level of ICP, level of seum transaminase or ammonia, or whether they had had peritoneal dialysis or hypothermia.

The ICP tracing of the 5-year-old boy with the mushroom poisoning is seen in Figure 1. This child became decerebrate 3 days after eating the mushrooms and both pupils dilated. A subdural pressure monitor was placed and the initial pressure was 50 mm Hg. The pupils responded to urea and he subsequently required 14 more doses of urea to control his pressure waves. He was neurologically normal on the sixth day of treatment. The child also had hepatic failure with a serum transaminase of 2300.

The 16-year-old boy with the meso-caval shunt and the duodenal hemorrhage also exhibited markedly elevated ICP (Fig. 2). The by became decerebrated with dilated nonreactive pupils 36 h after the onset of bleeding, and the initial ICP was 54 mm Hg. His pupils came down with mannitol and urea, but the left pupil again dilated 6 h later. This also responded to urea and he required 7 more doses of urea over the 9 days he was monitored. One month later he was neurologically intact except for moderate intellectual impairment.

Two young adults with presumed viral encephalitis showed only mild elevations of ICP, never rising above 23 mm Hg and with no evidence of plateau waves. No immediate effect of treatment was evident in these patients, but they were both functional with only mild neurologic deficits 3 months later.

Discussion

These cases substantiate the idea that patients with non-traumatic encephalopathies known to be associated with cerebral edema do have profoundly elevated ICP. They also demonstrated the spontaneous pressure waves described by LUNDBERG (8) and others in patients with neoplasma or trauma. Recognition of these waves has made the continuous minute-to-minute monitoring of the intracranial pressure essential for adequate therapy.

Reye's syndrome of encephalopathy and fatty infiltration of the viscera was reported in 1963 (12), and the mortality of the 83 cases in the literature by 1967 was 84% (2). The etiology of the disease remains unknown, and efforts have been unsuccessful to relate the encephalopathy to the ammonia level, the degree of hypoglycemia, or some toxic agent. Primary viral or fatty infiltration of the brain is believed to be unlikely, as the neuropathology consistently shows marked cerebral edema with little inflammation and no fatty infiltration (2, 3). These appear to be ideal candidates for monitoring, as many have marked cerebral edema with little necrosis or neuronal degeneration. PIZZI et al. (11) reported monitoring Reye's syndrome and decreasing ICP with exchange transfusions. Since none of our patients had exchange transfusions, our survival rate with ICP reduction alone might indicate that decreasing the ICP is an essential part of the treatment.

The child with the mushroom intoxication demonstrates that *any* encephalopathy must be suspected of having elevated ICP. The brains of patients reported as dying in coma with fixed pupils from mushroom poisoning have shown marked edema, with only mild lymphocytic infiltration (9).

The boy with portal vein stenosis and a meso-caval shunt was presumed to have had hepatic coma from rapid absorption of nitrogenous blood products which could not be detoxified by the liver. This is classified as the "exogenous" type of hepatic coma, and was brought on by the most common precipitating factor, gastrointestinal hemorrhage. The etiology of hepatic coma remains unclear, as 20% or more patients have normal venous ammonia levels (7). Various amino acids, phenols, indoles, and even glutamate neurotransmitters have been implicated as contributing factors (15). The neuropathology shows only proliferation and enlargement of protoplasmic astrocytes, and cerebral edema (7). THÖLEN (13) reported 16 of 20 patients dying with hepatic coma as having severe cerebral edema as the "immediate cause of death." WARE et al. (14) report 16 of 32 patients having cerebral edema and 4 with tentorial herniation as the cause of death. One of these patients died during lumbar puncture.

The patients with viral encephalitis had lower intracranial pressures, and were slower to recover from neurologic injuries. This correlates with the pathologic findings of severe neuronal loss, demyelination and marked inflammation, with only moderate cerebral edema (10).

Summary

Fifteen patients with cerebral edema not related to trauma underwent continuous monitoring and control of ICP. Their diagnoses included Reye's syndrome, mushroom poisoning, hepatic encephalopathy and viral encephalitis. We conclude that ICP monitoring can be vitally important in selected cases.

References

1. AOKI, U., LOMBROSO, C.T.: Prognostic value of electroencephalography in Reye's syndrome. Neurol. 23, 333-343 (1973).
2. BRADFORD, W.D., LATHAM, W.C.: Acute encephalopathy and fatty hepatomegaly. Amer. J. Dis. Child. 114, 152-156 (1967).
3. CHANG, L.W., GILBERT, E.F., TANNER, W., MOFFAT, H.L.: Reye's syndrome. Light and electron microscopic studies. Arch. Path. 96, 127-132 (1973).
4. GOSCH, H.H., KINDT, G.W.: Subdural monitoring of acute increased intracranial pressure. Surg. Forum 23, 405-406 (1972).
5. JAMES, H.E., BRUNO, L., SCHUT, L., SHALNA, E.: Intracranial subarachnoid pressure monitoring in children. Surg. Neurol. 3, 313-315 (1975).
6. KINDT, G.W., WALDMAN, J., KOHL, S., BAUBLIS, J., TUCKER, R.P.: Intracranial pressure in Reye's syndrome. Monitoring and control. JAMA 231, 822-825 (1975).
7. LOSCOWSKY, M.S., SCOTT, B.B.: Hepatic encephalopathy. Br. Med. J. 3, 279-281 (1973).
8. LUNDBERG, N.: Continuous recording and control of ventricular fluid pressure in neurosurgical practice. Acta Psychiat. Neurol. Scand. Suppl. 149, 1-193 (1960).
9. MARCOVITZ, E., ALPERS, B.J.: The central nervous system in mushroom poisoning. Arch. Neurol. Psych. 33, 53-71 (1935).
10. MILLER, J.R., HARTNER, D.H.: Acute viral encephalitis. Med. Clin. N. Amer. 56, 1393-1404 (1972).
11. PIZZI, F.J., SCHUT, L., BERMAN, W., HOLZHAPPLE, W.: Intracranial pressure monitoring in Reye's syndrome. Paper presented at the American Association of Neurological Surgeons Meeting, Miami/Florida, 1975.
12. REYE, R.D.K., MORGAN, G., BARAL, J.: Encephalopathy and fatty degeneration of the viscera. A disease entity in childhood. Lancet 2, 749-752 (1963).
13. THÖLEN, H.: Brain edema. A cause of death in endogenous liver coma. Klin. Wschr. 50, 296-301 (1972).

14. WARE, A.J., D'AGOSTINO, A.N., COMBES, B.: Cerebral edema: A major complication of massive hepatic necrosis. Gastroenterology 61, 877-884 (1971).

15. ZIEVE, L., NICHOLOFF, D.M.: Pathogenesis of hepatic coma. Ann. Rev. Med. 26, 143-157 (1975).

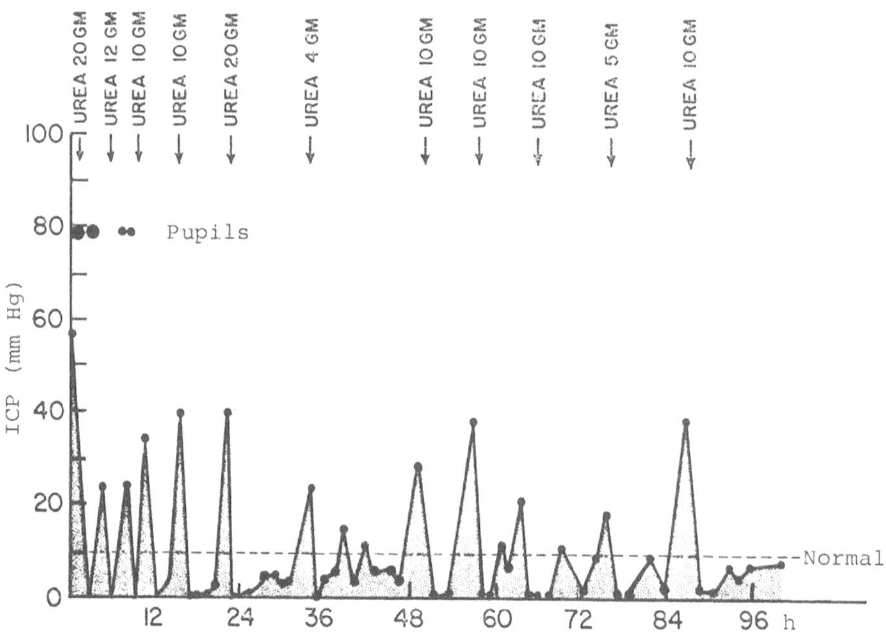

Fig. 1. Intracranial pressure tracing of child with mushroom poisoning

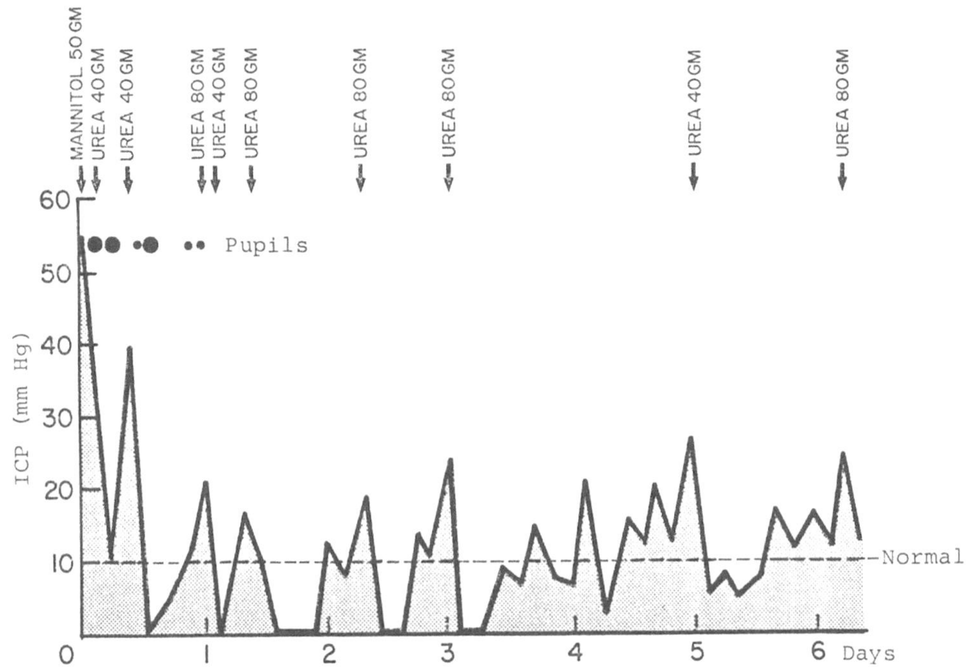

Fig. 2. Intracranial pressure tracing of boy with hepatic encephalopathy

Direct Measurement of ICP in Cases of Craniosynostosis as a Diagnostic Aid for Operation

W. Gobiet, E.W. Strahl, W.J. Bock, and W. Grote

Introduction

The most important indication for operation in cases of suspected premature craniostosis is the proof of raised ICP (1). Normally diagnosis is based on indirect signs of raised ICP, such as neurological and eye symptoms, or roentgenological findings (2, 3).

Since operation brought no success in some cases of clinically diagnosed craniostosis, we compared, in a group of children, the results of direct ICP measurement with the indirect signs of raised intracranial pressure.

Method

Investigations were carried out in 20 children aged 3 weeks to 12 years. All were admitted to our outpatient clinic with the tentative diagnosis of craniostosis.
When our clinical and roentgenological findings showed indirect signs of raised ICP, direct measurement of ICP was performed. All measurements were taken through a frontal burr hole and a ventricular catheter over a period of 24 h.

Results

Table 1 gives the results of direct ICP recordings. In 13 children very low pressure values between 0-10 mm Hg were found without any tendency to acute pressure rises. In 5 children ICP was raised between 15-50 mm Hg. Only 2 children showed pressure values over 50 mm Hg.

According to the different ICP levels, our cases were divided into two groups:
group I: 13 children with low pressure values under 10 mm Hg.
group II: 7 children with an ICP higher than 10 mm Hg.

Table 1. Results of direct ICP recording in children with craniostosis and suspected raised ICP. Only two children had very high pressure values over 50 mm Hg

ICP (mm Hg)	n=
0 - 10	13
10 - 25	2
25 - 50	3
> 50	2

The comparison between clinical symptoms and the level of ICP is given in Figure 1. It is clear that well-known clinical signs of raised ICP as seizures, spasticity, headache, mental disorders or microcephalus were found in the same frequency in children with a low ICP as in those with raised levels. The other symptoms such as impressiones gyrorum, protrusio bulbi or compression atrophy differ so little between the two groups, that diagnosis of raised ICP cannot be achieved with certainty by indirect signs (Fig. 2).

In contrast to this, papilloedema was exclusively found in children with raised ICP. From the group with low ICP, one child was operated. One year later its clinical status was found unchanged.

Six of the non-operated group remained unchanged, the other 6 showed slight improvement of their mental conditions 1 1/2 years later (Table 2).

In group II (higher pressure) all children were operated. In 5 of these children, whose ICP was higher than 25 mm Hg, the neurological status was improved. The other 2 remained unchanged. In 3 of the non-operated children with low pressure, measuring was repeated 1 year later. Again very low pressure levels were found.

Table 2. Treatment and clinical outcome, results of this study (group I = low pressure, group II = raised pressure)

	Group I		Group II	
	op.=1	not op.=12	op.=7	not op.=0
Improved		6	5	
Not improved	1	6	2	

Discussion

Direct measurement of ICP in 20 children with premature craniostosis and indirect signs of raised ICP showed that only in 7 cases was intracranial pressure really higher than usual. The other 13 had very low ICP values.
We can conclude that in most of these cases craniostosis and neurological deficit are a symptom of primary brain atrophy of unknown origin. Reduced brain volume leads to an early synostosis of skull sutures and to such typical deformities micro-, oxy- or dolichocephaly.

This is in accordance with the various other neurological symptoms found in this group, as there are spasticity, seizures, retardations, headache or atrophy of the papillae.

Thus, most of the children with the tentative diagnosis of raised ICP caused by premature craniostosis must be counted among the group of infantile cerebral palsy. In these cases craniotomy is not indicated, except for cosmetic reasons.

Raised intracranial pressure, found in the other group of children, indicates that they are patients with "real" craniostosis; i.e. brain growth is prevented by too early synostosis of cranial sutures.

Since clinical, neurological and eye symptoms differ so little among children with very low or with raised ICP, a clear indication for craniotomy can be achieved only by direct monitoring of ICP or proof of papilloedema.

The critical limit of ICP was found to be about 25 mm Hg. Children with ICP above this level should be operated on, for they have a good chance of improvement of clinical status, as the results of group II indicate (Table 2).

Summary

Direct measurement of ICP in 20 children with craniostosis and clinical signs of raised ICP showed that only in 7 cases was ICP markedly raised.

Since there was no clear correlation between the indirect signs of raised ICP and the values of direct monitoring, indication for craniotomy can be achieved with certainty either by measuring ICP or by proof of papilloedema.

References

1. ANDERSON, F.M., GEIGER, L.: Craniostosis: survey of 204 cases. J. Neurosurg. 22, 229-240 (1965).
2. GOBIET, W., GROTE, W.: Die direkte Hirndruckbestimmung als differentialdiagnostisches Kriterium bei Verdacht auf Hydrozephalus und Kraniostenose. Z. Kinderchir. 15, 273-278 (1973).
3. INGRAHAM, F.D., ALEXANDER, E.: Clinical studies in craniosynostosis. Surgery 24, 518-541 (1948).

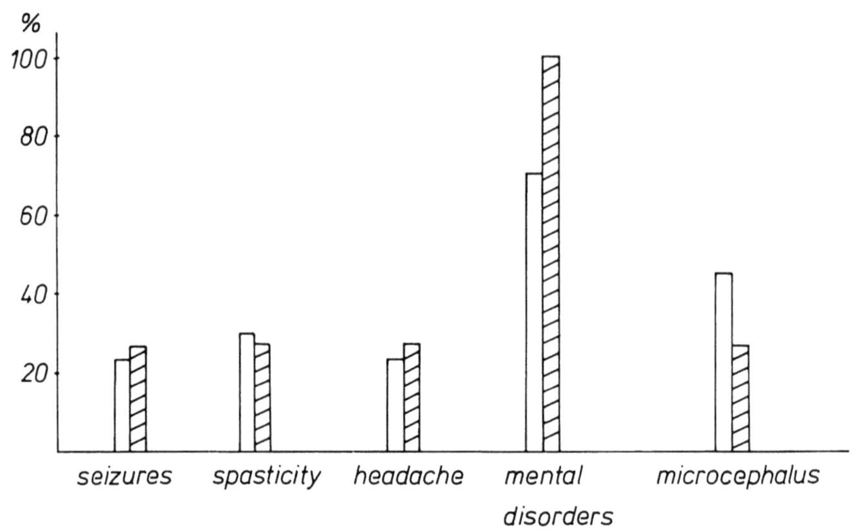

Fig. 1. Comparison between clinical symptoms and ICP level. There were no significant differences between the two groups

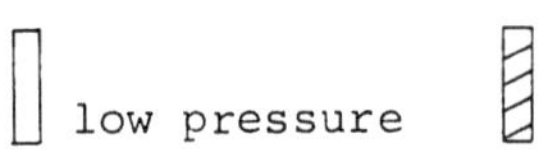

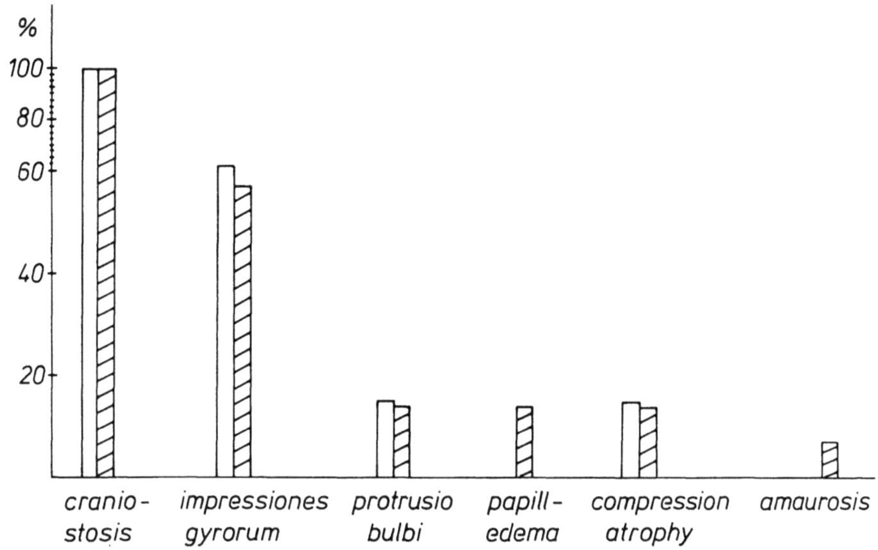

Fig. 2. Distribution of roentgenological and eye symptoms in the two groups. Papilla edema was only found in children wit elevated ICP

Summary

N. Lundberg and J.W.F. Beks

The first paper in this session by BRUCE and SCHUT reported experiences of ICP monitoring in children admitted to a pediatric intensive care unit. Among the 50 patients included in the material 15 had head injuries, 13 Reye's syndrome and 8 brain tumors. The choice of recording techniques in these series should be noted. In patients with head injuries and Reye's syndrome extraventricular measurements with a subdural screw were preferred, whereas the tumor patients (mostly posterior fossa tumors with ventricular dilatation) had a ventricular catheter for VFP measurements. This represents a practical demonstration of a policy implying that VFP measurements are preferred in cases of CSF obstruction and extraventricular techniques in cases of brain swelling - in our opinion an adequate policy.

The facility to diagnose brain edema and to estimate ventricular size by CT scanning was beautifully demonstrated by roentgen pictures. It is interesting that the majority of those children who showed a picture of diffuse swelling and obliteration of ventricles and cisterns had a clinical history of a mild injury followed by headache, vomiting, prostration and progressive obtundation.

The fact that plateau waves are a token of a "tight brain" is well established. The authors have observed that this relationship may be utilized for practical purposes by using the readiness of plateau waves to be triggered by tracheal suction as a sign of low intracranial compliance. It seems obvious that this observation might reduce the need for testing VPR by instillation or withdrawal of CSF. Another valuable observation concerns the correlation between the ICP and the clinical status. The authors found a good correlation between increased ICP and a poor neurological status in the head-injured children at the end of 2 weeks. They stressed the late appearance and long duration of ICP disorders in patients with traumatic and anoxic encephalopathy.

In consequence of the above observations, they are most positive concerning the value of monitoring ICP in head-injured children.

In Reye's syndrome a diffuse encephalopathy with brain edema is combined with fatty infiltration of visceral organs. It was first described in 1963; results of ICP monitoring were first reported at the Meeting of the American Association of Neurological Surgeons in 1975 by PIZZI, SCHUT et al.

In the first three papers of this session the results of ICP monitoring in a total of 34 cases of Reye's syndrome were reported (13, 11, and 6 cases, respectively). In their conclusions the authors of these papers agreed that ICP monitoring is a valuable, even necessary guide to treatment of patients with Reye's syndrome as well as similar encephalopathies connected with brain swelling.

These papers are important contributions because they show that intracranial (supratentorial) hypertension has a crucial importance for the course and outcome in many patients with encephalopathy connected with brain edema, both of traumatic and non-traumatic origin, and because they indicate that adequate pressure-reducing treatment guided by continuous recording of ICP may diminish mortality and cerebral sequelae in such cases. The authors should also be given credit for stressing the clinical importance of plateau waves and the similar rapid variations of the ICP. As expressed by KINDT et al. "Recognition of these waves has made the continuous minute-to-minute monitoring of the intracranial pressure essential for adequate therapy."

In the fourth paper of the session GOBIET et al. presented aspects on the diagnosis and indications for operation in craniosynostosis - aspects which differ from commonly accepted views. On the basis of ICP recordings in 20 children with the diagnosis of craniosynostosis they claimed that a low ICP means that the premature closure of the sutures is secondary to a primary brain atrophy, i.e., what is usually called microcephaly, whereas only patients with increased ICP have a primary synostosis. Consequently, they stated that the most important indication for operation in suspected craniosynostosis is the proof of raised ICP.

In our experience examination of the outer configuration of the head supplemented by neuroroentgenologic examination of the skull renders an early diagnosis possible. The diagnosis having been established, the deformity should be operated upon as early as possible, primarily for cosmetic reasons, but with the additional hope of giving the brain space for its normal growth. We think that the authors over-emphasized the significance of the ICP level for the pathogenesis of brain damage and of their ICP measurements for the clinical management (cf the combination of high elastance and low ICP in hydrocephalus). In any case, this paper certainly raises interesting questions concerning these problems.

Closing Comments

B. Jennett

To judge from the increasing numbers attending successive ICP symposia interest in the topic is steadily growing, especially among clinicians. An there is no reluctance to write about experience in this field - almost three times as many papers were submitted for this meeting as could be accepted. Nonetheless there was a sense of disappointment among some of the more experienced participants that few innovative ideas should have emerged, and that so many papers were still reviewing the use, or value, or role of ICP monitoring in a variety of different conditions or circumstances. Certainly the stage has now been reached when further reports of this kind will be justified only if based on large series of well-defined categories of patients - and if the criteria for entry to the study and the objectives of measurement are clearly stated. It is naive to look to the monitoring of ICP as a means of improving patient care in a heterogeneous group of patients. Such monitoring will help patients only if a clear plan of therapeutic action is based on the results of such measurements. Even then care must be taken to exclude (or to allow for) possible vicarious influences of the institution of ICP monitoring in certain patients and not in others. In some hospitals this decision may determine a different standard of care - this may be overt, because monitoring may require that the patient be moved to a special area; or it may be unrecognized, even by the physicians in charge of the patients, because it depends on some unspoken interpretation by nursing and paramedical staff of the physician's decision to monitor a given patient.
Several discussants referred to the need to accept more advice from basic scientists in biological and other fields - and some thought that our meetings would be enhanced by invited lectures from surch workers. More benefit is likely to accrue if we can capture their interest for longer than this, and if more clinicians were to engage in collaborative efforts with scientists and engineers in their own institutions. Substantial progress has been made in our understanding of the relationship between pressures in tissue and in various CSF spaces and about the gradients which can develop between them. There is much still to learn about the dynamic characteristics of these gradients, and the consequences of these, both functional (such as cerebral blood flow and neuronal activity) and structural (such as edema and brain herniation).

Controversy about elastance pressure/volume relationships continues; and the interactions between ICP and cardiovascular and respiratory function are by no means resolved. The role of formation and absorption of CSF, which had been discussed at length in Lund, were hardly mentioned at this meeting; perhaps it is time to look at this problem again, in the light of new methods and observations. Likewise methodology of measurement was given a rest at the meeting; most clinical reports seemed to be of intraventricular measurements, but the limitations and risks of this approach remain and probably account for the fact that it is still only a minority of neurosurgeons who regularly monitor pressure. It is apparent that those working in experimental laboratories have as much need as clinicians to standardise their procedures, and to be aware of reasons why discrepant results may be reported by different workers. In comparing experimental findings it is important to make due allowances for species differences, for the effect of the mode by which ICP is raised - whether acutely or chronically and whether diffusely by infusion or by a local mass; and for the possibility that certain relationships may be different under conditions of high pressure than within the normal range.

If we are to enter into productive cooperation with those in other fields we shall need to define more precisely what the problems are to which we are seeking a solution. The responsibility to take stock of the present situation, in the light of observations made so far, is largely one for clinicians - because intracranial pressure is primarily a clinical problem. Physiology text books usually deal with the topic in a few lines - about the Queckenstedt test. By way of stimulating interest in such stocktaking I have attempted a brief review of some of the outstanding questions - more as a reaction to the Groningen Symposium than as an academic exercise. It is not therefore comprehensive, and it reflects the clinical bias of this meeting.

It is now obvious that high ICP occurs in numerous circumstances; it is much less certain what causes it and what changes it may cause in the brain - and this confusion of cause and effect is at the root of much continuing controversy in this field. It can be epitomised in the question: Is high ICP *the reason for* a bad brain, or *a reflection of* a bad brain - or both? Probably there is often a vicious circle (see diagram), and not all factors in this circular equation are known in theoretical terms, let alone recognized at the bedside. Two kinds of interaction with ICP can be recognized - according to whether consideration is given to the effect which *ICP has on* various other factors (Table 1), or to the effect which other factors *have on ICP* (Table 2); these include those activities which are commonly carried out on patients in neurosurgical units and which are not quite directed towards influencing ICP - but which incidentally may do so (Table 3). It is likewise important to remember that some measures undertaken in order to control raised ICP have effects other than on ICP, both on the brain and on other systems (Table 4); clinical benefit resulting from such therapeutic endeavours may not therefore necessarily be attributable to the change in ICP - even when such a change is recorded. The relationship between the ICP and the clinical state of the patient is so variable that it is necessary to consider what aspects of ICP are of clinical significance. It is already abundantly clear that no one level can be defined as significant, or even as dangerous. Some of the other factors which determine whether a given level of high pressure 'matters' are already known; these include the compliance, or elastance or tightness of the brain, whether or not there is a focal mass producing brain shift, whether the state of raised pressure is due to engorgement, edema or an extrinsic mass, the rate of development of raised pressure and so on. Others have been proposed, but remain to be proved - such as the variability of the pressure and the significance of waves or peaks. What is certain is that ICP must not be considered in isolation, and a group of investigators gathered under the flag of ICP must be on their guard not to yield to the temptation to do so.

When it comes to considering the clinical value of, or indications for, clinical monitoring I can only repeat my previous suggestions (at Hannover and Lund) that a simple and useful set of headings is *diagnosis*, *treatment* (whether necessary and whether effective) and *prediction* (of response to treatment and of outcome). Given these broad applications it is still necessary to consider whether monitoring is justified or

Diagram

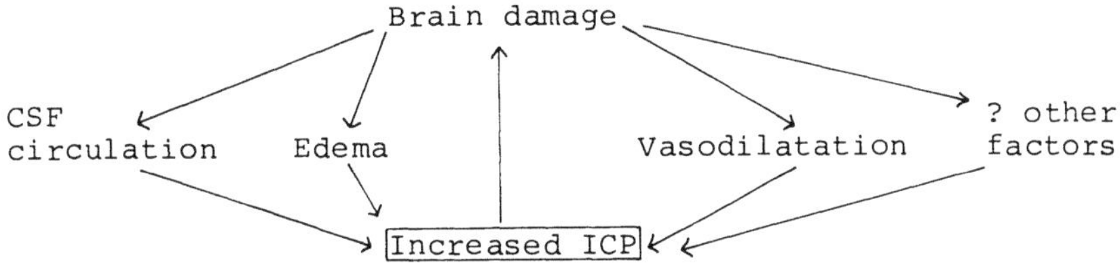

Table 1. Effect of raised ICP on:
Clinical state
CSF production/circulation/absorption
Cerebral blood flow
Electrical function
Cardiovascular system
Respiration
Outcome

Table 2. Effect on ICP of:
Primary lesion
Edema
Vasodilatation
Ventilation
Drugs
CSF circulation
Therapeutic activity

Table 3. Incidental therapeutic activity
Drugs
Anaesthesia
Neuroradiological procedures
Operative procedures

Table 4. Control of ICP	
Steroids	
Osmotics	
Hyperventilation	Vasoconstriction
	Cerebral pH
THAM	
Bony decompression	
Drain/shunt	

necessary. The decision depends upon the individual clinician, in the ambience of his particular surroundings and in different clinical circumstances. It must be accepted that the prediction which I made at the end of the Lund meeting that ICP measurements might soon become a routine part of clinical practice has not yet come about. The risk of infection remains, and it is the view of LANGFITT, of TROUPP and of myself that 3% is a more realistic rate than the much lower figure achieved by LUNDBERG in his carefully controlled study. We have therefore to consider both whether to measure ICP in a given patient, and if so for how long monitoring should continue - it being general experience that infection becomes more likely after 2-3 days. A balance must be struck between the returns and the risks, and opinions will continue to differ as to whether such measurements are motivated by curiosity, which is an admirable quality for a scientist, or by the clinician's belief that knowledge of ICP is sometimes crucial for good patient care.

Subject Index

MIX
Papier aus verantwortungsvollen Quellen
Paper from responsible sources
FSC® C105338

If you have any concerns about our products,
you can contact us on
ProductSafety@springernature.com

In case Publisher is established outside the EU,
the EU authorized representative is:
Springer Nature Customer Service Center GmbH
Europaplatz 3, 69115 Heidelberg, Germany

Printed by Libri Plureos GmbH
in Hamburg, Germany